# VEILED WARRIORS

**Christine E. Hallett** is Professor of Nursing History at the University of Huddersfield, Chair of the UK Association for the History of Nursing, and President Emerita of the European Association for the History of Nursing. She is a trained nurse and health visitor, and holds PhDs in both Nursing and History. Her main research focus for the last ten years has been on the work of nurses during the First World War. Among her publications are: *Containing Trauma: Nursing Work in the First World War* 2nd Edition (Manchester University Press, 2011); *Veiled Warriors: Allied Nurses of the First World War* (Oxford University Press, 2014); *Nurse Writers of the Great War* (Manchester University Press, 2016); *Nurses of Passchendaele* (Pen and Sword Books, 2017) and *Edith Cavell and Her Legend* (Palgrave, 2018).

## Praise for *Veiled Warriors*

'This book adds vastly to our body of knowledge, research and understanding of historical nursing'
**Jane Brocksom, *Nursing Times***

'[A]masterly account of a fascinating if horrific historical period.'
***Network Review***

'Military nursing was not only about winning the war, it was also about women gaining recognition for their profession and political rights for their sex . . . as this excellent book so amply demonstrates.'
***Good Book Guide***

'Immaculately researched, this is an authoritative and objective history of nurses both professional and voluntary in the First World War.'
**Baroness Shirley Williams**

'*Veiled Warriors* presents an eloquent appraisal of nursing's vital contribution to the care of wounded service personnel and its role in wider medical efforts. Christine Hallett has used some incredibly strong individual stories to illustrate her case and poses a masterful challenge to many of the myths that exist about nursing during the conflict.'
**Dr Peter Carter OBE, Chief Executive & General Secretary of the Royal College of Nursing**

'because Hallett is able to draw upon extensive clinical and professional knowledge to support her literary and historical research, she is able to bring a further dimension to her interpretation and analysis of these sources . . . The result is highly readable and will appeal to a range of audiences, general as well as academic.'
**Angela K. Smith, *American Historical Review***

# VEILED
# WARRIORS

## ALLIED NURSES OF THE
## FIRST WORLD WAR

Christine E. Hallett

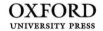

OXFORD
UNIVERSITY PRESS

# OXFORD
## UNIVERSITY PRESS

Great Clarendon Street, Oxford, OX2 6DP,
United Kingdom

Oxford University Press is a department of the University of Oxford.
It furthers the University's objective of excellence in research, scholarship,
and education by publishing worldwide. Oxford is a registered trade mark of
Oxford University Press in the UK and in certain other countries

First published 2014
First published in paperback 2021

Impression: 1

Published in the United States of America by Oxford University Press
198 Madison Avenue, New York, NY 10016, United States of America

British Library Cataloguing in Publication Data
Data available

Library of Congress Cataloging in Publication Data
Data available

ISBN 978–0–19–870369–3 (Hbk.)
ISBN 978–0–19–870370–9 (Pbk.)

Printed and bound by
CPI Group (UK) Ltd, Croydon, CR0 4YY

Jacket image: First World War postcard depicting a French nun-nurse
tending to a wounded French soldier; reproduced by permission C. E. Hallett.

Links to third party websites are provided by Oxford in good faith and
for information only. Oxford disclaims any responsibility for the materials
contained in any third party website referenced in this work.

*To*
*Margaret D. Hallett*
*and Keith Brindle*
*with love and thanks*

# Preface

The nurses of the First World War came from a range of national and cultural backgrounds; yet, they shared a common identity and purpose. At the outbreak of the so-called 'Great War' they were only just beginning to act in concert as a nascent global profession. In 1899, a group of prominent nurse-leaders had founded the International Council of Nurses, and in 1912 a meeting in Cologne, Germany, had brought nurses of many nations together in an atmosphere of mutual support. Within two years, these same nurses would be on opposing sides in the bitterest of conflicts. One of the main limitations of this book is its failure to capture the lives and work of nurses who cared for the wounded of the so-called 'Central Powers' (particularly Germany, Austria-Hungary, Bulgaria, and Turkey). My own limitations have dictated the parameters of the project. Even my attempt to fully capture the experiences and contributions of 'Allied' nurses (focusing particularly on British, French, Belgian, Russian, Romanian, Australian, New Zealand, South African, Canadian, and US nurses) is affected by my lack of skill in the Flemish, French, Russian, and Romanian languages. The history presented here is a partial and distorted one, written by an English-speaking historian from a highly Anglocentric perspective.

And the partiality does not end there. When I began to research this book, I believed it would be possible to capture the realities of the lives and work of Allied nurses. I was conscious that powerful ideas—or ideals—of First World War nurses pervaded the public consciousness, and I wanted to push aside the distorting veil of mythology and present a truer reality. Yet, even as I began to dismantle the representations created by both memory and imagination, I realized that I was only unearthing new layers of mythology. The project of separating myth from reality—a project I had believed would be so simple—came to resemble an attempt to pull apart two strands of DNA, and I realized that, even if the realities of nurses' lives could be disengaged from the myths by which they had been understood, the result would be so lacking in vitality that it would hardly be a history of human beings.

The writing and teaching of History is a dangerous occupation. As E. H. Carr pointed out, there really are no such things as historical 'facts'—there is only a historical record, which is subject to interpretation. But that does not mean we can do whatever we like with it. There are so many reasons why our knowledge of the past may be either deliberately or unconsciously distorted. Social and political elites have always been tempted to promote propagandist versions of past events. And media producers are under pressure to achieve commercial success—a pressure which does not lend itself to a detailed empirical unpicking of the historical record.

'Human kind cannot bear very much reality', wrote T. S. Eliot. It is, in many ways, easier to construct a coherent mythology than to grapple with an often-incoherent reality. But the most dangerous make-beliefs are those which are unconsciously propagated in the name of 'History'. In the twenty-first century, media representations of nurses are proliferating at a confusing rate. And our collective memory of the First World War is replete with distortions. As I write this book, broadcasting companies, museums, and publishers are preparing themselves to offer centenary commemorations of the First World War. Their aim is twofold: to honour the dead whilst at the same time feeding the hunger of a public whose consciousness has been blunted by a long-standing diet of soap operas, reality shows and instant news. Steeped as they are in such representations of human life, modern societies are ill-prepared to commemorate a series of events which are no longer within the reach of first-hand memory.

Twenty-first-century historians experience peculiar pressures. They find themselves caught between their own desires for discovery and creativity and external demands for 'outputs', 'income', and 'impact'. Such conflicts place integrity under strain, and historians need to be as aware as possible of the ways in which they may be feeding their own and others' expectations and desires. In my own case, I was attracted to the work of First World War nurses because it seemed to encompass the broadest possible range of healing practices. I could not help admiring the nurses' capacity to offer both fundamental nursing care and highly technical and scientific treatments. I found myself comparing them to modern nurses, who seem to struggle to express both the artistic and the scientific elements of their work. This is, perhaps, unfair—it certainly is unhistorical. But I could not help wondering how those who nursed the wounded of the First World War were able to offer such scope of practice under such difficult and stressful conditions. And I also wanted to offer a broad narrative of their lives and work: to tell their collective 'story'. In my attempt to complete this project, I found my thinking constantly enmeshed in the stories told by others: not just historians, novelists, and film-makers but the nurses themselves, through their letters, diaries, and semi-fictional accounts. Ultimately, my research was dominated by nurses' own personal testimonies, although it was complemented and balanced by a study of other archive sources, as well as a range of secondary materials. And, by immersing myself in their own writings, I came to argue that Allied nurses believed they were engaged in a multi-layered battle: for lives, for recognition, and for equality. I hope that it is, indeed, the voices of the nurses themselves that are heard most clearly in this book, and that I have been able to represent them in a way that openly and honestly fuses the reality of their experiences with my own interpretation of their lives and work.

# Acknowledgements

A project of this size and scope accumulates many debts. I am grateful to archivists, editors, colleagues, and friends throughout the world, many of whom were extremely generous with their time and energy.

I am very grateful for the support of the editorial staff at Oxford University Press, who have shown great patience and have been very helpful throughout the development and production of this book. Particular thanks to Matthew Cotton, Luciana O'Flaherty, Rowena Anketell, and Emma Slaughter. I am also grateful to The Wellcome Trust for a small research grant that supported some of the research work for this project.

A visit to Belgium in 2013 brought me into contact with several experts in the field of First World War Studies. Geertjan Remmerie of Talbot House Archives, Poperinge, Belgium spent hours unearthing and translating material on Allied nurses in Belgium. I am grateful to him and to his colleague Jan Louagie-Nolf for making the archives at Talbot House such a valuable and accessible source of research materials. Luc de Munck of the Belgian Red Cross Archives translated passages from the memoir of Jane De Launoy, and spent much of his own time offering me insights into the work of 'L'Hôpital de l'Océan at De Panne' [formerly La Panne] in Belgium. Lionel Roosemont, of 'Frontline Tours' in Ypres, went well beyond the bounds of his work as a guide, obtaining materials that would never have been available to me in the normal course of my research.

Much of the American material in this book was researched during two highly productive and hugely enjoyable visits to US universities. In 2009, I was awarded the Lillian Sholtis Brunner Fellowship by the University of Pennsylvania, and in 2010, the Barbara Brodie Fellowship by the University of Virginia. Both visits afforded me contact with individuals whose help was invaluable. They are too numerous to mention, but I would like to offer particular thanks to Julie Fairman, Patricia D'Antonio, Arlene Keeling, Barbra Mann Wall, Cynthia Connolly, Jean Whelan, and Linda Hanson. Barbara Brodie offered both intellectual support and warm hospitality in Charlottesville, and I will never forget the eggnog she prescribed and administered just before I departed for the airport following my first visit: it somehow symbolized her nursing values. Colleen and Dean Bowers showed great kindness and friendship by going to the trouble of producing a full photocopy of Alice Fitzgerald's Memoir, available only on microfiche at the Archives of the Maryland Historical Society, Baltimore. In the USA, I have also benefited from the support and friendship of Jane Schultz, of Indiana University-Purdue University, Indianapolis.

My understanding of the work of French First World War nurses has been greatly improved by conversations with Alison Fell, whose expertise in this field is unsurpassed. In similar ways, I have been aided by contact with Kirsty Harris and Ruth Rae, who, I am convinced, know everything there is to know about Australian First World War nurses; Pamela Wood, who supplied me with both material and insights into New Zealand nurses; Cynthia Toman, an expert on Canadian nurses; and Arlene Keeling whose understanding of US nurses and their practice was both impressive and invaluable.

Mark Harrison's book *The Medical War* permitted me to better understand the 'lines of evacuation' in the First World War, and enabled me to place the lives and work of Allied nurses into context. Peter Starling, of the Army Medical Services Museum, Aldershot was of help in making a number of primary sources and images available. His sane and calm support was of great help to me as this project was drawing to a close. Kate Luard's relatives showed generosity in allowing me to reproduce material from her books and letters. I would like to thank Caroline Stevens and Cathy Fry for sending me additional—and often very obscure—materials, and for directing me to academic sources relating to their great-aunt's life and work. I offer particular thanks to Tim Luard for supplying me with transcripts of letters held in the Essex Records Office, and for co-authoring, with me, a short piece on his great-aunt. The experience was an immensely valuable one. As this project was drawing to a close, I received very welcome help from Charlotte Smithson and Laura Wilson (The National Trust, Dunham Massey Hall, Cheshire) in accessing the notebook of Sister Catherine Eva Bennett.

Sue Light's encyclopaedic knowledge of First World War nurses is truly amazing. Even more impressive is the generosity with which she shares her knowledge and insights with anyone and everyone who asks for help. Her contributions to this book are many: she has offered insights; corrected errors; supplied images; and put me in touch with individuals who could provide me with materials which would enhance the work.

This work could not have been completed without the help of archivists and librarians throughout the world. I thank the staffs of the British Library, London; The National Archives, Kew; the Army Medical Services Museum, Aldershot; the Red Cross Archives, London; the Archives of the Order of St John of Jerusalem, London; the Imperial War Museum, London; the Royal College of Nursing Archives, Edinburgh; Talbot House Archives, Poperinge; the Belgian Red Cross Archives, Brussels; Library and Archives Canada, Ottawa; the Australian War Memorial, Canberra; the New Zealand National Archives, Wellington; the Alexander Turnbull Library, Wellington; the Archives of the Maryland Historical Society, Baltimore; the Barbara Bates Center for the Study of the

History of Nursing, Philadelphia; the Archives of the Eleanor Crowder Bjoring Center for Nursing Historical Inquiry; and the Claude Moore Health Sciences Library, Charlottesville. Thanks are due to the New Zealand Nursing Education and Research Foundation for permission to reproduce material from oral history interviews with New Zealand nurses.

My gratitude for their generosity in supplying images (and permission to reproduce these) goes to: Sue Light, Judy Burge, Talbot House Archives, the Belgian Red Cross Archives, the Army Medical Services Museum, the Claude Moore Health Sciences Library, the Archives of the Eleanor Crowder Bjoring Center for Nursing Historical Inquiry, the US National Library of Medicine, and the Wellcome Library. Images and permissions were also supplied in exchange for a fee by: the Imperial War Museum, London; the Australian War Memorial, Canberra; and the Royal College of Nursing Archives, Edinburgh. I am very grateful to Simon Offord of the Imperial War Museum, London; Anne Cameron, Fiona Bourne, and Teresa Doherty, of the Royal College of Nursing Archives; and Crestina Forcina of Wellcome Images for their help in sourcing photographs. Attempts were made to trace the copyright holder of the image of Queen Marie of Romania from her book: *Ordeal: The Story of My Life*. The author and publisher would be very grateful for any information that could be supplied on any current copyright held on this image.

My family have provided a combination of welcome distraction and intellectual support. Huge thanks to John, Steven, Melanie, Oliver, Dan, Pat, and Sami Hallett; Elliott and Benjamin Brindle; Shelley Tudor and Clare Holdsworth; Barbara, Geoff, Simon, Ruth, and Isabel Corfield. My mum, Margaret Hallett, is an unfailing source of support. Many of the ideas in this book have been 'bounced off' her sharp mind, and I am grateful for her kindness, positive outlook, and generosity of spirit. As always, my greatest thanks go to my husband, Keith Brindle, whose gallantry remains undimmed. His patience and tolerance of my obsessive tendencies; his cheerful acceptance of life in a house full of bulging book-shelves (though he has drawn the line at shelves in the kitchen); and his strength of character at times when this (and other) projects became a severe strain make him a true partner in this work—and in life.

# Contents

# List of Illustrations

# Glossary

| | |
|---|---|
| AANS | Australian Army Nursing Service |
| AGH | Australian General Hospital |
| ASN | Army School of Nursing (USA) |
| BEF | British Expeditionary Force |
| CCS | casualty clearing station |
| FFNC | French Flag Nursing Corps |
| NZANS | New Zealand Army Nursing Service |
| QAIMNS | Queen Alexandra's Imperial Military Nursing Service |
| QAIMNSR | Queen Alexandra's Imperial Military Nursing Service (Reserve) |
| QARNNS | Queen Alexandra's Royal Navy Nursing Service |
| RAMC | Royal Army Medical Corps |
| TF | Territorial Force |
| TFNS | Territorial Force Nursing Service |
| VAD | Voluntary Aid Detachment |

# Introduction

## War nurse: myths and realities

On 4 August 1914, the day her country declared war on Germany, a young woman named Vera Brittain was playing tennis. She was to reflect later that she did not know how she and her friends could possibly have played so calmly—and even taken an interest in the result.[1] The war that began that day would devastate their lives. Within four years, Brittain's brother, her fiancé, and two of her closest friends had died in the most horrific circumstances, and she herself had been both traumatized and transformed by sights and sounds in military hospitals which no young, gently-raised British middle-class woman could have expected to encounter. Her extraordinary memoir, *Testament of Youth*, like other war memoirs of the early 1930s, was written to expose war's realities and promote pacifism. It was an enormously successful project; the honesty and integrity with which its author told her story moved generations of readers, and when the book was made into a television drama series in the 1970s it was watched by tens of thousands of viewers worldwide.

One of the most powerful elements of Brittain's book was the story of her wartime nursing experience: it was nursing that enabled her to expose the trauma of war—to lay bare its destructive capacity through the sufferings of real, named human beings. Her writing brought the wards of the Royal Devonshire Hospital, the

First London General Hospital, and military base hospitals in Malta and northern France to life, and readers were invited to re-live with her the ordeals, sorrows and joys of the young volunteer nurse—the so-called 'VAD'. And yet, even as it exposed the truth about the war, Brittain's book also constructed a mythology of wartime nursing. The VAD is the book's heroine and, for this reason, readers throughout the world have come to identify the First World War nurse with the blue-and-white clad semi-trained volunteer—a snow-white scarf around her head, a blazing red cross on her breast. And even as the VAD has been brought to the foreground of the public imagination, the trained professional nurse has merged into the background, or, worse, has come to be identified as the bullying martinet who created some of the VAD's many personal ordeals.

The First World War Nurse is an icon, but, like most iconic fig-ures, her identity is obscured and distorted by the myths and nar-ratives of successive generations. Three of the most pervasive myths of First World War nursing are the myth of the courageous, mistreated VAD; the myth of the romantic nurse, who falls in love with her patient; and the myth of the nurse-heroine, who risks everything, not only to save individual patients' lives, but also to win the war. Vera Brittain's *Testament of Youth* perhaps encapsulates all three and is a classic illustration of how myth and reality can overlap. There can be little doubt that Brittain really did suffer personal hardship under the military regime of the First London General Hospital; the romantic intensity of her relationship with her fiancé, Roland Leighton, who she is 'nursing by proxy' when she cares for the war's wounded, is undeniable;[2] and the courage with which she faced tragic loss and personal danger has made her one of the recognized British heroines of the twentieth century.

The myths a society creates are as important as the realities it experiences. Myth contains an important kernel of truth, and any story that attains legendary status does so because the people of its time are powerfully struck by the truth at its heart.[3] Yet myths are not the same as realities, and most myths contain significant distortions. The stories from which they emerge are individual stories—told from individual angles or perspectives. The myth succeeds because the individual truths it conveys are taken to represent a more universal truth. The legendary status of writers such as Brittain has drawn a distorting curtain across the lives and experiences of tens of thousands of nurses—many of them highly trained professionals—whose experiences of the First World War were influenced by their position as female participants in a predominantly male world.

In their own time, nurses offered a significant contribution to their nation's war efforts and many saw themselves as patriots, offering their professional skills to the 'cause' of securing an Allied victory. Among them, however, was a small number of pacifists, who argued that a greater female participation in politics (which, for the time being, also meant engaging in war) would, ultimately, lead to the eradication of warfare. Their lives were full of contradictions. Some of those women who argued for peace also fought—sometimes with a degree of militancy—for the vote. Many of those who nursed the wounded, however, wrote little about the war itself or about either feminism or pacifism. They simply saw their work as a humanitarian service. They had come of age in an era when war was seen as an inevitable aspect of life—an unavoidable evil. They engaged in wartime nursing in much the same way as they would engage in a natural disaster such as a fire, flood, or earthquake. But even as they participated in a war which had been brought about by statesmen and would be directed by politicians and military commanders, nurses and volunteers also viewed themselves as fighting their own battles: struggling for the lives of their highly-traumatized and seriously-ill patients.

If all myths distort reality in order to present a deeper 'truth', then it is worth examining more closely those ideal forms over which nurses seemed to have little control: the courageous, bullied VAD; the romantic nurse; and the 'nurse-as-heroine'. This last form was the only one to which nurses themselves aspired, even though they realized that it too distorted the reality of their professional contribution to the war, by drawing attention away from their practice and towards their 'heroic deeds'. It is worth exploring, also, the myths nurses created—whether consciously or unconsciously—of themselves as 'fighters' or 'battlers' as well as humanitarians. These 'veiled warriors' believed they were fighting on three fronts: the 'second battlefield' of the military hospital ward, where patients were 'pulled back' from the brink of death; the dangerous territory of the 'war zone', in which all life was in danger; and the gendered and professional battlefield to which they would return, transformed by their experiences, after the war.

## The courageous VAD

Alongside Vera Brittain's *Testament of Youth* stand many other VAD writings. Two, in particular, have attracted attention. Irene Rathbone's *We That Were Young* and Enid Bagnold's *A Diary Without Dates* adopt and develop the theme of the courageous and much-put-upon VAD.[4] The military hospital sister is—almost invariably—an unthinking bully, who resents the presence of semi-trained but highly-educated and articulate VADs on her ward, and who therefore sends them at every opportunity to wash out bedpans in the sluice, sweep the floor, or clean out the grates. The VAD thus becomes the stereotypical victim-heroine, whose courage enables her to 'stick at' her duties, whose kindness and humanity makes her the patients' favourite 'nurse', and whose intelligence permits her, finally, to offer a truly reflective account of her experiences. She is, in fact, the female counterpart of those brave young men, the 'Lions led by Donkeys', who marched across no-man's-land to almost-certain destruction on the orders of foolish and callous officers.[5] But can a small corpus of VAD writings really tell us about the realities of the lives and work of those who nursed the wounded in the First World War? The memoirs of Brittain, Rathbone, and

Bagnold deal almost exclusively with the experiences of nurses in military hospitals on the home front (with the exception of Brittain's chapters on Malta and Étretat, which, significantly, offer much more positive images of professional nurses). Indeed, their accounts deal, almost entirely, with two London hospitals: the First London General Hospital, Camberwell, and the Royal Herbert Hospital, Woolwich. It is possible that these two institutions were among a minority of military hospitals in which discipline was particularly strict and senior nurses particularly determined to protect a hierarchy of command. Even if they were typical of military hospitals on the 'home front', there is evidence that trained nurses in casualty clearing stations and base hospitals overseas worked well with their VAD assistants, in a spirit of camaraderie and mutual support. There is also evidence that some wealthy and powerful 'volunteers' abused the trained skills of their professional counterparts, placing themselves in senior positions, while heaping work and responsibility onto their trained 'staffs'.[6]

The culture of early-twentieth-century nursing was a peculiarly restrictive one, in which 'discipline' of a quasi-military character pervaded the wards of most large teaching hospitals; and this is the context into which the experiences of VADs must be placed. All early-twentieth-century nurses began their training as first-year 'probationers': the lowliest of hospital personnel, who swept and dusted wards, cleaned out and laid fires, and spent much of their time mopping and scouring bedpans. It was not unusual for a junior trainee nurse to spend more of her time assisting the ward maid than nursing patients.[7] When volunteer nurses entered hospital wards, they were treated as first-year probationers—expected to serve their time carrying out the lowliest duties, before progressing to more responsible work. And it was not until they had several months'—even years'—experience that they were permitted to do anything 'technical' such as a dressing or a medicine round. Whilst VADs believed themselves to be singled out for the most mundane work, they were, in fact, being treated like any other inexperienced beginner.

One of the most significant features of the 'myth' of the VAD was age. Many VADs were in their early twenties, but others were much older. Yet, in novels, semi-fictional accounts, and films, they are depicted as young, idealistic, and enthusiastic. They are frequently seen as the embodiment of a new generation, challenging the views and norms of their elders.

The works of Brittain, Rathbone, and Bagnold—powerful writings by wealthy and influential women—ensured that the image of the VAD as the archetypal First World War nurse remained pervasive throughout the twentieth century. All three books were reprinted several times, and were, in the later century, promoted by the feminist press Virago as significant women's writings. And the image of the VAD was kept alive in other ways, too. In the early twenty-first century the most powerful image of the First World War nurse was that of 'Lady Sybil' in the highly popular British television drama, *Downton Abbey*, which was exported worldwide. Another VAD was at the forefront of the popular imagination: a young, kind, and beautiful woman (who also happened to be a member of the aristocracy and fabulously wealthy) once again captured the attention of a fascinated public.

## The romantic nurse

In 1929, Ernest Hemingway published what was probably his most successful book: *A Farewell to Arms*. Focusing on a love affair between American lieutenant Frederic Henry and British nurse Catherine Barkley, the book offers both a bleak portrayal of the First World War and a vivid and stylized depiction of the military nurse.[8] The novel—which was striking in its emotional intensity—became both a best-seller and a critically acclaimed example of a new, modern form of writing.

Hemingway's novel almost certainly drew upon his own experience as an ambulance driver on the Isonzo Front. He sustained severe shrapnel wounds to both legs in 1918, and was hospitalized for several weeks—first in a field hospital, and then in a base hospital in Milan, where he met and fell in love with American nurse Agnes von Kurowsky. When the two met, Hemingway was 19 and von Kurowsky 26. Hemingway appears to have been infatuated by his nurse, and wanted to marry her, but after corresponding with him for several months, von Kurowsky wrote ending their relationship, informing him that she loved him 'more as a mother than as a sweetheart', and confessing that she was planning to marry an Italian officer.[9]

Ernest Hemingway's later fame as a novelist evoked interest in his life and literary critics were fascinated to find that the emotional intensity of his writing seemed to be matched by the drama of his personal life. He married four times, each time disastrously, and his experiences seem to have prompted many to suppose that the emotional blow of losing von Kurowsky led him to form a pattern of relationships in which he abandoned his wives before they could betray him. Hemingway has become the subject of myth and Agnes von Kurowsky stands close to the centre of the myth, as the romantic—but somehow destructive—nurse. The fact that Hemingway himself fell in love with a nurse has prompted the supposition that the character and experiences of Catherine Barkley are accurately modelled on Hemingway's real-life nurse. And yet, it is highly unlikely that von Kurowsky resembled the somewhat overwrought and unfortunate heroine of Hemingway's novel. Like any fictional character, Catherine is more fantasy than reality. Not only does she fall completely in love with Hemingway's hero, she also becomes pregnant within months of meeting him and then dies following a stillbirth, prompting the—perhaps cynical—supposition that inventing her was an act of catharsis for Hemingway's feelings of unrequited love and betrayal.

Agnes von Kurowsky herself—although clearly a remarkable character—lacked the dramatic qualities of Catherine Barkley. The letter she wrote to Hemingway, ending their relationship, is striking in its simplicity and honesty. Her insistence that she loved him in a maternal way, rather than as a 'sweetheart', resonates well with the personal writings of other professional nurses of the time, who commented that they felt able to offer emotional containment to their traumatized patients, by developing relationships with them that were modelled on familial—sisterly or motherly—exemplars.[10] While von Kurowsky asserted her belief that she had been in love with Hemingway, her frank admission that she had fooled herself may well have been both demoralizing and infuriating for the young writer. Hemingway's fantasy—perhaps the result of his frustrated emotions—became one of the twentieth century's myths of the First World War nurse. *A Farewell to Arms* was published in several editions, and was adapted for stage, television, radio, and cinema. The 1932 and 1957 screen adaptations of the novel were highly melodramatic.[11] A recent 1996 film, entitled *In Love and War*, portrayed the relationship between Hemingway and von Kurowsky as a physical love affair, while, in reality, it is much more likely that, for professional reasons, von Kurowsky kept the relationship on a platonic footing.[12]

Whatever Hemingway's reasons for depicting the woman who nursed him in a base hospital in Italy as a tragic romantic heroine, his creation—Catherine Barkley—inspired generations of commentators, screenwriters, and directors to place a particular image of nursing before the eyes of a highly receptive public. The mystique of nursing—its intimacy and the fact that much of its work takes place behind carefully drawn screens—gives licence to portrayals which draw upon their audience's deepest fantasies.

Larissa Antipova—the war nurse with whom the eponymous hero of Boris Pasternak's *Doctor Zhivago* falls in love—is, in many ways, similar to Catherine Barkley; yet in others she is Barkley's antithesis. If 'Catherine' stands as the archetype of the highly-feminine but somewhat helpless nurse-heroine, then 'Lara' perhaps stands for a type of pure, noble womanhood who embraces nursing as both a duty and a form of self-expression. At the beginning of Pasternak's book the reader learns that Lara is from a genteel but impoverished background, and must tread carefully through life: 'people had to think well of you if you were to get on'. Yet she is also 'the purest being in the world'.[13] Pasternak goes on to confound the reader's expectations by drawing her fate as that of a 'fallen woman', who is apparently guilty of an attempted murder.

Lara goes on to marry a man who she loves more as a mother than as a wife. To her husband it is clear that she loves not him but 'the image of her own heroism', and he leaves her to join the army. When he goes missing, she trains as a nurse, and (somewhat improbably) joins an ambulance train, which will take her to that part of the front where he is serving, so that she can find him.[14] Here, she finally meets Yuri Zhivago, who is to become the love of her life. He—a married man—has seen her before, from a distance, and is already fascinated by her. Their joint work at the front brings them close together, both politically and spiritually. After a long time apart, they meet again in Siberia, where their relationship is consummated.

Pasternak's Nobel Prize-winning novel adeptly develops its theme of the survival of the individual human spirit in a world that has been destroyed by irresponsible power, ignorance, and squalor. But Pasternak's vision is that of a mid-twentieth-century male, who understands very little of the inner life of his female characters. Whilst Zhivago is a profoundly moral, spiritual, and intellectual character, Lara—for all her complexity—embodies many of the features of male fantasy: she is both angel and whore; mother and innocent child. As a nurse, she is described as embodying a spirit of sacrifice, and yet, her quest is not to alleviate the suffering of her countrymen, but to find and somehow make amends to the husband she should never have married. Her nursing is little more than a plot-device. Lara—like Catherine—is a classic nurse-heroine: beautiful and pure, yet driven by emotions and desires rather than by conscious morality or intellect, she exists merely as a foil to the hero's struggle.

## The nurse as heroine

When war broke out in the summer of 1914, it did not come as a shock to the people of Europe. While very few welcomed the conflict, most had been anticipating it for years, if not decades; and most had been preparing themselves for what they believed it would bring.[15] Thousands of British men had already joined the Territorial Force (TF), which had been formed in 1908 with the purpose of providing a home defence in the event of the British Expeditionary Force's (BEF) inevitable departure for the Continent. Men had been drilling, learning to use firearms, and preparing themselves mentally for combat for at least six years. Women's situations were more complex. Their wartime role was, traditionally, a passive one. They provided both the reason for the fight (the defence of women, children, and home), and the nurturing safe-haven to which brave fighting men would return. The vast majority of British women had accepted such roles for decades, throughout the many imperial wars of the nineteenth century. But the wars of the twentieth century were to be very different. No longer would women be content to wave their menfolk off to battle in remote parts of the empire. War now was being waged just across the British Channel, and women were determined to be among its active participants.[16] Some would even find their way to more distant battlefronts, such as the Eastern Mediterranean and Mesopotamia.

It was not only women's desire to participate that drove their actions. The First World War was a conflict of mass mobilization. Women were needed, as never before, to take the places of men in vital industries (particularly munitions), on the land as farmers, and in a range of vital services. Yet it was as nurses that their war service appears to have found its most patriotic expression. Since women could not be taken on as part of their nations' fighting forces, many sought work that might give them the opportunity to get close to the 'front lines' of battle. Sometimes geographical proximity to the front lines was not possible. 'Getting close' to the war might, in fact, mean a closeness to the wounds of war—a deep involvement in the suffering it entailed and a close contact with its combatants.

British women of the twentieth century's second decade were already very different from their Victorian and Edwardian mothers and grandmothers. Many had become increasingly dissatisfied with their passive and powerless roles in society, and some had joined the fight for female suffrage, through not only its recognized campaigning arm, the National Union of Women's Suffrage Societies (NUWSS), but also its more militant sisterhood, the Women's Social and Political Union (WSPU)—'the suffragettes'. Women had engaged in vociferous demonstrations, chained themselves to railings, and thrown stones at the windows of government offices in Whitehall. One, Emily Davison, had actually thrown herself in front of the king's racehorse, dying a martyr to the cause of 'votes for women'.[17] In America, the fight for the vote was gaining pace. In 1913, an influential parade for woman suffrage, held in Washington DC on the day before President Woodrow Wilson's inauguration, had attracted considerable notice—and a hostile reaction from some male observers.[18]

British and American women's claims to political participation were supported by their increasingly visible roles in society. Although employment opportunities for middle-class women were largely confined to 'traditional' female occupations, such as nursing, teaching and clerical work, their increasing autonomy in these roles—along with their early forays into traditionally male professions such as medicine—strengthened their argument for political power. Indeed, the claim that women could not participate in political life because they did not put their lives at risk in foreign conflicts was one of the last surviving arguments against women's suffrage—an argument that a small minority of women were determined to overturn through their direct participation in what was soon to be dubbed 'The Great War'. So female suffragists had powerful reasons for wanting to enter the First World War as direct participants rather than passive observers. Even those who were opposed to the suffrage campaign believed that women had the right to engage in what was believed to be a just fight against a dangerous aggressor. In 1914, Britain's Empire spanned the entire globe. As part of the nation which governed a large proportion of the known world, Britain's women felt a powerful sense of patriotic pride;[19] and this was a pride which seemed to be expressed even more powerfully in the self-governing dominions of Australia, New Zealand, Canada, and South Africa. In Canada, membership of an elite organization calling itself the 'Daughters of the Empire' had expanded dramatically during the first two decades of the twentieth century.[20]

Patriotic women wanted to play their part in what they saw as the great enterprise of war; but very few wanted to actually fight. Indeed, the tiny minority of Allied women who did fight in the First World War were confined to the Eastern Front, where armies were slightly more tolerant of female combatants; and, even here, the famous Russian 'women's battalion' met with opposition and abuse from its male counterparts.[21] In Western Europe, Flora Sandes, a British volunteer nurse who joined the ranks of the Serbian army, is believed to be a unique case.[22] The vast majority of women were seeking an 'acceptable' form of participation that would, nevertheless, take them close to the battlefields and enable them to feel that they were a vital part of the war effort. Nursing was their opportunity. For millennia, it had been seen as the archetypal—indeed the only—active role for women in wartime. Going well beyond the traditional role of sustaining a welcoming and nurturing home, nursing took women into the 'zone of the armies' and permitted them to exercise skill as well as care; courage as well as patience; and technical knowledge as well as sympathy and support. And because nursing was the obvious choice for all women, it became the privilege of the elite. Wealthy aristocratic and middle-class 'volunteer nurses' were amongst the first women to reach the Continent in August 1914—a fact that was openly deplored by many trained professional nurses.[23]

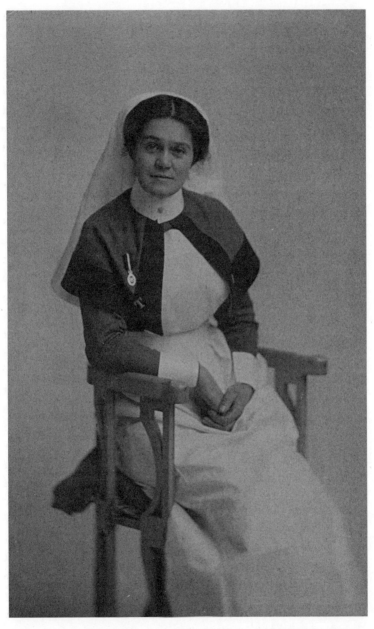

FIGURE 1 Sister Mabel Pearce, member of the Territorial Force Nursing Service (photograph reproduced with the permission of the Royal College of Nursing Archives)

Those women who wrote about their experiences of wartime nursing close to the front lines projected images of themselves as 'heroines'—the female counterparts of their brave, fighting brothers. The writings of some of the more influential and wealthy of these—women such as the aristocratic Millicent, Duchess of Sutherland, or millionaire Mary Borden—presented the efforts of those who nursed the wounded during the First World War as a battle in which clinical expertise and compassion waged war against trauma and disease. At the same time, the positioning of nurses on the side of 'right' against 'wrong' enabled them to see themselves as an integral part of the Allied war effort.[24] Eyewitness Mary Borden referred to her casualty clearing station as 'the second battlefield', and the writings of most nurses reveal a tendency to view their work as part of a great—and often heroic—struggle.[25]

The tendency for wealthy and influential women to claim a place at the forefront of the nursing services during the war was taken to its furthest extent by the royal families of Allied nations. In Britain, Princess Mary became a VAD member, attending a course of lectures and passing examinations at Buckingham Palace.[26] In Russia, Grand Duchesses Olga and Tatiana were closely involved in the work of the Anglo-Russian Hospital in Petrograd. Two of the most intriguing figures of the war, however, were the 'warrior-queens': Queen Elisabeth of the Belgians and Queen Marie of Romania. Both dressed as nurses and visited military hospitals; yet they appear to have been very different characters. Neither was a trained nurse, and Elisabeth, having acquired a shortened training at the beginning of the war, made a point of asserting that she had no formal nursing qualifications. She was instrumental in establishing one of the most famous hospitals of the war, L'Hôpital de l'Océan at La Panne close to the front lines in Belgium, where she frequently visited the wards and sometimes assisted head surgeon Antoine Depage in performing operations. She wore a simple white dress and a close-fitting headscarf, the purpose of which appears to have been to symbolize her commitment to the principles of cleanliness and discipline. She was closely involved in the work of L'Hôpital de l'Océan throughout the war.[27]

Queen Marie of Romania appears to have been a much more flamboyant character. She chose to dress in a dramatic Red Cross nurse's uniform and visited hospitals throughout the small corner of her country which remained in Allied hands. Although engaging in very little—if any—caring or clinical work, she played an important role in sustaining the morale of Romania's fighting force, taking sweets, cigarettes, and other small gifts to the wounded, and appearing alongside generals close to the front lines, to cheer 'her' troops into battle. She also played a very significant role in raising funds for the Red Cross.[28]

But if some women—particularly those from royal and aristo-cratic backgrounds—chose to deliberately cast themselves as 'war-rior-nurses', others found themselves reluctant heroines. One of the greatest heroic narratives of nursing is the story of Edith Cavell, a British nurse who assisted Allied combatants to escape incarceration, by helping to 'smuggle' them out of occupied Bel-gium. Cavell was shot as a spy on 12 October 1915. Her story might be read as the hijacking of individual accomplishment to serve a nationalist mythology. In her lifetime, Cavell had devoted much of her career to developing nursing education and professional practice in Belgium. But after her death this work was virtually forgotten—the reality of the past suppressed by a powerful propa-gandist project, which carved in stone on her monument in London the message that she had died 'For King and Country'. It was not until many years after the war that these words were supplemented with her own pacifist and conciliatory statement: 'Patriotism is not enough: I must have no hatred or bitterness towards anyone.' Edith Cavell was, first, a professional woman, and only second a reluc-tant heroine—an inadvertent martyr.[29] In 1939, just as a new war was beginning in Europe, a US 'biopic' film was made, which de-picted her as a saintly martyr and caricatured her German captors as cruel tyrants.[30]

Yet, nurses themselves promoted the image of themselves as heroines. Whether the impulse was conscious or unconscious, many seem to have wanted to portray their work as dangerous and themselves as fearless participants in warfare. Many of the classic tropes of wartime narrative can be found in the writings of trained nurses: from stories of escape from bombarded cities and torpedoed hospital ships; through memoirs of suffering and endurance in field hospitals; to narratives of both subversive war-work and overt heroism. Some of these key elements are particularly well rehearsed in the stories told about individuals such as Elsie Knocker and Mairi Chisholm—women who chose to work just behind the front-line trenches and came to be accepted as heroines.[31] Some trained nurses (and Elsie Knocker would be a particularly good example) deliberately portrayed themselves in their own published writings as heroines as well as technical experts. Others, whose writings remain hidden in the vaults of archives throughout the world, wrote in matter-of-fact ways about working in shelled-out casualty clearing stations or torpedoed transport ships. For them, the dangers of war were the necessary hazards one encountered in the course of duty.

## Nurses and volunteers of the First World War: the reality behind the myth

Behind the myths of courageous VADs, romantic nurses, and heroic front-line carers—and largely obscured by them—lie the realities faced by a nascent profession which was fighting its own hidden battles. Early-twentieth-century nurses, the vast majority of whom were women, were engaged in two struggles: for the vote and for a professional nurses' register that would recognize the training and experience of qualified nurses. But they were not united. Not all nurses wanted female suffrage; and the nursing profession was so divided over the issue of registration that some commented that it resembled an ideological battlefield.[32]

New Zealand and South African nurses had already acquired legally sanctioned registers for their professions, but in other countries the fight was becoming increasingly desperate.[33] In Britain, those who wished to see political recognition and a 'closed' professional register campaigned vigorously against an establishment which sometimes openly but more often furtively blocked its efforts. The campaign for registration was fronted by the volatile and irrepressible Ethel Gordon Fenwick, a former matron of the prestigious St Bartholomew's Hospital in London, who had retired from nursing following her marriage to Dr Bedford Fenwick. In 1887, the Fenwicks had founded the British Nurses' Association, and in 1893, they purchased the *Nursing Record*, a professional journal of which Fenwick was already editor, using it as the mouthpiece of their campaigns for both women's suffrage and the nurses' register, and renaming it, in July 1902, the *British Journal of Nursing*.[34] Fenwick was also, by this time, president of the International Council of Nurses and was working closely with its secretary, the influential US nurse Lavinia Dock, to promote internationalism within the nursing profession.[35]

Opposing the so-called 'registrationists' were hospital administrators such as Henry Burdett and Sydney Holland, who were anxious to prevent nurses from forming an *esprit de corps*. If nursing became a closed profession, hospitals would effectively lose control of their own staff who, as things stood, were both loyal and dependent. The 'anti-registrationists' had the support of a number of prominent matrons, among them the influential Eva Luckes of the London Hospital, who genuinely believed that a professional register would lower, not raise, standards. Their greatest asset, however, was Florence Nightingale, who, while never openly becoming embroiled in controversy, made it very clear that she did not support the formation of a closed professional register for nurses.[36]

In August 1914, the campaign for nurse registration was well into its twenty-seventh year, and, although Parliamentary Commissions in 1904 and 1905 had indicated their clear support, the securing of the much-desired register seemed as far away as ever. Members of

Parliament who were loyal to the anti-registrationists had blocked or delayed every bill for registration that had been brought before the House of Commons.[37]

When the British government declared war, campaigners for both women's suffrage and nurse registration suspended their activities in order to put their energies into supporting the war effort.[38] For most, their patriotism superseded their loyalties to gender and profession. Much space within the *British Journal of Nursing* was now devoted to publicizing the work—and sometimes the exploits—of nurses. The other two prominent nursing journals of the time, the *Nursing Times* and the *Nursing Mirror and Midwives Journal*, also paid much attention to 'war news'. Ethel Gordon Fenwick never fully abandoned her former campaigns, using the news of significant achievements by nurses to argue for both votes for women and professional recognition for nurses.[39]

At the outbreak of war, the nursing professions of most countries had still not succeeded in closing their professional ranks. Hence, the Allied military nursing services were a curious amalgam of highly trained elite professionals, semi-trained volunteers, and confident but largely untrained lady-nurses. In the British Dominions and the United States of America trained nurses dominated the services. The nascent army nursing services of Australia, New Zealand, Canada, and South Africa were very small at the outbreak of war, but were able, before their deployment in late 1914, to expand their ranks through the recruitment of fully trained nurses.[40] In the USA, the Army Nurse Corps, a small but effective cadre of highly trained and experienced nurses, had been created in 1901, following the Spanish-American War.[41] Because they did not enter the war at its outset, and because of their distance from the conflict, these elite cadres of trained military nurses were able to close ranks and exclude anyone who did not comply with their strict criteria for a full professional training.[42]

The British situation was very different. Here, the volunteer nurse was a significant and sometimes very powerful figure. The

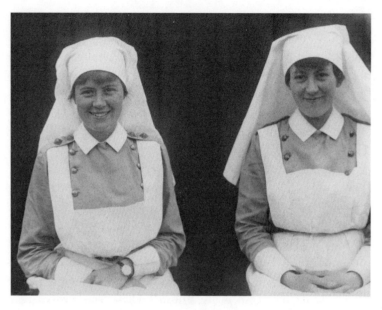

FIGURE 2 Canadian military nurses (photograph reproduced by kind permission of Talbot House, Poperinge, Belgium)

formation of voluntary aid detachments (VADs) in 1909, as part of the Haldane Reforms, had permitted the creation of small independent groups, usually governed by social elites, who came together for the expressed purpose of providing support for the wounded in time of war. They ran under the auspices of the British Red Cross Society, or the Order of St John of Jerusalem, and came to view themselves as the suppliers of elite, semi-trained volunteer nurses ready for a future national emergency.[43] Their volunteer-nurse members were, for the most part, drawn from the wealthiest families in their communities. Many were the daughters of industrialists and professionals; others were members of the landed gentry or aristocracy. Poorer, working-class women were effectively excluded by the requirement to buy one's own uniform and pay one's own expenses; they simply could not afford to join VADs. Voluntary aid detachments paid professional nurses to provide the training that would permit their members to acquire Red Cross or St John's Ambulance certificates in hygiene, home nursing, sick cookery, and first aid. Some trained nurses naturally resented the formation of cadres of semi-trained women, calling themselves 'nurses', at a time when the profession was struggling to gain recognition for its rigorous three-year training. Others, however, provided support and vital training to VADs, both through specially arranged 'classes' and through the supervision of apprenticeship-style experience on civilian hospital wards.

Britain did have a recognized military nursing service. The Queen Alexandra's Imperial Military Nursing Service (QAIMNS) and the Queen Alexandra's Royal Naval Nursing Service (QARNNS) had both been founded in 1902, towards the end of the Boer War.[44] The deaths of tens of thousands of men from infectious diseases had created an outcry in the national press. The avoidable deaths of so many British soldiers were viewed as a scandal rivalling that of the Crimea, half a century earlier. Many recognized that men were dying largely for want of adequate nursing care, and pressure was brought to bear on a reluctant military elite to support the formation of a dedicated female nursing service, which would work alongside the medical officers and orderlies of the Royal Army Medical Corps. Yet, by 1914 the QAIMNS still had a membership of only 297.[45] These numbers were augmented by a 'Reserve' numbering about 800 nurses, who were willing to be drafted for 'active service' at twenty-four hours' notice.[46] With only just over 1,000 nurses at the outbreak of war, the QAIMNS was about to find itself stretched to breaking point, as its members were rapidly deployed in field hospitals in France in support of the beleaguered British Expeditionary Force. During the course of the war, its 'Reserve' expanded dramatically, as over 10,000 additional members were recruited.[47] Its matron-in-chief throughout the war was Ethel Hope Becher, a highly experienced military nurse, and a veteran of the Second Anglo-Boer War (1899–1902).[48] To supplement and assist her central command, there was a matron-in-chief for each war front. On the Western Front this role was ably filled by Australian-born and British-trained professional nurse Maud McCarthy, who had also obtained extensive experience in the South African War (see Figure 3).[49]

At the outbreak of war, the Queen Alexandra's Royal Naval Nursing Service consisted of three head sisters, seven superintending sisters, fifty-six sisters, and five probationary sisters, all based at Haslar Hospital.[50] Like the QAIMNS, the QARNNS had a sizeable Reserve, upon which it could draw. Naval nurses formed the senior staff at royal naval hospitals throughout the war; they also served, alongside army nurses, on hospital ships.

In addition to the QAIMNS, QARNNS, and their Reserves, Britain also had a 'Territorial Force Nursing Service' (TFNS), which had been formed to supply nurses to a network of twenty-four 'Territorial hospitals' in the event of war. Large buildings such as schools, colleges, hotels, and public buildings had been earmarked to provide accommodation for Territorial hospitals. Sidney Browne, a trained nurse with extensive experience in the Second Anglo-Boer War, was at its head, and highly experienced matrons were recruited for its hospitals. These included Rachael Cox Davies, Matron of the First London General Hospital in Camberwell, the apparently strict and overbearing martinet who received such bad press from authors Vera Brittain and Irene Rathbone.[51] Nurses had been joining the TFNS since its formation in 1908. The organization had, by January 1911, recruited about 3,000 members, and was able to mobilize 2,784 within a week of the declaration of war in August 1914.[52] Criteria for enrolment were strict: all members had received three years' training in a recognized hospital and were between the ages of 23 and 50. Each had signed a declaration that she was willing to be mobilized in the event of war, and each had obtained the permission of her own matron to enrol in the service. By 1918, well over 7,000 members had served in military hospitals.[53]

With its QAIMNS, its Reserve, its TFNS, and its VADs, Britain's military nursing provision was highly complex, and perhaps mirrored

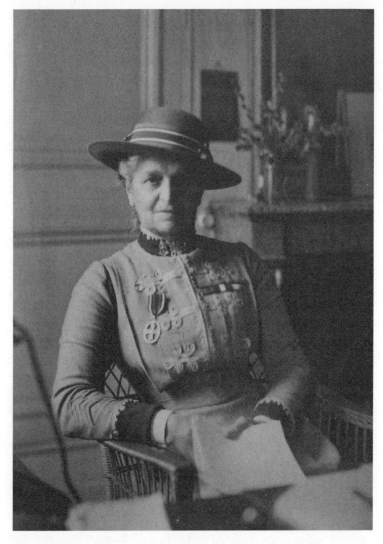

FIGURE 3 Maud McCarthy, Matron-in-Chief of the British Expeditionary Force in France and Flanders (photograph reproduced by kind permission of the Army Medical Services Museum, Aldershot, UK)

the complexity of early-twentieth-century British female society. The failure of trained nurses and VADs to work together has become one of the great myths of the First World War.[54] But the letters and diaries of both nurses and VADs belie the myth. Members of both groups expressed admiration and respect for each other, as well as occasional frustration and resentment. In reality, the two groups often worked well together.[55] Indeed, when the social class division between them and the context of their time is taken into consideration their cooperation becomes one of the remarkable features of medical provision during the First World War.

Adding a further layer of complexity to the military nursing services of all countries were the 'military orderlies' (in the USA known as 'corpsmen' and in Russia as 'sanitars') who maintained the hospital environment and offered fundamental care to the sick and injured. British nurses commented during the Second Anglo-Boer War that the existence of orderlies in military hospitals had discouraged members of the QAIMNS from providing as much hands-on care to their patients as civilian nurses.[56] The army medical services had their own turbulent history; military doctors had found it difficult, during the second half of the twentieth century, to gain full acceptance as army officers of equal standing to their combatant peers. In 1898, the Army Medical Department and the Army Hospital Corps had combined to form the Royal Army Medical Corps (RAMC).[57] The result was the establishment of a complex chain of command running from the most prestigious army doctors to the lowliest orderlies. Military nurses stood outside this system. Although they were responsible for the care of patients on their wards, they could not—at least on any official basis—give instructions to military orderlies. In practice they were usually able to command the respect of their fellow workers and to govern their wards. They were, nevertheless, vulnerable in situations where medical orderlies and doctors 'closed ranks' against them.

Many European countries had only nascent professional nursing services. In Catholic countries, nursing was still seen as largely the preserve of female religious orders. France and Belgium had begun to develop secular nursing schools, but these were few and had not been in existence for long enough to provide anything approaching a national nursing workforce.[58] Many French Red Cross nurses were skilled and experienced in volunteer work, and some had served in temporary hospitals set up in times of natural disaster. Nevertheless, France was experiencing a crisis in the provision of nursing care. Large numbers of nuns had been removed from hospital service as part of the deliberate secularization of public services under the Third Republic. However, due to the slow pace of reform and the difficulties associated with establishing an adequate number of training schools, their places had not, as yet, been filled by fully trained professional nurses. Secular training schools—such as those at the Salpetrière in Paris created by Désiré Magloire Bourneville, the École des Gardes-Malades established by reforming doctor Anna Hamilton in Bordeaux, and the *hospitalières* of the Lyons Hospices Civils—were few, and were hampered by confusion and conflict over the 'proper' place of nurses in society.[59] Doctors and politicians wished to replace nuns, who offered compassionate and attentive care to the sick but were said to take little interest in medical innovations, with women who would act as intelligent and proficient executors of the latest scientific treatments. Predictably, though, they hoped that such women would combine the scientific acumen of professional women with the humility and self-abnegation of the nuns. Essentialist notions of nursing as a 'mothering' and nurturing activity meant that both doctors and anticlerical politicians reacted with surprise when some nurses began to seek both rights as workers and status as professionals. Numbers of lay hospital staff in France had increased from 14,500 in 1880 to 95,000 by 1911, but not all of these were nurses, and very few had undergone a rigorous training programme.[60]

At the outbreak of the First World War, tens of thousands of volunteer nurses, recruited under the auspices of the three societies of the French Red Cross,[61] flooded military hospitals, and the image of the nurse underwent a dramatic transformation. No longer an occupation for the domestic class or a self-denying pursuit for those of a self-sacrificing disposition, nursing was now a highly desirable means of demonstrating loyalty to the Republic. The image of the nurse became one of patriotic femininity and women of wealth and social influence began to flock to military hospitals, their claims supported by certificates of proficiency, which some felt were awarded far too easily to women of wealth and status, following only three or six months' training. Suddenly, nursing was a respectable—even a desirable—pursuit. War had achieved 'what several preceding decades of reform had been unable to secure'.[62] But appearances were deceptive. It was not the skill, knowledge, and dedication but the romance of nursing that had captured the public imagination. And this was a romance that consciously drew upon memories of significant nursing contributions during the Franco-Prussian War, rather than upon a knowledge of the realities of modern nursing.[63]

The French nursing services were, therefore, ill-equipped to support the hundreds of thousands of wounded who began to arrive in military hospitals in the autumn of 1914. Their ranks were strengthened by the addition of fully trained nurses from Britain (where the military medical services were initially reluctant to make full use of their services) and the USA (which was not to enter the war until April 1917), but the confusion of roles within French hospitals made the work of professional nurses more difficult. Military hospitals were staffed by a combination of religious nuns, a small number of trained nurses belonging to the army's Service de Santé, military orderlies, Red Cross volunteer nurses, and women from overseas. Of the latter, most were British or American; some were highly trained, while others had even less training than the French Red Cross ladies.

In Russia, Italy, and Romania, military nursing services were dominated by three groups: military orderlies, members of female religious orders, and lady-volunteers. In Russia, almost all nursing care was provided by Sisters of Mercy, but 'war-training' courses (mostly of about six months' duration) were provided by the Red Cross at the outbreak of war, providing large numbers of 'military nurses' to staff the 'flying columns' that served the Russian army on a rapidly moving front, as well as the base hospitals in large cities, particularly Moscow and St Petersburg.[64]

## Conclusion

Those who nursed the wounded of the First World War were a complex and heterogeneous group. In each of the Allied nations there were those who regarded themselves as 'true' nurses: individuals who had undergone a carefully planned two- or three-year programme of training, and who believed they possessed not only the knowledge but also the experience to nurse well and safely. Then there were the volunteer nurses, many of whom—particularly in Britain and France—came from higher social classes than their professional counterparts. Every nation had far more volunteers than trained nurses; but proportions differed markedly, with Britain, its Dominions, and the USA having a greater proportion of 'professionals' than most other Allied nations. Further complicating the military nursing services were the 'orderlies', 'corpsmen', or 'sanitars', who worked alongside both nurses and volunteers. Of these, some were members of the armed forces who, because of either a lack of aptitude for combat or invalidity, had been detailed to care for the wounded rather than fight in the front lines; others were volunteers from a range of backgrounds. Following the introduction of conscription in Britain, some conscientious objectors became orderlies. Large numbers, particularly in France, were students or clerics. Trained nurses often appear to have found orderlies even harder to supervise than female volunteers, because the latter belonged to army medical corps, were subject to military discipline, and could, if they wished, ignore the directions of a ward sister.

Medical historian Mark Harrison has observed that the high status accorded to the British RAMC in the First World War had much to do with 'its potency as a symbol of the humanitarian ideals which had mobilized public support for the war and which continued to motivate British soldiers'.[65] The military nursing services, although existing alongside rather than as part of the army, were an integral component of this morale-boosting power. The nurse in her pristine uniform and white veil symbolized the care and security which would be offered to anyone injured in the line of duty. But the impression given by the nurses' apparently central role within the medical services belied their actual weakness as a fragmented service which existed alongside occasionally highly-chauvinistic medical professionals. Although belonging to highly-trained and dedicated cadres of workers, military nurses were, at times, treated as if their presence on the wards of military hospitals were a mere exercise in propaganda. And the presence of semi-trained volunteers and orderlies heightened their difficulties by making them responsible for the work of a group of individuals, some of whom were resistant to supervision.

When trained nurses wrote for their professional journals, they revealed a sense of confidence in their knowledge and skills and a recognition of the need to supervise closely the sometimes-inept performances of their volunteer assistants. Yet, history has accorded the 'VAD' a higher status than the professional nurse. The writings of nurses reveal an awareness of the dangers of crossing professional boundaries; yet portrayals of nurses in novel and film frequently focus either on emotional attachment and sexual involvement between nurses and their patients or on a cold and undesirable professional detachment. A simplified and strangely distorted image of the First World War nurse has been placed before the eyes of post-war generations.

Although they wrote assertively for their own professional journals, kept diaries, and were extremely conscientious letter-writers, trained nurses do not appear to have acted as apologists for their

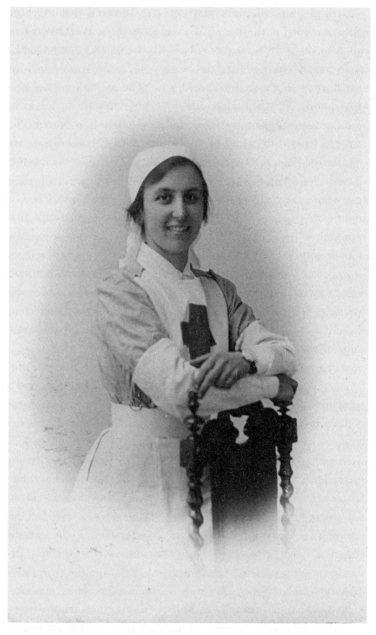

FIGURE 4 Postcard of a British 'VAD', signed 'Nurse Best' (photograph re-produced with the permission of the Royal College of Nursing Archives)

own professional expertise. Indeed, some of the best descriptions of professional nursing practice come from the observations of articulate volunteers such as Irene Rathbone and Florence Farmborough. There were probably several reasons why nurses themselves failed to address the significance of their work. As historian Janet Butler observes, writing about oneself was considered taboo for women in the early twentieth century; and there were very few exemplars of female writers for nurses to emulate.[66] Nurses may also have deliberately toned down the clinical content of their personal writings (particularly their letters home) for fear of provoking anxiety amongst friends and family whose sons and brothers were at the front.[67] For these reasons, the perspectives of nurses have been hidden from view. While the powerful outputs of wealthy and well-connected volunteer nurses were published in several editions during the course of the twentieth century and are still current today, the work of professional nurses (along with those of some of the most interesting volunteers) is, for the most part, languishing, unpublished and largely unread, in archives throughout the world. A few sources do offer an interesting perspective on the work of nurses. At the end of the war, Anne Beadsmore-Smith, then matron-in-chief of the QAIMNS, asked a number of nurses to write narratives of their wartime experiences. Some of these were collected into a book entitled *Reminiscent Sketches 1914 to 1919*. Others were simply stored in the QAIMNS archive, where they remain to be read today.[68] The work of Australian nurses is similarly represented in a series of 'Nurses' Narratives' collected by Colonel Arthur Butler to assist him in writing his official history of the Australian Army Medical Services during the war and complemented by notes on a series of interviews conducted by Matron Adelaide Kellett. Butler used very little material from the nurses' testimonies, but the originals can be retrieved from the Australian War Memorial Archives in Canberra, Australia.[69] The perspectives and emphases of the nurses are intriguing. Many took the opportunity to set out the importance of nursing work. Others stressed

the difficulties posed by conditions in military hospitals and high-
lighted what had to be endured by nurses on 'active service'. This
book uses these and a range of other sources in an attempt to bring
into view a fuller picture of First World War nursing—both professional and volunteer—to reveal the struggles of those who, although
they were not front-line combatants, were, nevertheless, fighters.

The war waged by nurses—both trained and volunteer—was a
multi-layered one. Above all, nurses saw themselves as fighting
against pain, disease, and death. Theirs was the 'second battlefield', where the wounded were drawn back from the abyss of
death.[70] And, by inhabiting that battlefield, nurses themselves faced
hardship, injury, and sometimes death. Beyond this, nurses were
fighting for recognition—for the right to exercise the freedoms and
responsibilities that were due to them as both citizens and professionals. For some, this was a fight for women's rights and, above all,
a fight for the vote. For others, it was a struggle for the recognition
of their skills and talents as not merely innate elements of their
femininity, but qualities that had been hard-won through years of
training and discipline. Finally, there was a battle going on within
the ranks of nurses themselves, between trained nurses and volunteers and between pro- and anti-registrationists. The serene image
of the nurse by the bedside of the wounded soldier belies the turbulence that infused the everyday existence of this 'veiled warrior'.

# A Call to Action
## August–December 1914

### Introduction: an army of nurses

When the British government declared war on Germany on 4 August 1914, young men volunteered in their hundreds of thousands, determined to be part of a war which many believed would be 'over by Christmas'.[1] Their expectations were cruelly dashed by a four-year conflict of attrition, which claimed millions of lives. The earliest months of the war were amongst the most lethal. In France, a series of highly mobile manoeuvres, punctuated by devastating battles, resulted in massive numbers of casualties. By Christmas 1914, military hospitals in France, and in the tiny strip of Belgium which was still in Allied hands, were caring for vast numbers of seriously injured casualties, many of whom were so badly damaged that they would never be able to return to normal civilian life—let alone rejoin the Allied war effort. The scale and seriousness of the injuries took the Allied medical services by surprise, as did the presence of devastating wound infections, such as gas gangrene and tetanus. Men were arriving at field hospitals with deep holes in their bodies or huge areas of lacerated flesh, caused by heavy artillery and machine-gun fire.

The lack of organization of the pre-war nursing services in Allied nations meant that nurses were mobilized for action only with difficulty. Many of the most highly trained were in a state of readiness, having offered their services to the 'Reserve' of the British Queen Alexandra's Imperial Military Nursing Service (QAIMNS) or to the Territorial Force Nursing Service (TFNS) prior to the war. These were quickly 'called up' for active service and began the work of establishing military hospitals in Britain and northern France. By the spring of 1915, their ranks had been swelled by members of the nascent military nursing services of the British Dominions, many of whom operated within their own medical units. In France, many towns, including Vichy and Troyes, designated themselves as *villes-hôpital* or 'hospital towns', offering many of their public buildings as auxiliary hospitals. Many French military hospitals were established in large hotels and casinos.[2]

During the early months of the war, the anxiety of continental Europe's military medical services to recruit trained nurses stood in striking contrast to the unwillingness of the British army to accept the services of female personnel. This anomaly led to the rapid recruitment of large numbers of fully trained British volunteers into French and Belgian field hospitals. The French accepted, with alacrity, the offer of a wealthy British woman, Grace Ellison, to establish a corps of British trained nurses willing to serve in their military hospitals. The 'French Flag Nursing Corps' (FFNC), as it came to be known, sent hundreds of women to the Continent during the course of the war.[3] Sarah Alice Claridge, in charge of the 'Foreign Service and Trained Nurses Department' of the St John Ambulance Association, had appointed 121 fully trained nurses for overseas service by 5 September 1914.[4] American nurses, too, travelled to the European continent in their hundreds—in spite of the dangers of Atlantic travel—eager to support the Allied war effort, long before their own nation entered the war.

British and American trained nurses, thus, often found themselves working alongside both nun-nurses and lady-volunteers in French- or Belgian-run field hospitals. Others became part of highly competent volunteer-units, such as the Scottish Women's Hospitals

(SWH), or of resource-rich, privately-funded field hospitals such as Millicent, Duchess of Sutherland's Ambulance and Hector Munro's 'Flying Ambulance Corps'.[5] Large numbers of nurses—both trained and volunteer—offered their services to the beleaguered Belgian nation at the outset of the war, only to find themselves trapped inside bombarded towns or made prisoners of war by the advancing German army.

## An excess of volunteers

Women—whether trained or untrained—were anxious to participate in what was seen as the great enterprise of war, and, for them, nursing—as a traditionally female occupation—seemed to be the most obvious contribution. Devonshire House was put at the disposal of the British Red Cross Society, and was quickly besieged by thousands of women demanding the right to serve their country. Everyone knew about Florence Nightingale's exploits in the Crimean War; and many were also aware that groups of wealthy and powerful ladies had served during the frequent colonial wars of the late nineteenth century. Rachel Williams, Matron of St Mary's Hospital, Paddington, had cared for the wounded of the Egyptian Crisis, marrying a medical officer while still overseas.[6] The wartime nurse was a romantic figure, and the highly feminine image of the white-clad nurse, soothing fevered brows, smoothing pristine sheets, and applying perfect bandages fuelled some highly unrealistic expectations.

London Hospital-trained nurse Violetta Thurstan was recruited by the British Red Cross Society to assess the applications of such hopefuls. She found many unsuitable: completely lacking in any training or preparation. There seemed to be a belief that women of the higher social classes somehow possessed the innate characteristics required of a nurse, and could practise with a minimum of preparation. Although many were conscientious and well-qualified 'ambulance workers', and others were highly competent managers, others seemed to believe that a middle-class upbringing naturally equipped them for nursing work, anticipating that the experience of running a wealthy household and overseeing the work of servants could be translated into the running of a hospital ward. Most failed to recognize that household skills were not enough. The nursing of seriously wounded men required both a technical training and experience in handling and supporting the sick. In her book *Field Hospital and Flying Column*, Thurstan expressed her shock at the behaviour of 'women who have a few weeks' or months' training, who blossom out into full uniform and call themselves Sister Rose, or Sister Mabel, and are taken at their own valuation by a large section of the public, and manage through influence or bluff to get posts that should only be held by trained nurses'.[7]

Writer Sarah Macnaughtan helped organize a voluntary aid detachment; she interviewed several enthusiastic would-be volunteers. In her book *A Woman's Diary of the War*, she commented wryly that they 'spoke of "Atthefront" as if it was one word', but had no idea of what nursing work would involve: they merely avowed that they would 'do anything'. In the early days of the war, she and her detachment had practised their bandaging techniques on 'little messenger boys' and marched in military fashion through the streets of London, enjoying the cheers of 'Sunday crowds'. Some months later, in Belgium, when she encountered the wounds of industrial warfare—the gaping holes and lacerations created by flying shrapnel—she recalled those clean, smiling messenger boys with their 'convenient fractures'.[8]

The British nursing profession felt itself overwhelmed by the sudden interest of socially-powerful and wealthy volunteers with little or no experience. Many nurses complained to their professional nursing journals about upper-class women with no training being encouraged by senior medical officers to establish themselves in charge of voluntary hospitals. Trained professional nurses were, understandably, made both anxious and indignant by such usurpation of their rightful place by untrained volunteers. Yet the efforts of voluntary aid detachments to form small, ad hoc convalescent hospitals in all manner of public and private buildings—including the stately homes of the gentry and aristocracy—did include small numbers of trained nurses in their ventures. These nurses supervised and supported the often naïve early efforts of their volunteer assistants and many VAD hospitals proved highly successful. Encouragement was offered by trained nurses who recognized the potential of well-educated and enthusiastic volunteers. M. N. Oxford, formerly a sister at Guy's Hospital, published a small textbook for VAD nurses in September 1914, in which she advised that 'only practice will show you the right way to handle a patient'.[9]

The French Red Cross—a collaboration of three highly influential societies—accelerated its programme of recruitment and training, attracting large numbers of wealthy ladies, who, it was assumed, would excel in nursing work because of their innate feminine qualities and abilities. Historian Margaret Darrow has commented on the conflicts that were created by the flooding of military hospitals with large numbers of semi-trained staff, some of whose motives seemed highly questionable. The propagandist ideal of the 'true nurse'—the self-sacrificing angel of mercy—powerfully promoted by both government and Red Cross, was countered by another compelling mythical image: the 'false nurse' who was interested only in romance or her own self-importance.[10]

The Belgian Red Cross, under the resolute command of Antoine Depage, began to take action, but both French and Belgian military services quickly realized that a lack of fully trained nurses was seriously handicapping their efforts to establish an effective system of care. There was no shortage of highly patriotic and very determined women who wished to nurse the wounded. But, although they accepted offers of help from both highly experienced nun-nurses and desperately inexperienced (and often totally untrained) lady-volunteers, they realized that their hospitals would function better with a higher ratio of trained to untrained nurses. Depage began to recruit British and American nurses to his vast military hospital, L'Hôpital de l'Océan, from the earliest months of the war.[11] Some of his British recruits were members of the FFNC.

### Getting to 'the front'

Some of the wealthiest and most powerful would-be nurses chose to circumvent the official vetting processes of the Red Cross Society and Order of St John of Jerusalem, by simply travelling directly to the Continent. Once there, they used their social influence and wealth to secure positions in French and Belgian field hospitals. Among these were astute and able individuals such as British aristocrats, the Duchesses of Sutherland and Westminster, and American millionaire Mary Borden, who quickly recognized the acute shortage of trained nurses in France and Belgium and decided to establish their own field hospitals, staffed by fully trained British, Dominion, and American nurses. Again using their considerable influence, they called upon members of the medical and nursing professions at home to select groups of doctors, nurses, and volunteers to send out to staff their hospitals. To their credit, they were astute enough to realize that an effective field hospital must have a high ratio of trained to untrained staff, and were careful to select doctors and nurses from the most prestigious hospitals in Britain, its Dominions, and the USA. They did, nevertheless, also appoint large numbers of volunteer nurses to act as assistants. In northern France, Lady Frances Belt Hadfield established and funded a hospital at Wimereux near Boulogne, which ran under the auspices of the Red Cross. One of its VADs, Dorothy Seymour, herself from a wealthy and influential family, found the hospital highly elitist and commented on Lady Hadfield's reception of the first wounded as 'heart rendingly pathetic in the best stage manner'.[12]

It was only those from the more elite sections of society who could circumvent the powerful veto of the British military medical services and insist on offering independent medical services to the war effort. Not only was vast wealth required to equip a hospital; the women who launched such remarkable enterprises also possessed 'social capital': their status as elite members of British society meant that they could persuade the military medical services in France and Belgium that their services would be of value. Their cause was helped by the shortage of fully trained professional nurses in these and other European countries. Allied propaganda had seized upon reports of German atrocities in towns such as Dinant, where 674 inhabitants had been massacred on 25 August 1914, or Louvain, where 248 were killed and dozens of public buildings—including the famous university library—were destroyed by fire.[13] The deliberate embellishment of reports from Belgium— stories of babies fixed to church doors by bayonets, or nuns raped and murdered—may have helped to steel the determination of nurses who eagerly grasped any opportunity to travel to Belgium with volunteer medical units. The fear of German brutality certainly does not seem to have deterred them. Millicent, Duchess of Sutherland's unit consisted of British-trained nurses, doctors, and volunteers. After being forced out of Brussels by the German advance, Millicent established her unit in a convent at Namur, where her nurses found themselves almost overwhelmed by 'rushes' of severely-injured and dying Belgian soldiers. In her published diary, Millicent commented on the 'coolness' of her nurses, and on how their calm determination inspired her to accomplish what would normally have seemed impossible: 'to wash wounds, to drag off rags and clothing soaked in blood, to hold basins equally full of blood, to soothe a soldier's groans'.[14] Soon, Namur was overrun by the German advance, and the town was 'fired'. Millicent and her nurses were forced to abandon their patients and walk to the Dutch border.

Following huge losses at the Battle of Liège in early August 1914, the Belgian army continued to put up fierce resistance to the German invasion—a resistance which, by delaying the movement of German forces into France, may have been a decisive factor in

the war's eventual outcome. Sarah Macnaughtan served as a volunteer nurse with Mabel St Clair Stobart's unit in Belgium. She
was in Antwerp during the German bombardment, an experience
she was later to describe vividly in her book, *A Woman's Diary of the
War*. The shelling began at midnight on 7 October, each shell
seeming to make a 'rending' noise, which increased in violence as
it approached. Macnaughtan commented on the 'unfailing pluck'
of the British nurses in her unit, who gave courage to their patients
by showing no fear. They even walked slowly through the bombardment, showing a 'British obstinacy...which refuses to hurry
for a beastly German shell!'[15]

Following the evacuation of Antwerp, the Belgian army retreated behind the River Yser, where it was reinforced by French
and British troops. The Battles of Ypres and the Yser proved decisive in halting the German advance and establishing the stalemate that was to last until March 1918. But the costs were enormous:
approximately 58,000 British, 50,000 French, and 18,500 Belgian
casualties.[16] Huge numbers of desperately injured men flooded
into Allied field hospitals and were carried to newly established
bases in northern France via hospital trains, to be cared for by
nurses who were only beginning to realize the horrific nature of
the injuries caused by industrial warfare.

Large numbers of independent units, operating under the auspices of the Red Cross or Order of St John of Jerusalem, were
overrun by the rapid German advance. Many became prisoners of
the German army and were put to work nursing German soldiers.
Violetta Thurstan was later to describe her experiences of dressing
the damaged feet of hundreds of German infantrymen.[17] Dorothy
Vernon Allen, based with the First Belgian Unit, wrote on 24
August of her experiences as one of the 'crowds of English nurses'
trapped in Belgium. At first, she and her colleagues cared for
German wounded at a château at Perke, about 20 miles from Brus-
sels. German soldiers mistrusted them, fearing them as enemies.
Later, they were allowed to work at a Red Cross ambulance station

'giving bread and water and doing any urgent dressings' for British prisoners of war passing through on their way to Germany. On 6 October, large numbers of British nurses, including Vernon Allen, were packed into third-class train carriages and taken under armed guard to Denmark via Hamburg—a journey which took four days and three nights. On arrival, their fortunes improved dramatically. They were treated as celebrities, and Vernon Allen commented that the sympathies of the populace appeared to be 'entirely English'.[18]

Even as untrained and semi-trained volunteers were making their way to 'the front', fully trained female professionals (both doctors and nurses) were finding their way barred by a patriarchal military medical service, which took a dim view of women's abilities. Louisa Garrett Anderson and Flora Murray, who were both trained doctors and members of the Women's Social and Political Union, founded the Women's Hospital Corps at the beginning of the war, but found their offers of help rebuffed by the military medical services. Their unit was taken on by the French Red Cross and located first at the Hôtel Claridge in Paris and then in Wimereux near Boulogne on the north coast of France. The value of their enterprise was to be recognized by Director General of the Army Medical Services, Sir Alfred Keogh, in May 1915, when they were permitted to open the 520-bed Endell Street Hospital as a British military hospital.[19]

When trained doctor and prominent member of the Scottish Federation of Women's Suffrage Societies, Elsie Inglis, offered a fully equipped hospital, staffed entirely by women, to the British Army Medical Services, she was famously told to 'go home and sit still'.[20] Her response was to offer the services of her 'Scottish Women's Hospitals' to the French and Serbian authorities; they were gratefully and immediately accepted. The most famous of Inglis's many hospital units was Hôpital Auxiliaire 301, located in the thirteenth-century buildings of the Abbaye de Royaumont, at Asnières-sur-Oise in the Chantilly region of France. Set amidst beautiful countryside near the forest of Carnelle, the hospital's Gothic buildings gave it an austere grandeur. In winter, its high, vaulted wards—which were given the names of famous women, such as Blanche de Castille and Jeanne d'Arc—were distinctly chilly, in spite of the large cast-iron stoves, which were repeatedly cleaned and fuelled by hard-pressed VADs. In summer, patients' beds were carried out into the courtyard, which was surrounded by cloisters and graced by a central fountain.[21]

By November 1914, the efforts of the unit's staff had transformed the abbey into a hospital equipped with cast-iron beds and the latest technology, ready to receive its first patients.[22] The hospital was to prove a success and fulfilled its founders' goal of demonstrating that women could mobilize and run a field hospital without male intervention. Yet, in spite of the remarkable opportunities it offered to women to work together in what would normally be regarded as a masculine military domain, the world of Royaumont was still a segregated one, in which doctors set themselves aside from nurses and VADs, sitting at their own table in the huge, vaulted dining room.[23]

Mabel St Clair Stobart was not a trained medical worker, but had run a highly successful hospital service during the First Balkan War in 1912. She took her 'Women's Sick and Wounded Convoy Corps' to Belgium, where she and her staff soon found themselves trapped behind enemy lines and obliged to negotiate their own release. Stobart herself narrowly escaped execution as a spy. After the invasion of Belgium, most volunteer units would turn their attention to Serbia. They were to experience extreme hardship and some of their members died in the typhus epidemics which affected large numbers of Serbian military hospitals in the early spring of 1915.[24]

### The 'little corner never conquered'

In the tiny strip of Belgium of less than 300 square miles that remained in Allied hands, Dr Antoine Depage, an experienced surgeon and the head of the Belgian Red Cross, was working to sustain a medical service for the shattered Belgian army. Queen Elisabeth of the Belgians invited him to create a hospital at La Panne, a small village on the Belgian coast. A large beachside hotel was used to form 'L'Hôpital de L'Océan', which eventually came to be recognized as a centre of excellence for wound management. By 1917, when it was taken over by the British military medical services, the hospital would have, in addition to the original hotel building, about forty temporary pavilions. It was one of the closest base hospitals to the German lines; shells frequently passed over it, the German range-finders deliberately missing it, in exchange for similar protection for their own military hospitals.[25] The King and Queen of the Belgians moved their residence to La Panne, which became 'the very heart and soul of Belgium,—the real capital of the country'.[26] Depage had worked with Edith Cavell at the Berkendael Surgical Institute in Brussels prior to the war, and had a particularly enlightened attitude to professional nursing. He staffed L'Hôpital de l'Océan, as far as he could, with trained nurses from Belgium, France, Britain, and the USA, supplementing these with volunteer nurses. In the early months of the war, he was also assisted by his wife, Marie, who was tragically drowned during the sinking of the *Lusitania* in May 1915. It is believed that more than half of those Belgian soldiers who were treated for injuries during the war, passed through L'Hôpital de l'Océan.[27]

Queen Elisabeth of the Belgians won extraordinary acclaim for her work at L'Océan (see Figure 5). A legend so powerful grew up around her reputation as the 'queen-nurse' that she found herself obliged to refute claims that she was, indeed, a nurse, by stating publicly that she had never undergone a full training and that, because of her royal duties, she was unable to work shifts. Her claim that she was unable to make a full contribution to the work at L'Hôpital was remarkably self-effacing, given that she was often at the hospital, and did, in fact, put her shortened war-training to good effect, caring for patients and assisting Antoine Depage in the

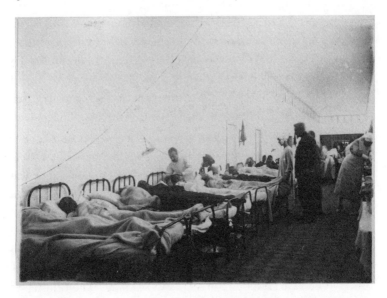

FIGURE 5  Queen Elisabeth of the Belgians visits L'Hôpital de l'Océan (Vinkem site) (photograph ©Archives Belgian Red Cross, Brussels)

operating room. More important than her nursing work, however, was her contribution in raising morale, by walking the wards, offering comfort and reassurance, and giving gifts of fruit and chocolate to both patients and nurses.[28] One Belgian soldier was moved to write a letter of thanks to the hospital: 'It will always be a very beautiful, consoling and enjoyable thing', he wrote, 'to think about all the love that was given to me in my days at the hospital.'[29]

Only two fully trained Belgian nurses worked at L'Hôpital de l'Océan throughout the war, moving with the hospital unit to its location further behind the lines, at Vinkem, when shelling drove the unit out of La Panne, and remaining there when the British medical services took over its site at La Panne. One, Jane De Launoy, kept a vivid diary of her experiences at L'Océan. She had trained at the Catholic School of Saint-Camille, and was clearly dismayed that so many of those who cared for Belgian soldiers should be foreign nationals:

26 December 1914: What I don't like is that on Belgian territory all nurses but 2 were foreigners. All orders and reports are given in English. Despite the draconian regime I heard that a lot of them refuse to do the night shift. I suppose that is the VADs...It has been necessary for me to devise for myself a programme—a code of behaviour—a strategy: 'Agree to do what others don't want to do'.[30]

De Launoy likened the British system of hospital governance to the running of an army: it was 'not amusing but perfect...a well-commanded service'. The head nurse on De Launoy's floor was the indomitable 'Miss Grant', who appears to have imposed an iron rule of discipline. Nurses were not allowed to remain in their wards beyond their duty-hours, and other wards were strictly out of bounds. No one must sit on any bed or have a conversation with a patient. If such a conversation began, Miss Grant invariably 'intervened'. De Launoy's comment was scathing: 'The British pretend that in matters of discipline the Belgians are nothing...No dinner at the hotel...no permission to go to restaurants...No...oh la la!' De Launoy's indignation was fuelled by her sense that Miss Grant and other British nurses misinterpreted the motivations of Belgian nurses, viewing them as frivolous when, in fact: 'We all have a very high ideal working for our country. Only a few seconds are enough to make a military hero, but a nurse at the front has to prepare herself to be a moral hero every hour.'[31]

## Mobilization

The British Expeditionary Force (BEF)—the established and fully-trained element of the British army—landed at Boulogne and Le Havre in early August 1914, and attempted, unsuccessfully, to hold back the German advance, first at Mons on 23 August and then three days later at Le Cateau. Meanwhile, the French forces had suffered serious setbacks in the Battles of Lorraine, the Ardennes, and Charleroi, with hundreds of thousands of casualties. Military medical services struggled to evacuate the wounded. In four days of desperate fighting on the River Marne in early September, the Allies succeeded in holding back a German advance which was coming dangerously close to Paris. Both forces then began to move northwards, each desperately trying to outflank the other, in a series of manoeuvres that became known as 'the race to the sea'.

In August 1914, Sir Henry Wilson, Director of Military Operations, decided that the wounded should be evacuated by horse-drawn wagon and train directly to the ports of France, where they would be embarked and brought to hospitals in Britain. Director General of the Army Medical Services, Sir Alfred Keogh, and his second-in-command, Sir Arthur Slogget, made provision for a chain of evacuation extending from regimental aid posts and field dressing stations close to the fighting lines, to distant base hospitals. The scheme proved impracticable, leading to a failure to evacuate the wounded sufficiently rapidly. Poor provision resulted in delays, which permitted severe wound infections to take hold. An acute shortage of motor ambulances worsened an already difficult situation, resulting in wounded men being left without expert medical or nursing attention for several hours—sometimes days.[32]

Members of the QAIMNS and its Reserve were mobilized for service overseas from the earliest months of the war. In the period of rapid mobile warfare, prior to the formation of the trench system on the Western Front, they found themselves coping with chaos, caring for very large numbers of wounded men in squalid conditions, with inadequate equipment. Sister Kate Luard (QAIMNSR) was posted to a railway station in France, where she and colleagues waited for each passing train to stop. The doors of the large railway carriages would be opened and they would board the train, to offer what care they could to wounded men inside. By the time the wounded reached the care of nurses such as Luard, many were in terrible conditions. Men with extensive injuries were lying on straw in their muddy, torn uniforms with their wounds covered only by first field dressings. The trains were travelling slowly; conditions were cold, and food and water were scarce. All the nurses could do was clean their patients' contaminated wounds, apply clean dressings, and offer what food and water was available, before the train moved on again to base.[33]

Luard, like many of her contemporaries, was an avid letter-writer. Many of her eleven siblings were still living in the family home, Birch Rectory, in a small Essex village. She wrote every day, sometimes penning letters to favourite sisters, sometimes to a select 'inner circle', and sometimes to all. She also, frequently, entered her thoughts and reminiscences into a series of 'journals' which she sent off to her family at regular intervals. Her observations of the courage, tenacity, and spirit of her patients were captured in her measured, yet lively, prose. The letters she received in return cast an interesting light on the perspectives of those left on the 'home front'. On 6 October 1914, her sister Daisy wrote to her:

> You are a lucky devil waltzing to the Front like that. The family is much amused because you're the 1st to get to the Front, 1st to go up in an air-yoplane [*sic*] & only one to get to the last war. Always so dashing...
> I suppose in spite of the horrors you are having the time of yr life—can't I come as a female orderly on yr train? Your exploits cause a gt sensation here—Florence Nightingale is nothing to it...Everyone is screaming to see yr letters...It's what we live for nowadays.[34]

Within weeks, the medical services were beginning to organize and Luard, along with others, was assigned to a designated 'hospital train'. She spent the last months of 1914 and the early part of 1915 caring for patients being transported from newly-established casualty clearing stations (CCSs), where many had undergone emergency surgery, to base hospitals, where they would be kept for several days or weeks before being either taken home to 'Blighty' or returned to the front lines.

Towards the end of 1914, as the trench system began to solidify, increasing numbers of qualified nurses were mobilized to base hospitals in northern France. In October 1914, Sister E. Dodd found herself posted to a wounded officers' hospital, which had beds for about 200 men. As injured men poured in from the First Battle of Ypres, she and her colleagues found themselves nursing twice that number. They could only accommodate the wounded by placing them on stretchers on the floor. 'We had to exercise great care in attending them', she commented when recounting her experiences later, 'as one might easily step on one patient in the effort to reach the next.'[35]

One matron described conditions at the sugar sheds near Boulogne's Gare Maritime, in October 1914 (see Figure 6):

> An indescribable scene met us. In the first huge shed there were hundreds of walking-wounded cases. (As long as a man could crawl, he had to be a walking case.) All of them were caked with mud, in torn clothes, hardly any with caps, with blood-stained bandages on arms, hands and legs, many lying asleep in the straw that had been left in the hastily cleaned sheds, looking weary to death...Dressings were being done on improvised tables; blood-stained clothes caked in mud, that had been cut off were stacked in heaps with rifles and

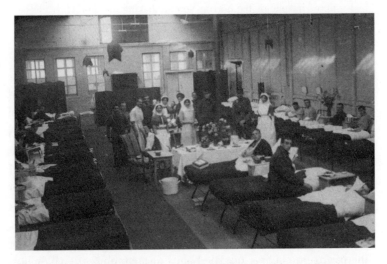

FIGURE 6 The 'Sugar Sheds' at Boulogne, following their establishment as a General Hospital (photograph from the collection of Sheila Brownlee, and reproduced by her kind permission)

ammunition. Further on, the sheds were being converted into wards; wooden partitions were being run up, bedsteads carried in, the wounded, meanwhile, lying about on straw or stretchers...As fast as one could get to them, the clothes were got off, and the patient washed, and his wounds dressed. Some had both legs off, some their side blown away—all were wounded in dozens of places. Doctors and nurses were hopelessly outnumbered, distractedly trying to meet the demands made on them. Here, too, we found the Matron-in-Chief helping and directing; under her supervision a miraculous change soon took place. Re-inforcements of nurses began to arrive, and the sheds took on the appearance of a well-ordered hospital.[36]

This anonymous matron's eagerness to give credit to both the dynamism and the organizational skill of her matron-in-chief, Maud McCarthy, perhaps belies the difficulties faced by the military medical and nursing services. Effective lines of evacuation were slow to form and nurses were forced to improvise for several weeks before anything like a clear strategy was developed.

## On the front lines

By the end of 1914 a network of CCSs, hospital trains, barges, base hospitals, hospital ships, and convalescent hospitals had developed—a process made easier by the fact that warfare had become static and entrenched on the Western Front. An initial process of apparent trial and error gave way slowly to a coordinated system of evacuation. Earlier wars, notably the Russo-Japanese War of 1904–5, had provided models, but the system which was developed on the Western Front during the First World War was, in many ways, unique. One of its most significant features was the establishment of CCSs within 6 miles of the front lines. By October, it was being recognized that many of the deaths which had taken place in the first weeks of the war on the Western Front had been avoidable. The bullet- and shell-wounds sustained on the muddy, manured fields of Flanders and northern France were almost always

heavily contaminated with anaerobic bacteria, which caused severe
life-threatening infections, such as gas gangrene and tetanus.[37]
These wounds needed to be treated—whether by the surgical excision of contaminated tissue, or by treatment with antiseptics—as
quickly as possible. The delay caused by transportation to base was
costing lives and there was a need for more small field hospitals
capable of performing emergency surgery near to the front.

Colonel Arthur Lee had been sent to France by Lord Kitchener
in the autumn of 1914 to report on the problems being experienced
on the lines of evacuation. Lee recommended that one motor
ambulance convoy should be assigned to each army corps to carry
the wounded from regimental aid posts to 'clearing hospitals', after
which hospital trains should convey them the rest of the way to
base hospitals. At first, only six clearing hospitals had been sent out
with the BEF; it became clear that these were unable to cope with
the numbers of casualties produced by battles such as those at
Mons and Le Cateau.[38]

Casualty clearing stations developed slowly during the autumn
of 1914, and the placing of female nurses in these was seen as
highly experimental and very dangerous. Male military medical officers had serious doubts over the wisdom of posting women so
close to the front lines, believing that they would be unable to cope
with the privations and stresses of life in the 'zone of the armies'.
Maud McCarthy, Matron-in-Chief of the British Expeditionary
Forces in France and Flanders, embraced the idea with some enthusiasm, and was supported by her senior, Matron-in-Chief of the
QAIMNS, Ethel Hope Becher. Both women had served as military
nurses with the nascent Army Nursing Service during the Boer
War, and even though wound infection in South Africa had presented nothing like the problems seen now in northern France,
both recognized the importance of rapid surgical intervention and
the impossibility of providing such intervention without nursing
expertise. There was, however, a problem: when CCSs were first
formed, small groups of nurses were drawn from base hospitals in

Boulogne at times when 'rushes' of casualties were already putting those hospitals under pressure. McCarthy urged the military medical services to allow for a sizeable 'reserve' of highly competent nurses at Boulogne and other bases, ready to be moved forward to CCSs at short notice.[39] Nurses were employed in CCSs for the first time during the First Battle of Ypres in October.[40] The development of this system would later permit recognized 'surgical teams'—each consisting of a surgeon and anaesthetist, a nursing sister, and orderlies—to move together as a unit from base to CCS, and also, as need arose, between CCSs.

Towards the end of 1914, McCarthy approved a decision to increase the number of nursing staff in each CCS from five to seven. The nursing staff of a CCS was to be composed of one sister-in-charge, two other sisters, and four staff nurses. In a letter drafted that winter, she affirmed that 'in selecting the nursing staff for CCS care has been taken to select the best workers, as well as the most suitable people, for the work, irrespective of ranks'.[41]

One of the earliest nurses to serve in a CCS was Glaswegian Jentie Paterson. Clearly a highly educated, professional woman, Paterson was confident in her skill and determined in her opinions. On 7 August she had travelled to her training hospital, Guy's, in London, to enlist for service as a member of the QAIMNSR. She was posted to No. 4 General Hospital, and left for France—one of a small contingent of Guy's nurses—on 22 August.[42] The diaries in which she recounted her wartime experiences were tiny, but her terse entries, clearly made contemporaneously with the events they describe, are vivid and arresting. At first, she was appointed sister to an acute surgical ward at No. 4 British General Hospital, Versailles. On 17 September, she commented on how some of her patients died soon after they reached her ward: 'Awful injuries! So thankful for anything we do...5.30: 400 wounded arrived. I got 26 as quick as lightning. Lord what injuries! One death young gunner 20 mins after admission. I left the Ward at 1.45 am!! All wounds dressed.'[43]

Paterson's work did not get any easier. On 18 September, after
four hours' sleep, she rejoined her ward at 7.30 a.m. and worked
continuously until her first short break at 2 p.m. Her next meal was
at 8.45 p.m., but 'all men thoroughly washed up blanket bathed all
redressed! Ward almost straight.' One of her patients was a Seaforth Highlander, with a wound the 'size of a saucer' in his back
and shoulder. Her terse and disjointed entry for the following day
speaks of the intensity of her experience: 'What a ward—busy all
day slog slog slog. Off 11pm no tea hour. Poor Seaforth died awful
brick. Got a bath!'[44] On 21 September she 'took in' fifty cases, several with compound fractures and concussion, and left the ward at
3.45 a.m. feeling 'Dead!' The next day she found that several of
her patients had contracted tetanus, and one had died of the disease in spite of having undergone an emergency amputation. Most
of her diary entries for late September refer to tetanus and gas
gangrene. It was clear to her—and becoming clear to the medical
services more generally—that patients were waiting too long for
the life-saving surgery which would remove infected material
from their bodies. In mid-September, Paterson commented that
anti-tetanus serum was to be given to all patients with wounds. By
the end of the month, heavy workloads, combined with misman-
agement of the hospital, were leading to 'rebellion in the camp'.
'We are so understaffed' complained Paterson, and *'matron is a
fool'*.[45] It was becoming clear that there were serious tensions between QAIMNS regulars and those nurses who had been recruited
at the outbreak of war: the 'Reserves' and 'Territorials'.

Paterson's ordeal at Versailles continued until December. Her
diary resonates with the horror of war: 'We see such sights!' she
exclaimed, as she wrote of one patient with 'half his head blown
away with a shell, and 2 with bullet wounds through lungs'.[46] But
in November, following a brief stay in Boulogne, Paterson was
given the opportunity to travel to 'within a mile or two of the lines'
to join No. 5 CCS at Hazebrouck. In a letter home, Paterson explained that she was one of 'the furthest up lot of sisters except

those on the trains', adding, 'we see the flashes of the guns and hear the roar day and night'.[47] She commented that the colonel had not wanted nurses at the CCS, believing that, not only would they be unable to cope with the dirt and squalor of a field hospital, but that they might actually be in danger. Stories of German atrocities against Belgian citizens were fuelling the indignation of the Allies, and Paterson herself recorded narratives of the mutilation of Belgian civilians by German soldiers in both her diary and her letter.

Paterson had volunteered for the most 'dirty' work going, but was not allowed to proceed to a CCS until she had made a written statement that she was accepting her posting voluntarily. Her ward was the huge hall of a monastery. At the approach of a convoy, staff would hear a whistle, and then a fleet of motor ambulances would arrive. On some days, the CCS took in 300 wounded men over a period of several hours and the nurses, assisted by orderlies, did what they could to make them comfortable. All wounds were dressed, and men were given food and drink. The 'walking wounded' were seated at long tables and given bottles of stout, cigarettes, and a meal of soup or stew. Some convoys could be kept overnight, making it possible for the nursing staff to wash them and 'at least change their socks most of which we cut off'. Often, the nurses found that their patients, who were 'alive' with fleas and lice, would beg them not to come near. Nurses had to offer reassurance that it was part of their job to clean hazardous dirt and vermin from their patients' bodies.

'Stretcher cases' were a more difficult matter (see Figure 7). These had to be carefully triaged, in order to decide which were in the most urgent need of operation. Paterson commented on how she had

> lost one man to-day. Poor chap, leg black, operation, died on the table. Another (as if to cheer us up) who seemed more desperate had mortified up to the level of R. Kidney. He has 17 incisions in his

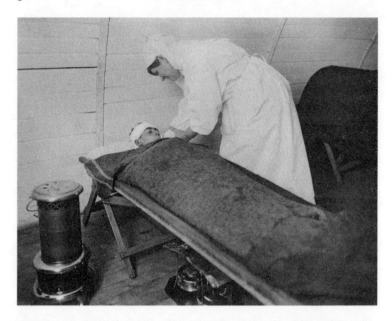

FIGURE 7 A stretcher patients is made comfortable in a casualty clearing station. Note: this image is of an Australian CCS and was taken after 1916 (photograph reproduced by permission of the Imperial War Museum, London, UK, and with the kind assistance of Talbot House, Poperinge, Belgium)

abdominal walls and is going to pull through, that is another reason we are up here. Such cases could not live without operation at once and they require careful nursing afterwards. Of course we have no beds only stretchers no air cushions, no sheets, so you use all your skill and ingenuity. I had a man last week who was almost pulseless for hours, today he is eating tinned chicken and travels to the base, tomorrow with a healthy stump! It is marvellous what can be accomplished amidst the din and dirt and dust of a convoy, and a good hot meal and sleep goes a long way. Nursing on stretchers on the floor is of course killing work and takes much more time…we literally nurse and improvise at the same time.[48]

Paterson commented on the remarkable changes that had taken place over the course of a few months. Rough horse-drawn carts had been replaced with motor ambulances, and trains with straw-filled cattle trucks were giving way to specially equipped ambulance trains with a regular staff of doctors, sisters, and orderlies. Yet, the military services still had their shortcomings, and Paterson lamented, in particular, what she saw as the inadequacies of the military orderlies, believing that they could '*never* take the place of women nurses', adding: 'they lack *education*, perception and conscience'. One of their greatest shortcomings, in her opinion, was their failure to understand the concept of 'surgical cleanliness'. She concluded that she would rather work 'with the most "fatheaded" woman probationer under me than a nursing orderly. They mean well and are kind to the patients *but*, oh, there are 100 buts!'[49] This view of the competence of orderlies was only one of the many strong opinions held by Jentie Paterson. On 9 December 1914 one of her letters from France appeared in a Glasgow newspaper. It praised the courage and heroism of the wounded, but deplored the need for the so-called 'car campaign' to induce men to enlist for active service:

> To think that free-born Britons who sing 'they never will be slaves' have to be induced to fight for their birthright...that it requires advertisements and decorated cars and posters of nurses ready to bind their wounds before they will take up arms to maintain their country's honour or to defend their own homes! We out here cannot understand how any self-respecting man, not required for home affairs, can remain in civilian garb![50]

Paterson's somewhat strident campaigning for enlistment sits awkwardly alongside her poignant descriptions of the horrific wounds and suffering of her patients. Historians such as Claire Tylee and Trudi Tate have commented on the susceptibility of nurses—and of women more generally—to Allied wartime propaganda.[51] From a twenty-first-century vantage point it is easy to judge those women who, although they may have worked close to the front lines and may even, at times, have found themselves under direct bombardment, never had to go 'over the top' and face the guns of their enemies. In the early twentieth century, the idea that women might participate in combat was completely alien to the vast majority of people, and Paterson undoubtedly felt that her 'front-line' experiences equipped her to comment from the perspective of a participant. She also seems to have been entirely convinced by stories of German atrocities against Belgian civilians, many of which were almost certainly exaggerated. To British nurses such as Jentie Paterson—steeped in the belief that the British Empire was the most civilizing force in the world—the need to fight against an apparently barbaric enemy was self-evident, and, for nurses, their work as healers was the greatest contribution they could make.

## Hospital trains

On Thursday 24 September, Kate Luard, having relinquished her work at a station in northern France, was travelling on a makeshift hospital train running from the front lines to Saint-Nazaire. The train was 'miles long' and had neither corridor nor special hospital equipment. The wounded lay on stretchers on the floors of its carriages, and the nurses could only reach them by 'clawing along the footboards'.[52] Every time the train stopped, Luard had a few of the most seriously wounded patients moved into one carriage where she could watch them more closely. Her haversack was lined with waterproof jaconet and filled with dressings, and she moved from patient to patient checking wounds, and offering food and water when it could be obtained. Luard's experiences were fairly typical of those of 'transport nurses' in the first few months of the war. It took some time for specially designed hospital trains to be provided in sufficient numbers to effectively transport the 'rushes' of wounded men who poured into the earliest CCSs back to base.

The provision of hospital trains in 1914 was, in fact, so poor that questions were asked in the House of Commons. As a result, the conversion of existing trains and the design and construction of new ones were commissioned not only by the War Office but also by organizations such as the Red Cross and by individual philanthropists who gave their names to trains they had funded. The 'Princess Christian Hospital Train' was one of the earliest in use.[53] Kate Luard commented in her diary that there was one 'swanky Ambulance Train' in her sector, which was properly equipped for transporting the wounded. She was delighted to find, on 27 September, that she had been placed on permanent duty on this train, which went 'up to the Front, to the nearest point on the rail to the fighting line'.[54]

Nurses who found themselves posted to ambulance trains considered themselves very lucky, because their posting permitted them to approach—albeit temporarily—as close to the front lines as any woman was permitted to be. It also ensured that they performed interesting and challenging work. Louise Bickmore wrote of the uncertainties of life on board such a train. The nurse never knew where she was headed, or where she would be at any given time. Indeed, one of the most difficult aspects of transport work was actually finding one's way to the train. The nurse would be ordered to wait at a particular station at a particular time; but these orders might change abruptly, and she might have to travel from station to station by ambulance, or be driven to a siding where 'a perilous foot journey...among and across railway lines' would bring her to 'a long, long Train—a shining vibrant, living creature of sinuous grace'.[55] Bickmore clearly relished her transport work, which took her through the devastated zones close to the front lines, where she could experience 'the booming of big guns, the rattle of machine guns, the hum of aeroplanes, the cram and crush and crowd of the high roads'.[56] Her somewhat florid prose conveys her sense of the drama and pathos of her work, and she chooses to pitch her account of train work at the level of a heroic narrative:

> Dashing at high speed 'Empty' to a far advanced Casualty Clearing Station (CCS) to gather a 'Crisis Load'; or returning at ten miles an hour, bearing within it the shattered remains of those, who so

proudly and bravely sallied forth against the foe, on the Battlefield a
few short hours before. Sometimes under shell fire, sometimes under
raiding or fighting aeroplanes it serenely 'carries on'.[57]

The epic narrative tropes of 'sallying forth' against a 'foe' and of
'serenely carrying on' in the face of extreme danger, belie the realities of nursing work in the cramped, confined spaces of railway
carriages. Bickmore's ambulance train was one of the more old-fash-
ioned models, and was poorly equipped. Patients lay on stretchers on
the floor of carriages, as well as on tiered bunks. Water for sterilizing
equipment, making fomentations, or preparing hot drinks had to be
boiled on small primus stoves 'in the midst of the crush'.

It usually took about two hours to 'load' a train at a CCS, and
then between six and thirty-six hours to travel to the base. Ambulance trains were given the lowest priority in the traffic schedule,
after trains carrying troops, ammunition, and supplies, and had
strict speed limits. Close to the front lines, they could be subjected
to air raids, and would stop and turn off all lights until the danger
passed. They sometimes took days to reach their destinations, but
patients were glad to sleep, even in cramped bunks, and nurses
could perform necessary tasks such as changing dressings and offering food and fluids. By the summer of 1915, even very complex
procedures such as wound irrigation could be performed—albeit
with difficulty, and, on upper bunks, requiring quite 'acrobatic'
techniques—by transport nurses. On arrival at the base, nurses
supervised the removal of blanket-wrapped patients on stretchers
to ambulances, and assisted the 'walking cases' from the train.

Many of the earliest ambulance trains were adapted French passenger trains; each carriage was self-contained, and was staffed by
two orderlies. Sisters and medical officers moved from coach to
coach as best they could. Usually, this meant waiting until the train
stopped at a station, when the nurse would move between coaches
in 'rain, wind or snow, unspeakable mud, daylight or pitch black
night'.[58] The alternative was 'foot boarding', a practice that proved

very dangerous. It was prohibited by the authorities, but continued throughout the war on trains without corridors.[59]

Life on board a hospital train was very restricted, because of the unpredictable nature of the schedules. Leave was always limited to two hours, and sometimes, when trains received orders to move suddenly, nurses were left behind. Yet many nurses seem to have relished their 'visits' to the front lines. One Australian nurse, Sister H. Chadwick, commented on how she and her colleagues had picked up some rather extraordinary souvenirs: 'We have some very nice shell cases...I have a nice lot of bombs too, some of ours as well as Fritz's. They are nice to take home and show what we threw at Fritz and what he shied at us...We are careful to get the boys to take all detonators and fuses out first as they are awfully dangerous toys.'[60]

## The British 'home front'

As members of the gentry and aristocracy were engaged in adventures on the Continent and fully trained members of the QAIMNS and its Reserve were struggling to establish the lines of evacuation on the emerging Western Front, professional nurses on the British 'home front' were working hard to perfect a network of 'Territorial Hospitals'—twenty-three at the outbreak of war—to which the wounded were being evacuated. Eventually, ten Territorial units would work overseas, but, in 1914, they were staffing important General Hospitals where patients could undergo treatment for injury and illness and could begin to rehabilitate. Patients were conveyed to them via ambulance trains and 'hospital ships' converted from existing rolling stock and passenger vessels. At first, most patients were either taken to the Royal Victoria Hospital, Netley, Southampton, or conveyed by hospital train to London. Territorial Hospitals soon opened in several major British cities, and, as the scale of the casualties became apparent, staff in even the smaller

auxiliary hospitals began to perform some surgery. As the provision
of care for the wounded became better established, most surgery
was performed in General Hospitals, while auxiliary units were
used for convalescence and rehabilitation. Some Territorial Hospitals were very large: the Second Western General Hospital in
Manchester, for example, had 6,700 beds by August 1917.[61]

Sister Louie Johnson, an experienced Yorkshire nurse, was appointed sister-in-charge of a surgical ward at the Second Northern
General Hospital in Leeds. Trained at Hull Royal Infirmary, and
invited to return there as a sister, Johnson had become engaged to
be married just before the outbreak of war, but her fiancé had enlisted and was later mobilized to Gallipoli. Feeling that she must do
something to support the war effort, Johnson 'signed on for the
duration' as a member of the Territorial Force Nursing Service.[62]
As a surgical sister, she began duty at 8 o'clock, taking a verbal report on her patients' conditions from the night-duty nurse and then
conducting a ward round before reporting briefly to the matron
and then returning to the ward to supervise a staff of trained and
untrained nurses. In an oral history interview conducted many
decades after the war, Johnson commented on how young many of
her patients were: they seemed like 'boys'. When they underwent
surgery, she personally accompanied every one of them to theatre,
recognizing their fear and need for support. Eventually, Johnson
was appointed 'night superintendent' of the hospital and spent the
last years of the war patrolling the eerily silent corridors of the Second Northern General, supervising and supporting her staff in
healing some of the most horrific wounds of war.[63]

On the 'home front' voluntary aid detachments 'mobilized' rapidly to staff a large number of ad hoc military hospitals. The scale of
the provision was enormous. There were, for example, eight wom-
en's detachments in the Kensington district of London alone, with a
joint membership of approximately 200 (which increased to about
1,300 by the end of the war). Most members had been 'in training'
for at least two years. The London/28 Detachment (Kensington)

provided volunteer nurses for a small hospital at White City, which was attached to a large military base. It was formed on 21 October, beginning with sixteen beds, which was rapidly increased to forty-six, and to which was added a separate sixteen-bed ward for soldiers suffering from an epidemic of measles. The hospital had a matron and two trained nurses; the rest of the staff were VAD members.[64] The rapid formation of this small hospital was typical of the creation of so-called 'war hospitals' in all manner of buildings. They were staffed by members of the voluntary aid detachments, who worked under the direction and supervision of a small trained staff. At the end of August, the British Red Cross Society and the Order of St John of Jerusalem had effectively joined forces, their efforts being coordinated by a 'Joint War Committee'.[65]

For fully trained British nurses it was an affront to their professionalism when wealthy, semi-trained volunteers were permitted to fund and take charge of hospitals overseas, staffing them with VADs and appearing, in some cases, to ignore the existence of the nursing profession. Yet, the majority of volunteers were both very aware of their positions as auxiliaries in the war effort and appreciative of any support and supervision that might be offered to them by fully trained professional nurses. May Cannan was a member of a voluntary aid detachment in Oxford, which had been founded by her mother in March 1911 at Oxford University. Prior to the war, Cannan had obtained a range of certificates from the St John's Ambulance Association and the Red Cross Society, some in first aid and others in home nursing, hygiene, and sanitation. Some members of the detachment had secured the permission of the matron at the Poor Law Hospital in the Cowley Road to gain some experience of nursing in the wards. Cannan commented that 'it was a beautiful little hospital and the sister there was most kind and helpful to us...We learned to make beds, give blanket baths, take temperatures, deal with feeding cups and bed pans, and a certain amount about the general work of a busy ward...We learned a lot and were very grateful for being allowed the experience.'[66]

In August 1914, the detachment established a hospital in a wing of Magdalen College School, but was informed that its hospital was not required and must close. Knowing that the nearest military 'base hospital' was not yet ready to receive patients, Cannan visited its commanding officer and offered him the VAD hospital as an auxiliary unit, an offer he accepted with relief. It was not, however, until 20 May 1915 that Felstead House, No. 23 Banbury Road was opened by the detachment as a unit in its own right—'an orthopaedic convalescent hospital under the base hospital and staffed by us...with two trained sisters'. Cannan later recalled with some amusement how different the sisters were. One was 'anti-VAD' and 'everyone was made unhappy and nervous by her'; the other was 'the exact opposite, and of course got far better work out of everyone'.[67]

One of the myths of the First World War focuses on the nursing care that was offered to soldier-patients in manor houses and stately homes throughout England. Initially, the intention had been to offer only convalescent care in such premises, but, during large 'rushes' of casualties such as that occasioned by the so-called 'Battle of the Somme' in 1916, they could find themselves caring for more acutely ill patients. Many large stately homes were converted into convalescent hospitals. VAD Margaret Van Straubenzee described how she managed to gain a posting to Clandon Park Hospital, the home of the Countess of Onslow, near Guildford, Surrey: 'the big hall and one of the drawing-rooms leading out of it were turned into wards I and Ia. The present Earl's study and the Green Ballroom leading out of it, on the right of the big staircase, were turned into Wards II and III, with a ward kitchen made out of part of the main hall and under the stairs.' Van Straubenzee enjoyed working with the 'very nice' matron and sisters. Many of the VADs belonged to 'old Surrey county families'.[68]

## Nurses from 'new worlds'

In the self-governing British Dominions, women volunteered enthusiastically to serve the Empire. The nascent Australian Army

Nursing Service (AANS) (which at this time existed only as a 'Reserve' service) began to mobilize at the beginning of the war, though nurses did not leave the shores of Australia until the last months of 1914. They travelled on hospital ships to the Eastern Mediterranean, where the Gallipoli campaign was already being planned. The service was organized into three Australian General Hospitals (AGHs), two of which were based in Egypt at Heliopolis and Ghezira, whilst the third was established on the Island of Lemnos.[69] The New Zealand Army Nursing Service was formed with some difficulty in the face of military and medical opposition. The efforts of its matron-in-chief, Hester Maclean, were thwarted until the spring of 1915, when New Zealand nurses were allowed to follow their counterparts in the other British Dominions into war service. The first contingent of fifty nurses left New Zealand on board the SS *Rotorua* on 8 April 1915, to join their Australian colleagues in the Eastern Mediterranean.[70] In 1915, a contingent from South Africa sailed for England, under the direction of Miss Jane Charlotte Child. After a time in Bournemouth this unit spent many months staffing the South African Hospital in France.[71]

In the spring of 1915, Canadian army nurses joined the Canadian Expeditionary Force, many of them mobilizing as part of already-defined hospital units. Trained nurse Dorothy Cotton travelled to France as part of No. 3 Canadian General Hospital, a unit formed by McGill University.[72] Unlike the Australian and New Zealand nursing services, the Canadian services decided to take volunteer nurses to Europe as part of its personnel. These came to be known by the British acronym, 'VADs'.[73]

## Mission of mercy: American Red Cross nurses in Germany and Austria

It was not only in the Allied lines that nurses found themselves overwhelmed with casualties and having to improvise care. Some American nurses spent the first winter of the war working long hours with very little equipment and supplies, caring for wounded

German and Austrian soldiers. One such nurse, Sara McCarron, graduated from Williamsburg School of Nursing in 1909 and became a public health nurse in New York City in 1910 (see Figure 8). Later described as 'deeply religious, courageous and loyal',[74] McCarron clearly possessed a strong spirit of adventure; she resolved to travel into dangerous war zones at a time when travel itself was hazardous, and to place her skills at the service of those in need. In July 1914 she applied to the National Committee on Nursing Service of the American Red Cross, hoping to be posted to Mexico. Instead, two months later, she found herself sailing the Atlantic on the so-called 'Mercy Ship', the SS *Red Cross*. American nurses had been promised to the military hospitals of both the Allies and the Central Powers, and McCarron was one of those chosen to serve in a German military hospital.[75] On 17 October 1914, she arrived in the town of Cosel, close to the Austrian and Russian borders. She was to remain in Germany until March 1915.

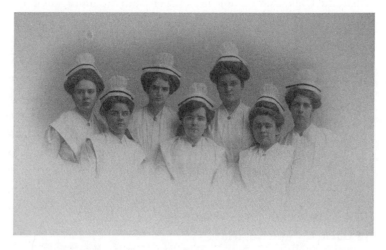

FIGURE 8 Sarah McCarron (centre, front row): Photograph taken during her graduation from the Williamsburg School of Nursing, New York, 1909 (photograph reproduced with permission of the Barbara Bates Center for the Study of the History of Nursing, the University of Pennsylvania)

McCarron began work at Ward 39 in the 'Garnisonlazareth' Hospital on 19 October, declaring that hers was 'the cleanest ward on that day'. On the 22nd, she received a large convoy of wounded and worked for thirteen hours. The forces of the Central Powers had won two decisive victories against Russian armies at Tannenberg and the Masurian Lakes. McCarron and her colleagues worked under extreme pressure for several weeks. On 26 November, she commented in her diary that the Germans had been 'very victorious today', capturing 65,000 Russians, 165 machine guns, and 60 cannon. Although the people were celebrating with flags and music in the town square, McCarron's soldier-patients were 'very restless'. Three days later she described a scene of great tranquillity—a strangely peaceful interlude in the midst of one of the fiercest phases of the conflict:

> 11/29/14: 2/30am standing at corridor window, looking out into the night. The moon is beautiful and the view is lovely. We can see the barracks and one of the Grey nuns who is on night watch sitting near window, apparently talking to a patient. It is certainly a picture.[76]

In her personal diary, Sara McCarron wrote of her German patients, their suffering, and her attempts to heal them. Her tone is remarkably similar to that used by nurses such as Kate Luard when writing of their brave British 'Tommies'. On 29 November, she described how she had walked in the cemetery close to her hospital, looking for the grave of 'Lampa', a patient who had died unexpectedly of a pulmonary embolism (a blood clot in the lung), just when his life seemed to have been saved. His wife, who had remained with him for weeks, had, just that night, decided to travel back to her home, confident that 'Lampa' was better. On departing, she had given McCarron a gift—a lily. That night, McCarron poured into the silent pages of her diary her sense of grief and shock at the death and bereavement she had witnessed.

Another diary entry, for 3 December, relates a more hopeful incident concerning a patient, expected to die, who recovered:

12/3/14...He was shot in the left leg; bled for 4–5 hrs on the field before he was attended to. Muscle and nerves were torn clean to the bone. Bone not broken but exposed (terribly pussy). Dr. Newman said if he amputated leg, he would die and if he didn't he would die anyway. When leg was fairly surgically clean, pt had septic chills <u>gray</u> previous to operation, fingers and hands edematous morning of operation color terrible—so white—never expected to see him leave the table alive. Well he did. That was about a month ago. Up to date he is doing fine and complains of some pain in stump. He is a great character, the life of the ward and my interpreter.[77]

Like Luard, McCarron often referred to her patients by name. She wrote of Lenhert, her 'fractured femur case' whose agony she tried to relieve with every remedy she could think of; and Pilzer, a 'pleurisy case', who was given morphine and a turpentine stupe (a hot compress) and had to be watched closely.

On 25 December, she joined the hospital staff—both American and German—for dinner, but commented in her diary that she 'did not enjoy it'. She had been shocked to find that the American flag had been draped beneath the German one underneath a portrait of the Kaiser, to whom the American medical director had proposed a toast. Her work in Cosel was becoming increasingly stressful: on 28 December, she received a convoy of desperately wounded men, many of whom had been left on a frozen battlefield for over thirty-six hours. Yet they considered themselves lucky; most of their regiment had died. One had had both feet amputated in a field hospital and arrived in great pain. McCarron's contract was drawing to an end and her time in Cosel was almost over. On 2 March, her last day in the hospital, she was given a bouquet of flowers by her patients. In return, she offered them cognac and cigars. Commenting in her diary on how she had 'certainly enjoyed taking care of these boys', she returned home via Vienna, Genoa, and Boston.

Of the ten units transported to Europe by the SS *Red Cross*, one—Unit No. 8—had arrived in Vienna on 14 October 1914 to staff the 'Imperial and Royal Reserve Hospital' on the Johann Hoffmann Platz.[78] Margaret Cowling, a 35-year-old graduate nurse from Virginia, joined its ranks on 31 May 1915, travelling to Austria on a USA special passport. Her stay was to be a brief one. That summer, the American Red Cross announced that (with the possible exception of those in Belgium) all of its hospital units were to be withdrawn from Europe. 'Financial difficulties' were cited as the cause, though it may be surmised that the rising tide of American support for the Allies following the sinking of the *Lusitania* in May might have influenced the decision. The Viennese unit was closed on 18 September, and, unable to travel through Italy (which had, in May, declared war on Austria-Hungary), its staff made their way back to the USA via Germany and Holland. Just before her departure for the States, 'Margarethe B. Cowling' was awarded the Silver Honorary Medal of the Red Cross with War Decoration' by the Austro-Hungarian monarchy.[79]

## Conclusion

By 1915 a complex system for the evacuation of the wounded through regimental aid posts, field dressing stations, casualty clearing stations, hospital trains, base hospitals, hospital ships, and convalescent hospitals was solidifying on the Western Front. Provision expanded gradually during the last months of 1914, and, as it became clear that the war was, for the time being, static, it began to be possible to place CCSs closer to the front lines in important strategic locations such as railheads or the confluences of several important roads. Soon they began to look like semi-permanent fixtures. By the end of the year there were eight CCSs in northern France and Belgium each capable of taking several hundred patients; within two years there would be fifty.[80] When a new assault was planned, teams consisting of surgeons, sisters, anaesthetists, and orderlies were moved to the nearest CCSs so that theatres could 'work' several operating tables at the same time.

From CCSs patients were packed into hospital trains, where transport nurses cared for them until they reached one of the main Allied bases, such as Boulogne, Étaples, Le Havre, or Rouen.[81] Here, they were once more conveyed by ambulance to base hospitals, where many would undergo further surgery before medical staff decided whether they should be evacuated across the Channel or remain in convalescence in northern France, before being returned to the front lines via a 'rest camp'. Those lucky enough to be 'shipped' to Britain underwent another long and hazardous journey to a General Hospital from where they were eventually moved to a convalescent hospital. Nurses in all treatment scenarios worked to minimize the trauma experienced by wounded and sick soldiers, to heal their wounds, and to offer them vital emotional support. Some openly questioned the processes that 'patched men up' only to return them to the firing lines, but others saw their work as a vital element of the war effort—healing wounded and broken men in order to give them back 'to the nation'.

2

# A Nursing Service on the Western Front

## 1915

### Introduction: trench warfare and its consequences

In its earliest months, the war in Western Europe had been highly mobile. Germany's strategy for a rapid invasion of France via Belgium had stalled in the face of vigorous Belgian resistance and the rapid mobilization of the British and French armies. A series of battles had culminated in the decisive Allied victory at the Battle of the Marne, resulting in the so-called 'race to the sea': a succession of attempts by each side to outflank the other. By the end of 1914, both sides had realized the deadly power of modern artillery and had learned that the only way to survive it was to 'dig in'. The trench system had emerged, and, with it, an evacuation system for the wounded, who were conveyed—via regimental aid posts and field dressing stations, casualty clearing stations (CCSs), hospital trains and barges, base hospitals in northern France, and hospital ships—to General Hospitals and convalescent hospitals in what became fondly known as 'Blighty'—Britain.

The deadlock was absolute. German troops were thinly stretched along a 450-mile 'Western Front', which consisted of deep defensive trenches, containing even deeper bunkers and protected by multiple rows of barbed wire. The year 1915 was to be spent in a series of devastatingly unsuccessful Allied attempts to break through these defences. Although most initiatives were launched by the British and French, the pattern of attack was established by a German assault at Soissons in mid-January, in which a heavy preliminary artillery bombardment partially destroyed the Allied defences and allowed a successful infantry attack.[1] For the next three years, fighting on the Western Front was to mirror this pattern of heavy bombardment (accompanied by aerial reconnaissance) followed by the movement of foot soldiers across the deadly territory known as 'no-man's-land'. Allied soldiers found themselves running (or even, sometimes, walking) across open ground—easy targets for an enemy which was able to cut them down in a hail of machine-gun fire.

In CCSs and base hospitals nurses found themselves dealing with the consequences of such horrific events. During an assault—which might last several days or weeks—CCSs were repeatedly inundated with huge 'rushes' of patients. Large numbers of casualties were retrieved from no-man's-land by stretcher-bearers, given the most cursory treatment in regimental aid posts, and then carried as quickly as possible by ambulance to CCSs. Often, these 'rushes' would occur during the darkest parts of the night—the only times when it was safe to retrieve the wounded from no-man's-land. Even in 'quiet' periods, CCSs treated victims of shell-blast and sniper-fire. Soldiers in defensive trenches were never completely safe. The enemy might fire an artillery shell into—or near to—a trench at any time. Flying shrapnel caused devastating injuries or instant death, depending on how close the blast was. Sniper-fire resulted in a more controlled form of destruction, but could cause deep injuries which rapidly became infected; bullets carried fragments of muddy uniform deep into the body, creating the perfect oxygen-free environment in which 'anaerobic' bacteria could thrive.

During 1915, nurses on the Western Front at CCSs, on hospital trains and barges, and at base hospitals nursed tens of thousands of casualties, particularly during the failed 'pushes' at Neuve

Chapelle, Festubert, and Ypres. They lived and worked in harsh conditions. During the year, their clinical practice developed to deal with a range of new and deadly forms of warfare, and they created new systems that would cope with 'rushes' of shocked and desperately wounded men.

On 23 May 1915, Italy declared war on Austria-Hungary and many volunteer nurses found their way to the Italian Front to support a limited and inexperienced Italian nursing service. Alpine warfare carried its own unique problems. In addition to the injuries caused by shellfire and bullets, soldiers were exposed to the risks of fighting across one of the most rugged terrains in the world, in conditions that, in winter, were truly desolate. Nurses in Italian base hospitals became adept at caring for patients suffering from exhaustion and exposure.

## Crisis-management on the Western Front

The early days of war had been characterized by a rapid and almost ad hoc development of field hospitals, which were often overwhelmed by the numbers of casualties produced by modern warfare. The military medical services worked to create a system to allow patients to receive the life-saving treatment they needed as quickly as possible, and yet still be moved rapidly 'down the line' to safety.

In Belgium, L'Hôpital de l'Océan at La Panne was functioning as a highly disciplined military machine—taking in huge numbers of casualties from the Belgian front lines at the northernmost point on the Western Front. Vague rumours were circulating that 'scandalous things' were going on at the hospital, but no specifics were ever mentioned. Of greater credibility were reports of conflict between British and Belgian nurses. Estelle and Thérèse Bieswal, stationed in a hospice at Furnes, commented that 'there is not much entente ... the English nurses have much more experience of medical matters; they complain that the Belgian nurses are always tired. The Belgian nurses feel that the English nurses do not offer the

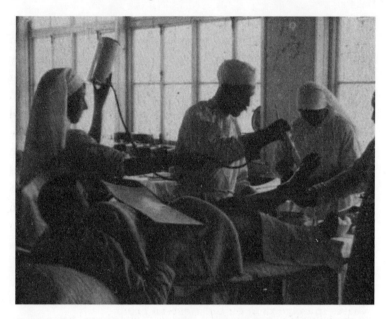

FIGURE 9 Jane De Launoy (far left) at L'Hôpital de l'Océan, La Panne (photograph ©Archives Belgian Red Cross, Brussels)

patients enough comfort, and that they follow orders too strictly.'[2] Jane De Launoy (see Figure 9) commented on 29 April that her English nurse-colleagues were 'authoritarian and difficult...but what services they render! The organization is perfect.' On 20 June, she wrote: 'Everything goes here as in an army.'[3] Yet the inscription on the medal that was issued to nurses at La Panne also implies that compassion was recognized as a fundamental nursing value: nurses were exhorted to 'Sometimes Cure; Often Comfort; Always Console'.[4]

L'Hôpital de l'Océan was an important patriotic symbol for the Belgian people, who attached great significance to its role in supporting the wounded and returning 'Belgian heroes' to the battle lines. On 6 June, when a fire broke out at the hospital, local villagers are said to have hurried to the beach with their buckets, pots, and kettles, to form a 'human chain', transferring water up the beach from the sea, over half a mile away. It took until midnight to extinguish the fire, and two months to make the wards habitable again.[5]

For the French, one of the biggest trials of 1915 was what came to be known as the First Battle of Champagne, but was really a series of failed assaults which lasted from late December 1914 to mid-March 1915. French field hospitals receiving the wounded were well equipped but lacked trained nurses. Their nursing services were strengthened by the support of a number of fully-trained British and American nurses. The 'French Flag Nursing Corps', formed by Grace Ellison in the autumn of 1914, was staffed by trained British nurses, many of whom were deeply frustrated by the British military medical services' refusal to accept their offers of help.[6] The so-called 'American Ambulance' in Paris was staffed entirely by volunteers from the USA, many of whom were also fully trained. Their motives for offering their services to the French were varied. Ellen La Motte, who had undergone the rigorous training offered at the Johns Hopkins Hospital, Baltimore, may have been inspired by her French Huguenot ancestry to offer her services, firstly to the American Ambulance and then (finding that institution to be overly bureaucratic) to a field hospital known as L'Hôpital Chirurgical Mobile No. 1, located within 5 miles of the French lines in Belgium.[7] Many nurses in French field hospitals found themselves caring, for the first time, for members of their nations' colonies; some commented on the cultural differences between indigenous 'Tommies' and 'poilus' and patients from colonies such as India or Morocco. Often, the comparisons they drew out in their writings emphasized the greater stoicism and bravery of the former.[8]

Among the most unusual of the French field hospitals were those units donated by the Scottish Women's Hospitals. The Abbaye de Royaumont, near Senlis, had been formed at the end of 1914, and by the spring of 1915 was a fully functioning hospital located about 30 miles from the front lines (see Figure 10). It was staffed almost entirely by British women. Volunteer nurse Evelyn Proctor wrote home to her mother of how 'clever' the staff were: 'the standard of

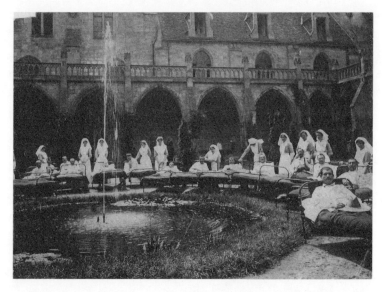

FIGURE 10 The Cloisters at Royaumont (image from Marian Wenzel and John Cornish, *Auntie Mabel's War* (London: Allen Lane, 1980), reproduced with the kind assistance of the Department of Documents, Imperial War Museum, London, UK)

intelligence is so much higher than in an ordinary crowd of women anywhere'.[9] One Canadian volunteer, Marjorie Starr, who worked as an 'orderly' at Royaumont from 6 September 1915 to 9 January 1916, wrote a detailed and moving diary of her work there. At the end of September she was having problems with her feet, which were becoming increasingly sore, from constant standing to assist with dressings. She was also frequently finding lice and fleas inside her clothing. In early October, she confided to the pages of her diary that the quaint sounding of the horn, which signalled the arrival of *blessés* (wounded men), was losing its appeal. She was being woken up at 4.30 every morning to assist the night staff with new arrivals and then worked with only a few short breaks until 4 p.m. The wounds were terrible—many gangrenous—and a man with tetanus on her ward was slowly dying. Eventually, when she was called she 'simply wasn't able to get up', having been sick all night.

She still managed to get on duty at 7.30, but was sent to bed by the sister at 1 p.m. On 8 October she walked to a nearby village to see if the exercise would 'stop my nerves jumping and so get to sleep', but eventually she was given a sedative by one of the hospital's doctors and sent on leave. On her return she was placed in the kitchens to enable her to avoid the stress of ward-work. She commented:

> I just want to rest my mind and get away from the horrors for a little. Several of the girls have given up completely under the strain, but I hope this change will just pull me up in time, and I won't mind the hard work if I have no responsibility...I am terribly amused at people writing to me not to overdo it and take care of myself; one simply can't think of oneself at all; one's little ills are nothing at all in comparison to the wounds about us, and it matters more if they are neglected than if I am tired, but, however, now I am compelled to think of myself when I have come to the end of my tether.[10]

Among the nursing sisters at Royaumont was Mabel Jeffery, a 31-year-old professional nurse from a wealthy steel-producing family in Sheffield. Jeffery, who had apparently not enjoyed her training because she found most of the work to be unpaid 'domestic grind',[11] wrote home from Royaumont: 'Wasn't it strange I "trained" as a nurse and now I feel quite satisfied.'[12] Her work at Royaumont was clearly rewarding, and yet soon after joining the Scottish Women's Hospitals and travelling to Royaumont, Jeffery began to send extraordinary postcards home to her family, sometimes with quite macabre scenes of death and destruction, but containing mundane messages on the reverse side, requesting that flea pads should be sent, asking about seaside holidays, or thanking her mother for cakes or hampers. In describing her aunt many years later, Jeffery's niece had commented that Jeffery had 'a morbid streak', which the family believed was the result of a serious head injury she had suffered as a child. Life at Royaumont was clearly exhausting, and Jeffery commented that it was not possible for her to rest in her room at any time during the day, as it was occupied by the night staff. In July 1915, she told her family that she had better not come home on leave, or she might never be able to find the strength of will to return, and in August she said that she hoped to be able to last out until the end of the war, at which time she 'might sleep for ever'.[13] She was not to know that the war would last another three years.

Jeffery did, in fact, take a period of leave that autumn. While she was at home a romantic picture-postcard found its way to her. On the back was a carefully composed message: 'In affectionate remembrance and friendship from one of your patients. When will you return?? Marcel Renard.'[14] Jeffery and her nursing colleagues were clearly very popular with French soldier-patients, who made them rings and other trinkets out of pieces of German shell, wrote them poems, gave them flowers, and corresponded with them from the trenches, following their recovery and return to the front lines.[15]

In the British lines a system of CCSs, hospital trains, and base hospitals had become well established by early 1915. This was made easier by the deadlock which existed on the Western Front. Armies were entrenched—'dug in', rather than mobile—hence routes for the evacuation of casualties could become well established, and systems of treatment and evacuation could become stable and well organized. When first treated at their regimental aid posts, the wounded were given a 'specification tally' or 'field medical card', which was attached to their clothing.[16] This stated the nature of their wounds and the preliminary treatment given, including whether they had received anti-tetanus serum. At the CCS, patients were 'triaged'—a process of rapid assessment during which a decision was taken about what treatment should be offered, and how soon it must commence. Triage was often performed by nurses, particularly during 'rushes' of patients when all surgeons were occupied in the operating theatres. Patients were moved either directly onto trains (if lightly wounded), into the resuscitation ward (if shocked), or directly to the operating theatre (for those with the most dangerous wounds). Wound-shock was a particularly dangerous condition, which, if ignored, would lead rapidly to death. Patients with shock were treated with hot alkaline drinks, warmth, rest, and reassurance. In severe shock the blood vessels were depleted and the circulation was slow and weak; in these cases fluid had to be replaced rapidly. The transfusion of saline solution using large needles inserted into the groin or armpit was used in most CCSs; in others, the 'Murphy' method, whereby saline was introduced via a tube into the rectum, from where it could be absorbed into the bloodstream, was common. Blood transfusion, first used by Canadian surgeons in 1917, was rapidly adopted throughout the Western Front. Blood was drawn into a sterile tube directly from the vein of a healthy volunteer, into that of the shocked patient. It was only in 1918 that techniques for preserving blood (using sodium citrate to avoid coagulation) were developed.[17]

Early in 1915 a system of hospital barges was established to convey casualties from CCSs to base hospitals. These were said to have been inspired by the barges run by associations of the French Red Cross, in particular the Union des Femmes de France (see Figure 11).[18] There were five 'flotillas', each with six barges, which travelled in pairs, towed by steam tugs. On board each barge was a nursing sister, a staff nurse, a medical officer, and a staff of orderlies. The centre of each barge was a large ward of thirty beds, with a hand-lift to load and unload patients. The exteriors of the barges were painted grey, with large red crosses on the sides and roof. In summer the hatches could be removed, and awnings would protect the patients from the glare of the sun, while each bed was protected by a mosquito net. At such times, the environment on board a hospital barge could be quite pleasant, but during wet or cold weather, with all hatches shut, it could be stifling. Even in summer, hatches often had to be closed at night to ensure that internal lights could not be seen by enemy aeroplanes. Millicent Peterkin, a member of the QAIMNSR, commented later on the dilemmas that could be faced by the sister in charge of a hospital barge: 'The

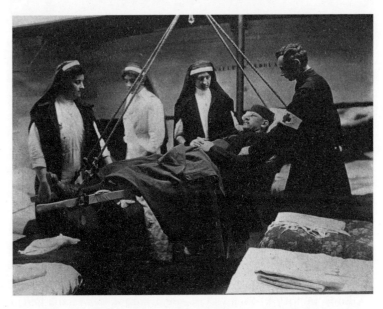

FIGURE 11  A stretcher patient is taken on board a French hospital barge (photograph reproduced by kind permission of the Wellcome Library, London, UK)

only alternative, after settling the patients for the night was to put out the lights, and open the ventilators, but this was not very satisfactory when one had bad cases on board, requiring much attention. This meant juggling with a carefully shaded electric torch at frequent intervals, or to sit in inky darkness and meditate on the number of patients liable to haemorrhage at any moment.'[19] She added that during large 'rushes' of patients, stretchers would be wedged close together and it could be difficult to reach some of the patients, adding, however, that she 'never lost any of my patients en route, though we sometimes had a hard fight to keep them alive'.[20]

As the so-called 'Battle of Champagne' drew to a typically indecisive close, a British assault commenced in the Artois sector, close to the small village of Neuve Chapelle. The British were determined to capture the Aubers Ridge, just beyond the village; they succeeded in reaching their objective, but were pushed back by a

German counter-offensive. Nurses in CCSs behind the British lines found themselves inundated with 'rushes' of severely wounded men. Kate Luard, on an ambulance train taking wounded 'down the line' to the base, commented on how bad many of their 'loads' were—many still in a shocked state, with severely infected wounds, some dying before they could reach the base.

At the end of March 1915, Luard was posted to a casualty clearing station taking wounded from the Second Battle of Ypres. Her style of writing offers a remarkably personal account of her work with the war's wounded, and she is clearly more concerned to educate her readership of the bravery and endurance of her patients than to inform them of her own work. When caring for the wounded from the Battle of Festubert, she writes of how 'last night a stiff muddy figure, all bandages and straw, on the stretcher was brought in. I asked the boy how many wounds? "Oh, only five", he said cheerfully. "Nice clean wounds,—machine-gun,—all in and out again!" '[21] She also writes of an officer, hit by a shell, who crawled around no-man's-land in a disorientated state for twenty-four hours, being further wounded before being found by stretcher-bearers. Her comment, 'I don't know how they live through that',[22] probably sums up the feelings of nurses who received severely damaged casualties in CCSs.

Luard's letters home revealed the complexity of her professional—and yet also profoundly personal—relationships with her patients:

> I'm writing in the ward. Opposite me is a boy of 22 w his shoulder, left arm and left leg all in shell holes—he has curly hair, blue eyes and a serene face, and says 'oh rather' to whatever you want him to do...I look upon it as a great privilege to be a mother to these young heroes, wouldn't you?[23]

She added that her family must not be shocked if she used the expletives 'Good God', 'Hell', or 'damned swine' when she came home on leave, adding 'if I ever get there out of this damned war'. She went on to describe the Second Battle of Ypres as 'another gory gassy mess—u.b.c. [utter bloody chaos] all over again. Isn't it funny to think of Frank fighting hard these days?' Luard's brother, Frank, was killed in action at Gallipoli, just a few weeks after she wrote this letter. Towards the end of May, perhaps at about the time she received the news of her brother's death, she wrote to the bereaved wife of one the patients she had been unable to save. The grieving widow replied, expressing her thanks: 'If it is possible to gain any comfort in my agonizing loss, you have given it me. I sent flowers addressed to you for his grave because I felt that you would of your goodness lay them on my hero's grave.'[24]

Later that year, a happier letter arrived, expressing thanks for work Luard had done at a base hospital in Le Tréport, earlier that year:

> Dear Sister, I am afraid you have little time for reading letters but felt that I must send to say how deeply grateful I am to you and the nurses who did so much for my dear son, Aubrey Baltec, in nursing him w typhoid in the critical time of his illness, and getting him well enough for his journey home. He is now improving each day in the military hospital, Looting [*sic*]. He...feels deeply the untiring care and attention that he received while at Le Triport [*sic*] and often wishes he was back again with you. You can hardly realise what a source of consolation it is to we mothers to know our dear lads fall into such loving hands in their terrible sufferings. God bless your noble work.[25]

On Tuesday 13 June, Luard wrote in her journal: 'This war is sitting very heavily on one's chest tonight.' Five days later, a letter from her sister, Nettie, offered condolences to the 'poor girl', who, it seems, had 'come down with trench fever'.[26]

Luard's later book, *Unknown Warriors*, published long after the war, in 1930, offers further eyewitness testimony of the suffering of her patients during her experiences from October 1915 to the late summer of 1918, when she was obliged to resign from active service in order to care for a dying father. In it, she describes her patients by name: 'my Reggie, Walter, Joseph, Harry and Billy, and the armless, legless ones, who won't tell their mothers'.[27]

Soon after the largely unsuccessful first British assault at Neuve Chapelle, the horror of war on the Western Front was intensified by the first use of chemical weaponry. On 22 April, during the Second Battle of Ypres, the Germans opened hundreds of canisters, releasing chlorine gas across a 4-mile section of the front. Military meteorologists had assessed the wind conditions that day, ensuring that the gas would be carried rapidly to the Allied lines.[28] A strange green vapour flowed eerily across no-man's-land, turning yellow and destroying vegetation as it moved towards its waiting victims. French colonial troops—Algerian and Moroccan soldiers—were taken completely by surprise, as the gas flowed into their trenches, killing many of them instantly, and completely disabling thousands more. Those who tried to escape were killed by machine-gun fire.

In nearby CCSs, nurses and doctors were shocked by the arrival of huge numbers of seriously ill patients, who seemed to be suffering from both pneumonia and blindness. The chlorine had attacked their airways, causing swelling and inflammation and making it almost impossible for them to breathe. A yellowish, thin, frothy liquid was pouring from the noses and mouths of those worst affected: these men were drowning in their own secretions. Others were suffering acute congestion of the lungs, leading to heart failure: their struggles for breath stopped suddenly as their hearts simply 'gave out'.[29] Those who managed to survive the first few hours continued to experience partial suffocation, until the initial effects of the gas wore off. They then experienced temporary relief, before the damage caused to their lungs led to an acute form of bronchitis. Soon, they began to cough up thick greenish phlegm and run a high fever. Many suffered such severe and permanent lung damage that they endured chronic bronchitis and, in some cases, heart failure, for the remainder of their shortened lives. Violetta Thurstan advised, in *A Text Book of War Nursing*, that nurses could be called upon to administer a wide range of treatments—some of them quite 'heroic' and experimental.[30] These included the administration of stimulants such as strychnine, to support the action of the heart; and salt and water emetics, which were believed to relieve lung congestion, although this was discredited as a treatment later in the war. Amongst the nurses' most significant interventions, however, were the provision of rest, calm, and reassurance. Later, when their patients were beginning to recover from the initial life-threatening effects of toxic gases, nurses provided total nursing care—feeding, hydrating, washing, and toileting patients whose breathlessness made them virtually helpless. Such work was enormously labour-intensive, and could not have been achieved without the assistance of orderlies and volunteers.

In a letter of 7 May 1915, Maud McCarthy, Matron-in-Chief of the British Expeditionary Force (BEF), expressed her concern about the understaffing of casualty clearing stations during 'rushes' of casualties. There were now fourteen such units all located close to the front lines. At quiet times, the work could be done by five sisters, given that an improvement in the provision of ambulance trains had ensured that evacuation was more rapid. But during an assault, staffing levels had to be increased at very short notice, thus depleting the already overworked bases. McCarthy's solution to this problem was to establish a 'reserve' of base nurses prepared to move to CCSs at short notice.[31]

During the summer of 1915, the Allies' focus on the campaign in the Dardanelles meant that the Western Front was relatively quiet, but in September the French launched a prolonged series of assaults, which came to be known as the Third Battle of Artois. The British supported this offensive at the town of Loos, where, on 25 September, they released chlorine gas, poisoning many of their own soldiers in the process. Historian Mark Harrison has observed that the Battle of Loos was 'an important turning point in casualty disposal': CCSs in the Loos sector had become overwhelmed by the large numbers of casualties from the assault. Soon after this, CCSs began to operate in pairs, each taking turns to admit the wounded. When one was full the other would take over, while the first focused on care, treatment, and evacuation.[32]

## Nursing 'at the base'

In the early months of the war, hospitals had been established at military bases in the northern coastal towns of France to receive the wounded from the battlefields. These rapidly became established as large 'base hospitals' where seriously wounded patients might spend several weeks—or even months—before being either sent home to 'Blighty' or returned to the front lines via a rest camp. The most significant were at Boulogne, Étaples, Wimereux, Le Havre, and also further inland at Rouen. Many of the hospitals in these centres housed well over 1,000 beds. The bases of Étaples and Rouen were each accommodating 14,000 patients by the autumn of 1915.[33] In June a unit staffed by medical and nursing personnel from the Harvard School of Medicine in the USA began work under the auspices of the British medical services.[34] In addition to the 'official' base hospitals belonging to the BEF, there were also large numbers of Red Cross hospitals, many housed in large municipal buildings in the Channel ports. The Allies' unsuccessful attempts to break the German defences at Neuve Chapelle and Ypres resulted in huge pressures for the nurses at base hospitals, as patients were moved rapidly 'down the line', sometimes with the mud of the battlefield still on their bodies and clothing. These patients were often severely debilitated, suffering from exhaustion, and often experiencing pain from multiple wounds.

Once the network of CCSs and hospital trains had been established, the most seriously injured arrived at base hospitals with their wounds already operated upon. They were often swathed in bandages and still recovering from the debilitating combined effects of injury and surgery. Whatever their condition, patients were received into the wards by nurses, who began by making them comfortable and giving food and hot drinks. Many patients commented on the joy of being put into a clean, comfortable bed and allowed to sleep, and many did sleep—for over twenty-four hours—waking only when hungry.

Most patients with wounds and gas injuries would have received some treatment at the CCS. The role of base hospital nurses was to continue those treatments, prepare the patient for further surgery, and monitor his condition. In the earliest days of the war, before surgeons had perfected the technique of extracting debris and excising infected tissue from wounds in CCSs, nurses in base hospitals cared for large numbers of patients with severe life-threatening wound infections. Among the worst of these was gas gangrene, which could be recognized by the 'mousy' smell given off by the wound, and by the fact that the tissue around the wound 'crackled' with gas bubbles, when pressed by the fingers. Although appearing mild in its early stages, a gas gangrene infection would eventually cause a wound to break down, become blackened with dead tissue, and exude a thick green or yellow pus, which soaked even the bulkiest dressings.[35]

Patients with anaerobic wound infections required frequent dressing changes to remove pus, apply antiseptics, and give the wound a chance to heal. Gas gangrene could often only be halted by amputating the infected limb. In some cases, nurses found themselves in the heartbreaking situation of dressing an amputation stump only to find it infected with gas gangrene. In some cases, patients returned to theatre several times, to have more and more of a limb removed as the deadly infection spread. Vigilance was vital, and it was part of the nurse's role to report signs of infection immediately, to permit rapid surgery, which would, hopefully, halt the spread of the disease. If the infection were lodged in a wound of the abdomen or chest it was often fatal.

Even worse than gas gangrene was tetanus, another anaerobic infection, which, as it moved into the bloodstream and through the body, caused agonizing muscle spasm. The disease was commonly known as 'lockjaw' because, as the infection invaded the muscles of the jaw, it caused them to contract, pulling the mouth up into an uncontrollable rictus grin. As the disease progressed, the muscles of the back would contract, resulting in a dramatic and excruciatingly painful arching of the body. The death rate for the disease was high, with patients dying from a combination of the toxic effects of the bacteria themselves, and the exhaustion of constant muscle contraction. Patients with tetanus were often put in the care of one single nurse, in a process known as 'specialling'. Screens were placed around the patient's bed; the nurse supported him by feeding with small frequent amounts of soft or liquid food and drinks. Only in this way could his strength be sustained. Meanwhile, she attempted to maintain the absolute quiet and rest that was required to prevent sudden muscle-seizures.[36]

Jentie Paterson was based at No. 3 General Hospital at Le Tréport from December 1914 to May 1915, nursing casualties of the failed 'pushes' in the British sector of the front. She was working under huge pressure, with the assistance of orderlies and VADs whose abilities she doubted. She also appears to have felt rather scornful of what she saw as the inadequacies of the 'regular' members of the QAIMNS. On 23 February, she 'found' a Canadian soldier with a fractured tibia, who had been left in bed for five hours without a splint. Her comment—confined to the secret pages of her private diary—was scathing: 'Idiot of an army staff nurse.'[37] Two weeks later she was expostulating on the failures of 'well meaning but blundering' orderlies who were caring for her typhoid patients, adding: 'what can you expect from the class they are drawn from?' On 15 March, however, she appears to have been happier with her colleagues' work: 'Convoy 210 cases detrained and in bed 1hr 15 mins! Good.' Later that month, she had an 'awful night' caring for a man with a temperature of 105.4 degrees Fahrenheit, but felt that she had 'really got him nursed'. At the end of March, she was sent to a new surgical unit of a hundred beds, staffed by only three nurses and five orderlies. After a twelve-and-a-half hour shift in which the work was not completed, she confided to her diary: 'this is terrible work'. This pattern of overwork and dissatisfaction continued throughout April, as colleagues became sick and staffing levels dropped further. She began to receive convoys—always containing very large numbers of seriously wounded men—from the attempted push at 'Hill 60', exclaiming, on 25 April: Ye Gods, will they never end?' Her final entry from Le Tréport reads: '14 May: Lazy slack orderlies makes me sick.'[38] In May Paterson was granted special leave to care for a sister at home who was seriously ill. Because her sister's condition continued to be 'serious' and 'extended leave' was not permitted, she was obliged to resign her service with the QAIMNSR on 1 June.[39]

In the early spring of 1915, the British military medical services, realizing that hospitals on both the home front and at bases in France were severely stretched, decided to permit VADs to work in military hospitals. Ruth Manning had joined a voluntary aid detachment at the beginning of the war, and had covered the work of the district nurse in her home village of Diss, Norfolk, who had been called up on 'active service'. This had involved 'some washing and occasional first aid work, which I thought was tremendous fun'. In March 1915, she had been 'proud and pleased' to be taken on by the First Eastern General Hospital in Cambridge, part of the Territorial system. She had found the work physically draining and emotionally disturbing, but her spirit of adventure remained undimmed and when the First Eastern was asked to send a complete unit to start a new military hospital on the cliffs above Boulogne, she volunteered, enjoying the 'very thrilling farewell' her unit was given as it set off from Cambridge Station.[40] Dorothy Seymour, an upper-class VAD from a highly influential military family, was moved to the Rawal Pindi Military Hospital in May. At that time, the hospital was receiving its first cases of gas-poisoning, and Seymour was horrified to see them 'all black and grey in face and men of 20 looking between 50 and 60'.[41] In October 1915, she declined the offer to run a ward of her own, because it was 'one where tiny scratches of wounds go and I didn't think I should be learning anything'.[42]

The work of VADs was mundane and some of their duties were apparently very basic. Much of the work involved washing patients, emptying bedpans, and maintaining a clean and safe ward

environment. The military nursing services worked hard to instill in
them a sense of the significance of such work. In the first two decades of the twentieth century, one of the first things trained nurses
learned was that disease and injury were damaging not only to that
part of the body which was immediately affected but also to other
surrounding tissues and organs. Disease and injury presented, furthermore, a danger not only to the immediate sufferer, but also to
all those around him. Germ theory was well established as part of a
body of medico-scientific knowledge but neither sulphonamides
nor antibiotics were yet available to tackle the bacteria. Disease processes were clearly associated with parasitic microorganisms—living
enemies, so tiny that they were invisible—which established themselves insidiously in one part of the organism, then spread to others,
rather like an invading army. Disease itself, in a pre-antibiotic era,
was seen as a process of invasion, and its eradication was a form of
active warfare. Volunteer nurses were a vital component in the
battle against infection. Towards the end of 1915, a new manual of
war nursing for probationers and VADs focused on the 'dignity'
of ward work, interpreting the dusting of lockers and the mopping
of floors, as part of the 'hand to hand fight against disease germs'.[43]
Sister Edith Appleton, based at No. 1 General Hospital at Étretat,
commented on her VAD colleagues:

> The VADs are a source of great interest to me—taking them as a
> bunch they are splendid. They may be roughly divided into 4 sorts—
> 'Stalkers', 'Crawlers', the irrepressible butterflyers and the sturdy
> pushers—At the moment I am thinking of a butterfly one who is on
> night duty on these wards & says with a little light-hearted laugh—
> 'It's rippin' nursin' the men great fun, when I was in the Officers'
> ward I did housework all the time—great fun—but there men are
> really ill—great fun'—When I show her how to do anything fresh,
> she twitches to get at it & says 'oh do let me try—I'd love to do that
> simply love to'. She is an aristocratic little person most dainty and
> well groomed—& the thought of her scrubbing and doing dusting
> all day—makes me smile. The 'Stalkers' are nice girls very lordly

with high pitched cracky voices—they look rather alarmed at some
of the jobs they have to do, but do them well and with good grace.
By 'Crawlers' I mean the little people…who think they are un-
worthy to do anything at all—with an expression of 'Stand on me if
you like I should be pleased to be your door mate [*sic*]. There is little
to say about the sturdy pusher ones—they are not remarkable for
anything, but are quite reliable—very strong—never forget—& are
always ready to do every bit of work[44]

Most patients were treated at bases in France and then returned via
rest camps to military service. There were those, however, whose
wounds were severe enough to warrant further treatment. There were
also some who were so badly damaged that they would never return to
the front lines. These were moved further down the line to General
Hospitals in Britain. Patients often anxiously asked their nurses
whether their wounds were so-called 'Blighty' ones—wounds which
would allow them to be 'ticketed' for home by the medical officer.

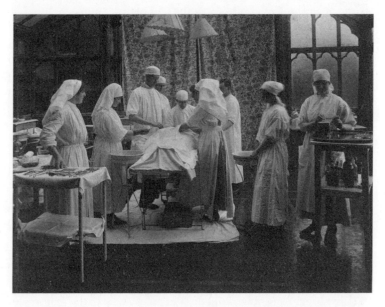

FIGURE 12  The operating theatre at Mount Stuart Royal Naval Hospital (photograph reproduced by kind permission of the Wellcome Library, London, UK)

## Healing the wounds of war

Nothing in their previous experience could have prepared nurses for the wounds created by the industrial weaponry of the First World War. Veteran army nurse Kate Luard commented that the rifle wounds of the Boer War seemed like 'pin pricks' compared with the damage inflicted during the battles of Neuve Chapelle and Ypres. After the war, soldier-writers were to comment on incidents in which men had been almost completely obliterated by exploding shells. Edmund Blunden wrote of the horror of shovelling the remains of a lance corporal into a small sack—of retrieving an eye from beneath a duckboard. But many survived—in badly damaged states. The force and speed with which shrapnel could strike was such as to cause destruction of vast swathes of tissue, or to tear completely through a limb. Similarly, machine-gun fire could cause extensive damage, leaving behind bullets and debris to act as seats for infection.

By the time he arrived in the reception hut of a CCS, a wounded man would invariably have endured a long and painful journey. Having been taken from the battlefield to his own regimental aid post, where he would have been given morphine and his field dressing assessed, he would have been put into an ambulance and bumped over the rough pavé roads of northern France or Belgium. In the reception hut, he would be 'triaged' by a doctor or nurse. During the 'rush' of patients created by an assault on the Western Front, surgeons would be so busy in the operating theatre that most triage work was undertaken by nurses. A decision was made quickly about whether a patient needed to go straight to theatre, remain in the reception hut to await less urgent surgery, be sent to the 'resuscitation ward', or be put into an ambulance train for base.

During the early months of the war, most patients had been taken straight from the battalion first-aid post or field ambulance to a base hospital, possibly as many as 30 miles away. In the majority of cases—whether the wound was caused by shrapnel or bullet—debris of some sort was still lodged in the wound, and was not removed until the patient underwent surgery at the base. By the end of 1914, it had become clear that the incidence of so-called 'anaerobic' wound infections, such as tetanus and gas gangrene, on the Western Front was truly shocking. A deep wound-bed, wherever it was located in the body, was the perfect environment for the growth and proliferation of 'anaerobic' bacteria. The longer the debris remained in the wound, the more time the infection had to take hold and spread—often leading to fatal septicaemia (infection of the blood). It did not take military surgeons long to realize that their patients would have a much better chance of survival if all debris and shrapnel were removed from their wounds before they were moved 'down the line' to the base. The CCS thus became the most significant treatment scenario on the Western Front.[45] Nurses often confided in their letters and diaries a strong desire to work in a CCS—not only because it was close to the front lines and 'in the thick of the action', but also because it was where the most heroic surgery took place; it was the place where most lives were saved.

Surgery was designed to make wounds safe—to remove anything that could cause an infection. But in doing so, it also extended and expanded the wound, often cutting away vast swathes of already-infected tissue in order to leave behind a wound-bed that could heal. In small, simple wounds, healing took place by what was known as 'first intention', but these wounds were rarely found in CCSs. Most were deep and complex and could only heal by 'second intention'—that is, from the base up, closing only when the whole cavity of the wound had successfully filled with healthy tissue. This type of wound replaced skin with scar-tissue, which could cause distortion and pain.[46] In addition to the surgical treatment of wounds, the army medical and nursing services were also, by the end of October 1914, giving anti-tetanus serum to all wounded men.[47] The first injection was given as early as possible, at the regimental aid post, followed by subsequent doses at regular intervals in CCSs and base hospitals.

The avoidance and treatment of wound infection had become a subject of great controversy by the spring of 1915. Initially, when confronted with the combat-wounds of the First World War, surgeons had implemented a conservative treatment, which had proved successful during the Second Anglo-Boer War, consisting of a sterile dressing which was left undisturbed for several days. It soon became clear that wounds contracted on the muddy fields of France and Flanders were very different from those associated with the dry, dusty South African veldt. Some surgeons such as William Watson Cheyne and Sir Anthony Bowlby began to advocate the rigorous and unsparing use of antiseptics to combat these virulent infections. Sir Almroth Wright argued vociferously for the use of a hypertonic saline solution, which would draw serum through the wound, mobilizing the body's own defences against disease.[48] Probably the most successful treatment was that recommended by H. M. W. Gray: the excision of large areas of tissue around the wound, removing all infected matter.[49] Nurses—as the practitioners most likely to dress patients' wounds—found themselves at the centre of controversy and having to exercise considerable diplomacy in following doctors' orders while ensuring that their patients had the best chances of survival. Violetta Thurstan advised nurses in her *Text Book of War Nursing* never to 'give the impression that they disagree with the surgeon for whom they are working', adding: 'The soldier is one of the quickest people in the world to discover any want of harmony, and certainly the feeling that the best possible is not being done for him would react on his mental condition, retard his recovery and make him anxious and suspicious.'[50]

Wound-care had, since the later nineteenth century, been the joint responsibility of nurses and surgeons, but it was, increasingly, becoming part of the nurse's domain. Surgical nurses were highly experienced in such work and many had cared not only for clean, surgical wounds, but also for those caused by industrial accidents, which could be large and were often infected. In CCSs and base hospitals, it was usually the most highly trained nurses who dressed wounds, although many experienced VADs were allowed to assist their work and might, during times of great pressure, find even the most complex wound dressings delegated to them.

In the wards of military hospitals, much of the patient-care was performed in a highly routinized way, and this was especially true of wound-care: dressings were performed as part of a 'round'. Sisters and staff nurses would wait until all patients had been awakened, washed and made comfortable, and had their breakfasts before commencing dressings. They would also wait until ward-maids, or- derlies, and VADs had completed all of the cleaning routines—the dusting and mopping of floors—that had to be performed every day. Only during the later part of the morning, when the ward was tranquil and the environment free of dust, would the dressing round begin. VAD writers commented on the ritualistic nature of these rounds. Wound-care was a complex matter; vast numbers of different antiseptics were available, and these were used liberally on wounds which were infected, or seen as being at risk of infec- tion. They included tried-and-tested compounds such as iodoform, hydrogen peroxide, and perchloride of mercury; and innovations developed under the stress of war, such as flavin, picric acid, and most famously a range of variations on sodium hypochlorite, in- cluding the so-called 'Dakin's solution' (named after its inventor) and 'Eusol' (named after the institution—Edinburgh University— in which it was developed). The liberal use of antiseptics undoubt- edly saved many lives in the short term, although most were dropped from clinical practice during the decades following the war, because of their toxicity to healthy tissues and organs.[51]

It took two individuals—a nurse and a VAD—to perform the most complex dressings. The qualified nurse would wash her hands in carbolic solution and perform the dressing procedure under strictly 'aseptic' conditions. The VAD would prepare a trolley and fetch and carry instruments as required; once the dressing com- menced, she would handle the dirty dressings and support the pa- tient while the trained nurse performed the more intricate work.

The division of labour between the 'clean' nurse using an aseptic procedure, and the assistant whose hands were contaminated permitted dressings to be performed safely.

Typically, a mackintosh sheet would be placed under the wound to protect the bed; then the old bandages and dressings would be removed. Once the wound had been exposed, the nurse would clean it with antiseptic solution, often using irrigation techniques— washing and draining the wound with a continuous stream of antiseptic poured from a sterile tube, or forced onto the wound under pressure through a syringe. Once the wound was clean, the nurse would use a sterile probe to remove any remaining pieces of debris—including bits of bone and shrapnel—which had worked their way towards the surface since the last dressing procedure. Finally, a sterile dressing would be put in place and secured with a bandage. A complex dressing might take at least half an hour to perform—and 'perform' was the operative word here, as the procedures often required a remarkable degree of artistry.[52]

In the spring of 1915, two scientists invented a new system of wound irrigation which came to be widely used on the Western Front. British scientist Henry Dakin discovered that sodium hypochlorite could act as a powerful antiseptic, killing the causative organisms of the most dangerous wound infections—including gas gangrene and tetanus—and French surgeon Alexis Carrel invented a method for delivering it into deep, infected wounds.[53] The two men developed what became known as the 'Carrel-Dakin' method of wound irrigation at a field hospital in Compiègne, and many nurses were sent there to learn the technique. It soon came to be applied in CCSs, hospital trains, and base hospitals across the Western Front, and its fame spread to other war fronts, until, for a time, it was the most widely used method for the treatment of infected wounds. L'Hôpital de l'Océan at La Panne claimed status as one of the foremost centres for Carrel-Dakin treatment.[54]

The technique was highly labour-intensive, involving a huge amount of work for nurses and VADs. The apparatus consisted of a glass bottle which was placed on a stand high above the patient's bed; a long piece of rubber tubing which ran from this bottle and was divided into several smaller tubes at its end; a series of tiny glass tubes, which were fitted onto the rubber ones; and, finally a number of narrow rubber tubes, the ends of which were placed in the bed of the wound. Each piece of equipment had to be washed, dried, and sterilized by boiling (or in a steam autoclave) at regular intervals. Every two hours, a nurse or VAD would do a 'round' of the ward, going to each patient receiving the Carrel-Dakin treatment, opening a valve on the rubber tube, and allowing the sodium hypochlorite to flow through the wound. Sometimes the fluid would be literally 'squirted' into the wound under pressure.[55] The aim was to keep the wound constantly bathed in antiseptic, and sometimes a completely free flow of Dakin's solution was maintained—a technique that, if it went wrong, could result in patients' beds became completely flooded with sodium hypochlorite.

The irrigation and dressing of a wound was, invariably, an intensely painful experience for the patient, but patients were not routinely given painkillers prior to these procedures. In an era when the 'stiff upper lip' was highly prized, patients often endured painful procedures with great stoicism.[56]

Military surgery on the Western Front became more sophisticated during the course of 1915. The administration of military medicine at all levels and in all scenarios was beginning to be dominated by a new focus on 'managerial rationality'. A new emphasis on 'efficiency' began to be expressed through specialization by surgeons. Individual wards—and even whole CCSs—began to 'take in' only certain cases, cooperating with their neighbouring units to ensure that particular surgeons became experienced and highly proficient in dealing with particular types of injury. As a result, surgical and ward nurses also attained specialist skills in the care of limb, abdominal, thoracic, head, or other surgical cases. Specialization appears to have had a highly beneficial effect. In 1914, for example, most abdominal cases had been declared 'moribund' but, by the end of 1915, many were being treated successfully. Even cases who had several feet of shrapnel-riddled intestine removed were able to survive. In orthopaedic units new innovations—such as the 'Thomas Splint' designed by Robert Jones and Hugh Owen Thomas, which immobilized wounds to better promote healing—had highly beneficial effects.[57] The availability of expert and experienced nurses in CCSs was an important element in the survival of wounded men whose conditions would previously have been considered hopeless.

It was not only on land that nurses provided life-saving wound-care to patients. Mary Clarke, a qualified Navy nurse, worked on board the hospital ship *Plassy*, taking on wounded from the Battle of Jutland.[58] Amongst the most dangerous wounds were the severe burns caused by explosions on board ships. These had to be dressed with the greatest of care, using the most meticulous aseptic technique; most were treated with picric acid, a powerful antiseptic. Severe burns were already life-threatening, and any wound infection would dramatically reduce the patient's already compromised chances of survival.

### The hardships of trench warfare: caring for sick soldiers

Wounds were not the only types of damage suffered by those who fought in the First World War. Even on the Eastern Front, soldiers lived in trenches for many weeks at a time, enduring the dirt and filth of their subterranean surroundings. They existed among lice, fleas rats, and even—on occasions—the partially buried corpses of their fellow men.[59] Many soldiers became dangerously ill simply as a result of being forced to live in such squalid conditions. CCSs and base hospitals could become particularly busy at times of cold and wet weather, when already-muddy trenches became water-logged with icy or slushy water. Soldiers were obliged to wade through whatever mud or water lay in the bottom of their trenches.

Some recounted tales of trenches which were waist-deep in mud. This, combined with the interruption of the blood-supply by tight puttees, could lead to a condition known as 'trench foot', which was believed to be a fungal infection existing concurrently with frostbite and made worse by poor circulation. Trench foot could be highly dangerous; it often resulted in the loss of toes, and sometimes led to more serious infections such as gangrene. For some sufferers the only solution was the amputation of the foot. Many soldiers lost both feet to the disease. It was not until November 1915 that the scale of the problem was recognized; literally thousands of men were being lost to front-line service from trench foot. Special wading-boots were sent to the front, and instructions were given to commanding officers that no man was to stand in water for more than eight hours at a time.[60] The notion that men could be left standing in cold water even for eight hours illustrates how desperate conditions had become in the front-line trenches. When nurses received these patients in CCSs, once they had treated wounds and offered shock-treatment and pain-relief, they worked to remove layers of mud from patients' bodies and to offer the warmth and rest that would assist a return of circulation.[61]

Conditions in the trenches—including a shortage of water for drinking and washing—also placed soldiers at risk of diseases such as dysentery (caused by contaminated food and water) and typhus fever (transmitted by lice). In the winter of 1915, large numbers of casualties were transferred to base hospitals with severe fevers, and nurses had to take care that they were nursed under the most hygienic conditions possible, to avoid the transmission of infection to other patients. Special wards, and some whole base hospitals, were set aside for patients with infectious diseases. Although enteric diseases were fairly common, epidemics of the more dangerous typhoid fever were avoided by the inoculation of troops.[62]

One of the most mysterious diagnoses of the war was 'disordered action of the heart' or 'soldier's heart', also referred to as 'effort syndrome',[63] which appears to have emerged as a result of the harshness of trench life and the exertion of carrying a heavy soldier's pack. Cases of previously-unrecognized congenital heart malformations and heart failure emerged as the exertions of trench life began to take their toll.[64]

## Emotional wounds: 'shell shock' and its treatment

The assault in October 1914, which later became known as the First Battle of Ypres, was probably one of the most destructive battles of the war's opening year. For the British Expeditionary Force, which lost a third of its men, it was undoubtedly one of the most costly; and for those who experienced the dreadful advance towards Passchendaele Ridge, into the teeth of enemy artillery, its horror could never be forgotten. As casualties streamed into military hospitals in northern France, nurses and medical officers noticed a peculiar phenomenon. Many of the 'wounded' actually had no physical wound, but were, rather, suffering from a range of strange and disturbing symptoms: some were blind, others deaf, and still more unable to taste or smell; some vomited uncontrollably; some could not speak; many had 'the shakes', while others were completely paralysed. And accompanying their physical symptoms was a profound emotional depression. Nurses offered hot drinks, comforted them, and settled them into beds, hoping that rest would relieve their symptoms; but their physical debility continued, and their emotional states, if anything, worsened. At night they suffered from long periods of insomnia; and when they did manage to sleep, many experienced terrifying nightmares. Nurses soon learned that it was unwise to wake such men suddenly; many wrote in their memoirs of being attacked by disturbed patients who were reliving their battle-front experiences.[65]

Towards the end of that year, one of the few psychologists on the Western Front, Charles Myers, who was based at the Duchess of Westminster's Hospital at Le Touquet, began to take a close interest in these cases. At the end of the year, he published a paper

in *The Lancet,* labelling their condition 'shell shock'. British newspapers seized upon the term, popularizing it until it became part
of the new vocabulary of a wartime population. Myers was appointed 'Specialist in Nervous Shock' to the British army in France,
and moved to a base hospital in Boulogne, where he continued to
work with 'shell-shock' cases.[66] But the subject rapidly became
highly controversial. Many medical officers believed that, while a
small number of soldiers did genuinely suffer from a debilitating
conditions associated with shell blast, many more were using the
label 'shell shock' to escape the Western Front and return home
'sick'. Shell shock came to be inextricably linked to malingering,
and shell-shock victims were increasingly accused of 'funk'; some
were even court-martialled and shot for desertion.[67]

It was only after the war that a real understanding of the psychological pressures under which soldiers had lived began to
emerge. Memoirs such as Edmund Blunden's *Undertones of War,*
Robert Graves's *Goodbye to All That,* and Erich Maria Remarque's
*All Quiet on the Western Front* began to bring home to a horrified
readership the realities of trench warfare.[68] But some of the most
shocking stories are told in the least well-known autobiographies.
Douglas Bell, a member of the BEF, who was injured three times,
wrote of how, in Flanders during April, he had a 'bad time with
shells and trench mortars'. He described how 'terrific' the concussion of the shell could be, and how it could sometimes demolish
whole stretches of trench: 'you hear the faint thud of the discharge,
look up, see it coming, whirling and twisting in the air, and scuttle
along the trench away from it. But this gets on your nerves after a
while; it is so tiring dodging up and down the trench like that.' In
addition to exhaustion, he and his fellow sufferers were becoming
'engulfed in slime' every time they ducked, because their trench
was a 'moving river of mud'.[69]

The contrast between Bell's descriptions of trench life and his
experiences of hospital care are striking and offer a poignant illustration of the comfort that could be offered in a base hospital.

After being wounded in the leg, and having caught 'a slight chill with catarrh, the latter perhaps due to a whiff of gas' just outside Ypres, he was conveyed by ambulance to a CCS at Poperinge, 'feeling rather shivery and empty', but by the time he had been transferred by hospital train to Boulogne where 'some dear sister' was in charge, and then by steamer and another train to Guy's Hospital, he felt that life was 'luxurious; everybody most kind'.[70] Bell was even more seriously wounded later that year, in October. This time he was taken to the Duchess of Westminster's Hospital at Le Touquet, 'a spacious beautiful place' where he 'received the greatest kindness from everyone, from the Duchess herself to the ward orderly'.[71] Douglas Bell was one of the many who endured hardship and terror without succumbing to 'shell shock'. Yet his experiences place into context the suffering of those who became seriously mentally ill. They also illustrate the sense of well-being which could be experienced by a patient in a military hospital.

By the end of 1915, Charles Myers had serious doubts about the value of the label he had invented. During that year, two competing definitions of shell shock had emerged: one which saw it as a physical disease, 'shell concussion', caused by the bursting of a shell close to the sufferer; and one which viewed it as a 'psychic' condition resulting from terror and loss of control. The terms 'hysteria' and 'neurasthenia'—terms that were current in psychological thinking before the war—began to be reused, in an attempt to release the hold of the idea of 'shell shock' on the popular imagination. But the label stuck. A profound dispute emerged, between scientists such as Frederick Mott, who insisted upon a physical cause for the disease (be that damage to the brain tissue from minute particles or gases, or just the blast itself) and those such as Harold Wiltshire, who explained the physical symptoms of the disease in terms of 'disassociation' between mind and body, created by extreme fear. For nurses, these debates were largely academic. The nature of their work meant that they would offer comfort, rest, and support to a 'shell-shocked' patient whichever explanation proved to be the 'correct' one. Their training had not taught them to distinguish between physical and mental causes in the same way as a medical training. The measures they implemented were not designed to search out and treat a 'lesion', but to support the entire system—physical, psychological, and emotional—to care for the human being as a whole person.

Very few nurses recorded their views on shell shock. But few could avoid being influenced by the labels which were applied to victims: whilst some were labelled 'Shell-shock, W' (for wound), others were labelled 'Shell-shock, S' (for sickness).[72] Later in the war, yet another diagnosis emerged, designed to avoid giving an early diagnosis of shell shock to those who might be fit to return to the front after a short period of rest. This was 'Not Yet Diagnosed Nervous' ('NYDN'), a label designed to conserve manpower. A patient who had received this label would be sent to a specialist medical unit close to the front lines where his condition was carefully assessed.[73] Nurses had already noticed that the wounded were treated with respect by a grateful public, while the sick were viewed with some suspicion. Some commented that it seemed sad that those who had fallen seriously ill as a result of their war service— many of whom would probably never recover—received neither the status of 'the wounded' nor a pension. For them, it made sense to treat shell-shock cases as 'wounded' men. In her *Text Book of War Nursing*, Violetta Thurstan chose to adhere resolutely to the theory that shell shock was, indeed, caused by the 'percussion' on the brain and nervous system of shell blast. She advised nurses to give carefully any calming drugs, such as bromide or chloral, that might be prescribed by doctors and to ensure that patients were able to obtain 'complete mental and physical rest in bed'.[74]

### Wounded nurses

In 1915, a young middle-class British volunteer, Alice Essington-Nelson, secured a position as assistant to Lady Gifford, the Head of House at Princess Louise's Convalescent Home for Nursing Sisters. The home—a beautiful country mansion midway between the bases of Étaples and Boulogne—had been donated to the Red Cross by the Duchess of Argyle, and was being used to house nursing sisters who had fallen ill or been injured on the Western Front. Patients were encouraged to rest and recuperate before returning to their duties in base hospitals, CCSs, and hospital trains and ships.[75] Essington-Nelson described the 'base' of Boulogne as being 'like a huge hospital'. Most of its large buildings had been converted into either base hospitals or military headquarters. Several hospital ships lay at anchor in the harbour and ambulances were moving constantly through the town, taking patients from hospital trains in the station to base hospitals or straight to the quay for embarkation. It was 'from this city of intense work and nerve strain' that she and her colleagues took 'the sisters to our house of rest away out in the country'.[76]

Enthused by her new responsibilities, Essington-Nelson spent much time with the 'sick sisters', listening to their stories, many of which were truly remarkable. Some described how, in the earliest days of the war, they had slept on the floors of their billets and spent their days cleaning the hotel rooms that were to become their hospital wards. Others told of nursing on the earliest hospital trains, with no furniture or bunks of any kind. After the establishment of base hospitals and evacuation lines on the Western Front, many found themselves overwhelmed with rushes of patients. For Essington-Nelson, their devotion to their patients was 'magnificent'.

Perhaps the most dramatic story she was told was that of Sister Walton, who had been on the hospital ship *Anglia* when it was torpedoed in the English Channel in November 1915. Walton was caring for fifty 'cot cases' in a lower ward, when one patient began to suffer from such intense pain that she went upstairs to an officers' ward to find some aspirin. Just as she reached the medicine cupboard, there was a 'most awful explosion'. Walton lost consciousness for several seconds. When she recovered, she found that her legs were pinned beneath a heap of iron cots, water was flowing into the ward, and the officer-patients were 'drowning before her eyes'. Before she could even begin to free herself, another massive explosion dislodged the debris from above her. She found herself free, but under water. Seeing light above her head, she swam towards it, eventually reaching an upper deck. For several minutes she assisted other nurses, orderlies, and sailors to free patients from their splints, tie them into lifebelts, and throw them into the sea; most survived, as they were very quickly pulled from the water by the crews of several destroyers, which had hurried to the scene of the disaster. The matron and other sisters slid down a rope into the sea, but Walton felt she could not leave her desperate patients. At the point where she had given her lifebelt to an injured patient and had decided that death was inevitable, she was picked up by two men, a stoker and an orderly, and thrown 'like a ball' across 8 feet of water into the arms of a group of sailors from one of the rescue ships nearby. After spending three days in hospital, she returned to duty in a base hospital. It is not possible to know whether the story of Sister Walton was in any way embellished in the account of Essington-Nelson, who declared the subject of her story to be 'one of the unknown heroes of the war'.[77]

The 'sacrifices' of nurses were being recognized from the spring of 1915 onwards. An appeal for funds for nurses 'who have suffered, or may suffer, from attendance upon the sick and wounded during the war' was published in *The Times* on 27 March 1915. Elizabeth Haldane took the opportunity to publicize the importance of nurses' wartime contributions and to argue for a formal pension system:

> Ought the public to permit of their sacrificing themselves on the altar of patriotism even if they recognize their debt by founding a fund to assist them later on? We seem just lately to have wakened up to the value of the splendid work done by our trained nurses because their numbers are so limited and the demands made upon them at

this time of stress are unlimited. Let us see that our gratitude, which is very real, is expressed in a proper way.[78]

Some nurses contracted serious, life-threatening illnesses as a result of nursing patients with infectious diseases. Clementina Addison, a British nurse who had trained at the Leicester Royal Infirmary, joined the French Flag Nursing Corps and left England to work for the French Service de Santé on 9 April 1915 (see Figure 13). She served close to the front lines at Verdun, and in 'Hospital No. 4 de la Butte, Besançon'. On 3 March 1916, eleven months after her departure, she returned to England—to her family home in Caton, Lancashire—'utterly broken down by the arduous tasks she had so willingly undertaken'.[79] She appears to have contracted a serious infectious disease—possibly typhus—and she died, at the age of 26, a week after her return home. Her coffin, draped in both the Union Jack and the French Tricolour, was followed by a long procession of mourners as the cart on which it was carried climbed the long hill to Caton parish church. Her grave in the churchyard is unmarked, yet her name is engraved on Caton War Memorial alongside her male soldier-comrades, followed by the words: 'By Their Sacrifice We Live'. A report in the *British Journal of Nursing* recorded that 'the death of this gentle Sister is the first to be recorded in the ranks of the French Flag Nursing Corps, though we regret that the health of several of the Sisters has suffered severely in consequence of their arduous duties'.[80]

There can be little doubt that nursing the wounded of the First World War was an arduous—and at times a dangerous—occupation. Some women's historians have emphasized the trauma suffered by nurses themselves. Working close to the firing lines and enduring danger and hardship could create a sense of anxiety and a loss of control which could predispose nurses and other women-workers, such as ambulance-drivers, to their own forms of war neurosis—their own type of 'shell shock'.[81] But, even if they were not in direct danger, nurses experienced the distress of witnessing

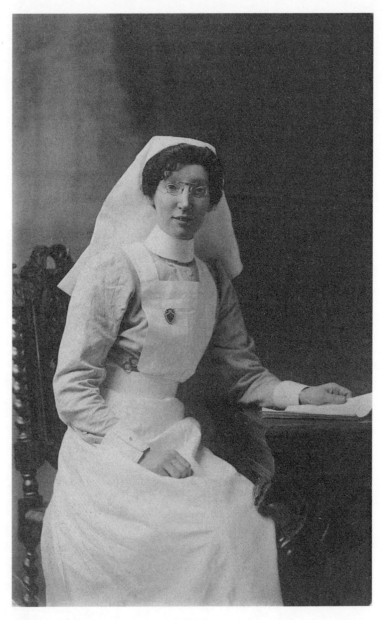

FIGURE 13 Portrait photograph of Clementina Addison taken at the Leicester Royal Infirmary (photograph reproduced by kind permission of Leicester Royal Infirmary Museum)

the suffering of their badly-injured and sometimes irreparably-maimed patients. Those who wrote later of their wartime work described feeling 'haunted' by their experiences.[82]

## Conclusion

The 'Western Front' in the First World War has become synonymous with horror. Even when not in direct danger of injury, soldiers endured hardship. Many sustained extensive and seriously infected wounds, and experienced an emotional strain which would result in grave mental illness. Nurses in CCSs, on transport services, and in base hospitals received these badly damaged men and put into action a range of measures to clean, comfort, calm, and heal them. During large assaults, patients arrived in CCSs in 'rushes' several hundred at a time. Those who needed it underwent emergency surgery, while the walking wounded were placed into trains for base. As the 'lines of evacuation' did their work, 'waves' of wounded men were moved rapidly outwards from the front lines towards bases on the north coast of France. Many of the most seriously wounded were moved further, across the Channel to Britain.

Their work placed enormous strain on nurses, some of whom found themselves succumbing to stress and requiring recuperation in 'sick sisters' wards' or rest homes. Others braced themselves against the strain of wartime work, seeing their contributions as important elements of the 'war effort' and believing that, if their soldier-patients could only expect rest and relief when damaged, then they too must push themselves to breaking point.

# 3

# Nursing on the Russian
# and Serbian Fronts

## 1914–1916

### Introduction: mobile warfare on the Eastern Front

The First World War's 'Eastern Front' campaigns stand in stark contrast to the stagnant entrenchment of the West. Rapidly moving armies fought decisive battles in several regions simultaneously, resulting in huge numbers of military casualties and creating a humanitarian catastrophe, as millions of families were driven out of their homes as refugees. For nurses, the Russian and Serbian Fronts presented enormous challenges. In Russia, severe bullet and shrapnel wounds were incurred many hundreds of miles from base hospitals located in cities such as Moscow and Petrograd, and the military medical services were forced to devise methods for attending them rapidly and effectively close to where the fighting was taking place. Instead of casualty clearing stations, the Russian military medical services had much more mobile units: 'letuchka' or flying columns, which followed advancing armies (or joined their retreats). Once they had stabilized their patient's conditions, medical officers and nurses in these units applied occlusive dressings containing salt packs or iodine swabs, which would remain in place during the long train journey back to base.

In the first months of the war, the Central Powers launched attacks on a number of sectors of an enormously lengthy 'Eastern

Front'. In the south, their forces, led by the Austro-Hungarian General Franz Conrad von Hötzendorf, invaded Russian Poland in mid-August 1914. After fighting a number of indecisive but costly skirmishes they found themselves badly outnumbered and forced to retreat. The Russian forces enjoyed early successes in the north too, and were able to push into East Prussia, before being decisively defeated at the Battles of Tannenberg and the Masurian Lakes in late August and September. They suffered huge numbers of casualties and were pushed back in the north, although they managed to hold on to most of Galicia in the south. Between September and November the Central Powers launched two unsuccessful counter-attacks on Warsaw and both sides found themselves under intense pressure and losing hundreds of thousands of casualties.[1] A bitter conflict in the Carpathian mountains during the winter of 1914–15 resulted in intense suffering for troops who were forced to fight in sub-zero temperatures over mountainous terrains. Historian Graydon Tunstall has referred to the 'Carpathian Winter War' of 1915 as 'one of the most significant—and, in terms of human sacrifice, most tragic—chapters of World War I military history'.[2] Resulting in the deaths of over 1 million Russian, Austro-Hungarian, and German soldiers, it was to be dubbed 'the Stalingrad of World War I'.[3] Many of those who survived were severely debilitated both physically and emotionally by dire conditions in the high mountains, where wolves could be heard at night and supplies froze solid. Conditions such as trench foot and hypothermia led to heavy workloads for flying columns.

The brief stalemate on the Eastern Front ended in May 1915, when the Central Powers won a decisive victory at the Battle of Tarnow-Gorlice. The Russian armies in the south were forced out of Warsaw. They retreated deep into their own territory, their flying columns alongside them, taking what wounded they could, but forced to leave behind many injured and dying men.

Following their successes in the summer of 1915, several German divisions headed south into the Balkan region in order to join with Bulgaria and effect a decisive victory over Serbia. As German and

Bulgarian armies swept into their country from the north and east, Serbian troops and civilians were forced to retreat westwards. Their headlong flight took them into the hostile Albanian Alps in the middle of winter, resulting in thousands of deaths from starvation and exposure.

Meanwhile, the complexity of the situation had been increased by the entry of Italy into the war. Its government had, in April, signed a treaty with the Allies, and had declared war on Austria-Hungary on 23 May. Thus began a series of campaigns along the Isonzo which would extend into no fewer than twelve bloody 'battles', creating enormous pressures for the Austro-Hungarian armies, most of whose divisions were already committed on the Russian Front. In the Alps, limestone shrapnel created severe injuries, whilst the ruggedness of the terrain made it difficult to bury the dead, resulting in desperately unsanitary conditions.[4]

## Russia's 'Sisters of Mercy'

Imperial Russia's nurses belonged to a culture and a society that were steeped in a powerful sense of religious devotion and deference to authority. To become a nurse during the second half of the nineteenth century was to join one of the communities of 'Sisters of Mercy' (*obschiny sester miloserdiya*) and become part of a recognized order of caregivers. Although they were not 'closed' or subject to strict rules of self-denial like convents, these communities were imbued with an atmosphere of service and sacrifice, and acknowledged the supreme authority of the Russian Orthodox Church. Their members received no formal training, but learned the art of nursing by working closely with their seniors. The foundation of the earliest known community took place in 1844 and by the outbreak of war there were about 150 in total.[5] Clearly, there was a serious shortage of experienced nurses.

In Russia, a 'nursing profession' had never developed. Nursing was not seen in any way as falling under the auspices of the state, and was, rather, both controlled and supported by wealthy patrons, who saw it as their private, philanthropic concern. Nor had Russian Sisters of Mercy chosen to organize themselves on any national basis. Their focus on self-abnegation and their refusal to take control of their own work meant that they had created no national societies or unions and had no journals or textbooks. During the crisis of 1917 they were to form the 'All-Union Congress of Russian Sisters of Mercy' (*Vserossisskii Soiuz Sester Miloserdiya*) in Petrograd, but their organization was to be short-lived and would be disbanded by the Bolsheviks in 1919, following the establishment of so-called 'red sisters'—nurses who were sent to the Civil War front following two-month training courses and would later be defined as 'middle medical workers' alongside midwives and *feldshers* (surgeon's assistants).[6]

The history of Russian nurses during the early twentieth century is one of deference, self-denial, and perhaps missed opportunity. This is not to say that the development of a better-established and more independent organizational structure would have enabled them to take control of their own destinies. All existing national organizations were crushed during the crisis period of Bolshevik rule, the Civil War, and the succeeding totalitarianism of Stalin. Russian nurses appear never to have sought personal power or influence. They did, however—in a way very similar to nurses in other countries—gravitate towards existing sources of political influence. Members of the aristocracy, the Russian royal family, and the Empress herself offered them patronage and support, and, following its foundation in 1867, the Russian Red Cross gave the movement coherence and a sense of common purpose, as many communities were brought under its auspices, some through the All-Russian Union of *Zemstvos* (local government bodies).

## Mobilizing a wartime nursing service

The mobilization of Russian men for war in the summer of 1914 was accompanied by an upsurge of enthusiasm among women determined to play a part in protecting 'the motherland'.[7] While patriotic motives and the desire to serve appear to have been uppermost in the minds of 'war nurses', some also saw participation in war as an opportunity to enhance women's rights to equal status with men as citizens.[8] The presence of women in military hospitals aroused great anxiety among military men but the nurturing and compassionate image created by the Sisters of Mercy, with their nun-like uniforms and carefully deferential modes of behaviour, did much to allay these fears. Workers in flying columns were able to cast aside some of the conventions of the traditional nurse-like image, dressing when necessary in breeches and jackets, riding on horseback, sleeping under canvas, and enjoying both the freedoms and the privations of the 'campaign' life.[9]

At the outbreak of war the Russian Society of the Red Cross rapidly mobilized nurses to serve in military hospitals and flying columns. The need to expand the size of the existing nursing workforce led to opportunities for women to undergo a shortened war-training. Florence Farmborough, an English governess to the two teenage daughters of a Moscow doctor, decided to offer her services to the Russian state. In her book, *Nurse at the Russian Front*, she recounted the rigours of her training and the devout and emotional religious blessing which took place as part of her graduation as a Russian nursing 'sister'.[10] Similarly, Mary Britnieva, a young Anglo-Russian woman living a life of wealth and privilege in Moscow, described in her memoir how she became enthused by a patriotic desire to serve Russia and enrolled in a war-training course. The ranks of the military nursing services were further swelled by Western women, like British nurse Violetta Thurstan, who travelled independently to Russia to offer their services to the Russian Red Cross.[11]

## Nursing Russia's wounded

It was Russia's alliance with Serbia which had helped escalate what began as a local conflict between Serbia and Austria-Hungary into a 'world war'. The Triple Entente between Russia, France, and

Britain ensured that all three nations declared war in quick succession. And yet, in the earliest years of the war, the Allies were worried that Russia would shift its allegiance to the Central Powers—an event which did actually take place after the Revolution of 1917. Recognizing the need to support the Russian war effort, and keen to develop a project that would both be of obvious service to the Russian army and symbolize the 'entente' between the two nations, the British created a hospital unit which travelled to Petrograd at the end of 1915 to join Russian medical and nursing colleagues and form what became known as the 'Anglo-Russian Hospital'.[12] Although directly supported by the British Red Cross and the Order of St John of Jerusalem, the Anglo-Russian Hospital also had many of the overtones of female philanthropic movements such as the projects of Millicent, Duchess of Sutherland and the Duchess of Westminster. Its two co-directors, Lady Muriel Paget and Lady Sybil Grey, were extremely well connected: Lady Muriel was already well known for charitable work in Russia, while Lady Sybil was daughter of a Canadian Governor General.[13] Also joining the unit that November were Dorothy Cotton, a Canadian nurse serving in Europe with the Canadian Army Medical Corps, and Dorothy Seymour, a British VAD. The 200-bed hospital opened in the palace of Grand Duke Dimitri Pavlovich on Nevsky Prospect in the centre of Petrograd in January 1916, with much ceremony, and in the presence of several members of the Russian royal family.[14] Its official patroness was the Tsar's aunt, Alexandra, who was the dowager queen of Great Britain. The hospital was, indeed, a powerful symbol of entente, and its organizers could not possibly have known that the Russian elite which supported it would soon be swept away. Its nurses—particularly those from upper-class backgrounds—were treated as honoured guests. Dorothy Seymour, an upper-class VAD from a highly influential military family, wrote home to her family of the many dinners and ballets she enjoyed.[15]

The Anglo-Russian Hospital was one of many military hospitals in Petrograd and it was rarely overcrowded with patients. It did, however, from time to time, provide support and hospitality to other foreign units. Katherine Hodges, an ambulance driver with the Scottish Women's Hospitals, was travelling through Petrograd following the evacuation of the organization's First Serbian Unit from the Romanian Front in December 1916; she commented that 'the Anglo-Russian people were very kind to us, and used to let us have any number of meals there, and baths'.[16] Another guest at the hospital was trained British nurse Margaret Barber, who had travelled to Armenia with the Lord Mayor's Armenian Relief Fund in April 1916, via Stockholm, Petrograd, and Moscow, and had worked at a civilian hospital in Van. In August, as the Turkish army approached the town, her unit was forced to join crowds of refugees. On reaching Petrograd, she was offered hospitality by the Anglo-Russian unit, remaining to work with them for several weeks. In October she joined a 'Friends' War Victims Committee' Unit travelling to a remote village in the Samara Government, where she stayed until May 1918.[17]

Dorothy Cotton was in France, serving with the No. 3 Canadian General Hospital, when she was selected by Matron-in-Chief Margaret Macdonald to join the Anglo-Russian unit.[18] She, along with twenty other nurses, ten volunteers, three doctors, and four orderlies, boarded the SS *Calypso*, which departed for Russia on 4 November 1915. She remained with the Anglo-Russian Hospital for eight months from its opening in January 1916 until September, when she went home on leave, following the deaths of her two brothers in France.[19] She rejoined the unit in January 1917, this time staying until August, by which time the increasing disorder created by the Revolution was making it almost impossible for Westerners to remain. She left Russia to become the matron of an officers' hospital in London, remaining there until August 1918, when she returned to Canada to nurse in a military hospital in Halifax.[20] In acknowledgement of her status as a member of the Canadian Army Medical Corps, Cotton was allowed to wear her own uniform. She was, in fact, the only member of the unit who was accorded this privilege, her colleagues being ordered to dress in the uniform of a Russian Red Cross nurse.[21] This gave her a very distinctive 'look'; the Canadian military nursing uniform was particularly martial in appearance, with a formal, tailored style and rows of brass buttons across the chest. The contrast between Cotton and her Russian (and other) nursing colleagues could not have been more marked. Her military appearance was very different from their classic nun-like robes. Nor were such appearances deceptive. Canadian military nursing sisters were afforded an officer-equivalent status at the time of the First World War. The recognition that they were members of the military, along with their somewhat militaristic appearance, provided a dramatic contrast to the low-status Russian Sisters of Mercy, with their deliberately self-sacrificing demeanour.

Trained British and Dominion nurses were fascinated by the marked differences between their own and Russian approaches to care. Violetta Thurstan marvelled at the meticulousness of the aseptic dressing techniques of Russian sisters, but deplored what she saw as their failure to perform the more holistic work of making patients truly comfortable. She, like others, commented on the practice of removing patients from their beds to a 'dressing room'— a space where complete asepsis could be more readily guaranteed— for the performance of wound dressings.[22] This did have a number of advantages. Apart from offering a better environment for the performance of an aseptic technique, it also permitted VADs or sanitars to make the patient's bed and clean his bed area before his return. The disadvantage of the procedure was that it required all patients—even the very sick and severely wounded—to be moved, a process which could be both intensely painful and detrimental to recovery.

This tendency to concentrate on the 'wound' rather than the whole person was one of the things which, Thurstan felt, distinguished Russian from British nurses. The performance of dressings was one of the most striking features of wartime nursing work, and

the term 'performance' is significant. The ritualistic, almost cere-
monial way in which dressings were done served two purposes: it
protected the wound—and the patient—from infection or other
harm; and its certainties provided comfort and a sense of security.
British VAD Irene Rathbone, in her semi-fictional account *We That
Were Young*, offers an almost reverential account of the ritual surrounding the performance of 'the dressing round' at the First
London General Hospital during the war, elevating the removal of
soiled dressings and the application of new ones almost to the level
of a quasi-religious ceremony.[23] And it was believed, by those who
saw and wrote about it, that this awed, almost spiritual, atmosphere
was captured par excellence in the 'dressing rooms' of the Russian
nursing sisters. Similar procedures were used in French military
hospitals, with the *salle de pansements* being a protected environment,
almost on a par with the operating theatre, but it was the work of
Russian nurses that seemed most to impress commentators.

Cotton had trained at the Royal Victoria Hospital, Montreal,
and was clearly confident in her own skills as a nurse. She, like other
Western nurses, adopted the routines and procedures of the Russian sisters only insofar as she believed that these were both safe
and practical. Her diary speaks of her fascination with the horrific
wounds of war, and her respect for her surgical colleagues, who
seem able to save the lives of even the most 'hopeless' cases. She
wrote, for example, of

> a man who had a glancing shrapnel wound across the chest, about
> four and a half inches long which at one place exposed the chest
> wall—so that the heart could be seen, plainly, pulsating. He was dis-
> charged at the end of two months, no complications having set in,
> and his wound was well healed.[24]

Another extraordinary 'case' was that of a 20-year-old, admitted
with a shrapnel wound in his leg, just below the knee, and two
severe head wounds—one the entrance and the other the exit of
a single bullet. The head injuries caused great concern, because,

although the only debris to be found at operation was loose bone, a very large amount of his skull was cracked, and the pieces could be moved with a pair of forceps. Brain tissue was protruding from both wounds, and both 'hernias' worsened over time, yet the wounds remained 'wonderfully clean'. At first the patient was very drowsy and 'seemed dazed' when spoken to. His wounds were dressed by 'moist Eusol dressings'.[25] 'Eusol' (Edinburgh University Solution of Lime) was a version of the sodium hypochlorite solution which was used as 'Dakin's Solution' on the Western Front. The fact that these wounds never became infected attests to the nurses' skill in aseptic technique. Shortly after admission, the young man's leg wound did, however, begin to show signs of infection, becoming more painful and exuding pus. It was operated upon; a small piece of shrapnel, which was clearly the seat of the infection, was removed and a large drainage tube inserted. The patient continued to recover well, although his speech remained slow and laboured. After a few months, his temperature rose rapidly, and he began to experience pain in the side of his face, around the area of the mastoid bone. Emergency surgery was once again performed and, by the time Cotton left the hospital on 10 June, he was 'sitting up in bed, gaining strength every day'.[26]

Dorothy Cotton's diary offers insights into the suffering of the Russian people in wartime which also features in other Western nurses' writings. She writes of a young 'soldier' who claims to be 15 years old, but who she believes cannot be 'a day over 11'. Both his hands are badly wounded, and one will probably have to be amputated. She is also horror-struck by the suffering of the tens of thousands of refugees, pouring into Petrograd from the provinces. Their numbers, she comments, are enormous, and in their loss, grief, and hunger, they are 'one of the saddest sights you can conceive'.[27]

The unit had its own mobile field hospital, which travelled close to the front lines in order to offer more immediate support to the Russian Guards.[28] Cotton was part of this unit when, towards the end of her first 'tour of duty' in Russia, it travelled in a special

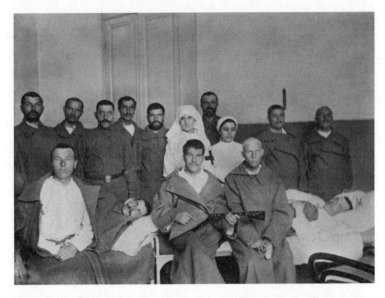

FIGURE 14 Staff and patients at Princess Golitsin's Hospital, Petrograd, 1914 (photograph reproduced by permission of the Imperial War Museum, London, UK)

train of forty-one carriages to a small country village near the town of Polock, 15 versts from the front.[29] The unit was soon moved on to the village of Maledetchona, even closer to the front lines. On the journey, Lady Sybil Grey was injured in the face by a stray piece of shrapnel during a visit to the trenches, and had to be evacuated to Petrograd for urgent surgery. At Maledetchona, the booming of heavy artillery could easily be heard. They were in a devastated zone, which had earlier in the war been in the hands of the Germans, but was now 'a mass of trenches and wire entanglements'.[30]

## Work in flying columns

Very little is known about the work of Russian nurses in 'letuchka', or flying columns. These highly mobile units, consisting of doctors,

nurses, and orderlies, travelling in fleets of motor vehicles supplemented by horse-drawn carts, saw themselves as the elite of the
military medical machine. Everyone knew that the most important
work was performed 'at the front'. Here, effective therapy to
ameliorate physiological shock could pull a patient back from the
brink of collapse and make the difference between life and death.
And if wounds could be operated upon early, cleaned up, cleared
of infection-forming debris, and carefully dressed before the patient underwent the long and gruelling journey to base, they were
much less likely to become dangerously infected. It was 'at the
front' that the difference was made. But in 1914 and 1915 it was
difficult to know where the front was. Multiple campaigns were
being fought and, although techniques of trench warfare were
being employed, armies were not becoming 'entrenched' in
the same way as those on the Western Front. Flying columns were
aptly named: they moved fast, often over difficult terrain, and
employed highly skilled orderlies who could construct (and just as
quickly dismantle) a field hospital in almost any type of temporary
accommodation, or under canvas where no suitable buildings
were available. They did manage to remain in close proximity to
the rapidly moving Russian front lines, during the advances of
1914, the retreats of the summer of 1915, and the last great push
of 1916–17.[31]

The nurses employed by the letuchka were a combination of
Russian Sisters of Mercy, Russian women who had undergone a
shortened Red Cross war-training, and volunteers from overseas,
many of whom were highly trained and very experienced. One
such volunteer was Violetta Thurstan, who wrote a heroic narrative of her experiences on the Polish Front.[32] For Thurstan, the
opportunity to put her meticulous London Hospital training to use
in such dramatic circumstances was something she clearly relished,
though another member of her unit, Elizabeth Greg, commented
that Thurstan was really 'over-qualified' for such highly-improvised
emergency work.[33]

The letuchka with which Thurstan was stationed, was run by two members of the Russian aristocracy, the Prince and Princess Volkonsky, and, under the influence of Thurstan's pen, its work takes on a highly romantic quality. Its members clearly cared deeply about the successes and defeats of the Russian armies and seem to have been intimately involved in the work of the military units they served—even to visiting the front-line trenches one night and listening to bullets pattering against the trees around them. Thurstan's work in and around Warsaw during the terrible war of attrition that was taking place in the winter of 1914, is vividly recounted, as is her surgical work in a series of highly improvised field hospitals, including one in a disused theatre in Skiernevice.[34] But Thurstan's career as a flying-column nurse was cut short by pleurisy, brought on by overstrain, poor food, and exhaustion, which forced her to return to England in the early spring of 1915. Although desperately disappointed, she also counted herself lucky to be alive. A stray shell had exploded right next to her days before she had fallen ill, and she had only survived because it had somehow planted itself deep into the clay earth and exploded upwards rather than sideways.

Florence Farmborough, a young woman who had been working as a governess in Moscow, and Mary Britnieva, a young and privileged member of the Anglo-Russian elite, also joined letuchka serving the southern campaigns. When the Central Powers took Warsaw in the late spring of 1915, both were forced to flee, and Farmborough writes movingly in her memoir, *Nurse at the Russian Front*, of her despair at having to leave behind desperately wounded and dying men:

> I turned from the doorway and stepped inside over the littered floor and paused by that row of silent figures stretched out on their straw beds. Two were already dead, one with eyes wide open as though looking attentively at something—or someone; I closed them and laid his hands on his breast. To his left a man was lying; great convulsions ran every now and then down his long frame and a queer gurgling noise was audible in his throat; Death had taken his hand

too. And he—in the corner—was lying as before, with strangely contracted limbs and eyes still dull and glazed, but his lips had ceased
to move.[35]

When she was interviewed sixty years later by Peter Liddle, Farmborough's memory of her experiences in Russia were still raw:
'I shall never, ever forget the feeling that one had when you came
to a hopeless case and he would look at you not able to speak but
all his longing was in his eyes. "Help me, I want to live," and you
just passed him by.' Liddle found Farmborough to be 'a very fine,
lively, kindly, lady'.[36]

Mary Britnieva's early experiences of work in a flying column
were very similar to those of Florence Farmborough. Enrolling as a
volunteer nurse, with a shortened, six-month war-training, Britnieva was desperately inexperienced when she first travelled west
as part of the letuchka of the Council of State, a unit consisting of
'three doctors, seven sisters, a dispenser, a house-keeper and about
twenty orderlies'.[37] Britnieva's account is highly romanticized—
if unconsciously so. Her experience of working for the letuchka,
clearly, was one she remembered with great fondness. During
her time on the Polish Front, she enjoyed the camaraderie of
her unit, fell in love with and married its head doctor, lived
in some remarkable accommodation (including the 'fairy tale'
palace of Teresino), and performed work she considered to be of
great value.

During the winter of 1914–15, the unit was based in Poland,
taking wounded from the battles that were raging in the region of
Warsaw. It gained a reputation for excellence: its mortality rates
dropping over time as transfer-times from front-line dressing stations and surgical techniques at the hospital were improved. Britnieva's obvious pleasure at being a part of such a unit was poured
into the pages of her published diary, as was her enjoyment of the
emergence of springtime in the lovely Polish countryside. Even
during the retreat, she revelled in the freedom offered by the open-air

lifestyle of the letuchka, with its long marches and evening camp-
fires. But joy was to be short-lived. The breakdown of army discipline which followed the March Revolution of 1917 was to lead,
eventually, to the dismantling of the letuchka. Britnieva and her
'head doctor' were to marry at the beginning of 1918, but their
lives under Bolshevik rule were full of hardship and deprivation.
Britnieva was to compose her memoir of her experiences in 1934,
at a time when her memories of the war's horrors were undoubtedly softened as they were filtered through recollections of Bolshevism
and Stalin's 'cultural revolution'.[38]

## Volunteer units in the Serbian campaign

When the British government declared war on Germany in August
1914, its citizens' attention was focused on Belgium, which was perceived as a tiny, almost defenceless nation which had fallen victim
to the might of the 'Prussian hordes'. Inculcated into a profoundly
positive view of their nation as the guardian of freedom against
oppression, the vast majority supported their government's intervention in Europe as a matter of 'justice' and 'right'. But Belgium
was not the only nation to be cast in this role. Serbia too was seen
as a small yet noble nation, facing the oppression of a large and
belligerent neighbour. The nation whose feud with Austria-
Hungary had been the spark which ignited the war, was considered
a worthy ally, evoking an emotional response from a British people
who still held the ingrained belief that their empire stood for lib-
erty and civilization. And, as in the case of Belgium, it was wealthy
philanthropists and campaigners who chose to rush to the aid of
the Serbian nation. A number of volunteer units made their own
way to the Balkans in 1915—many fresh from their retreat from
Belgium—determined to offer what support they could. Among
them were four units of the Scottish Women's Hospitals, led by
their chief medical officer, Dr Elsie Inglis; a unit headed by Sir Ralph
and Lady Paget; and the so-called 'First British Field Hospital',

which was said to be 'the only unit officially attached to the Serbian Army'.[39] In April 1915, Mabel St Clair Stobart took a unit of her 'Women's Sick and Wounded Convoy Corps' to Serbia under the auspices of the Serbian Relief Fund. She established a camp hospital on a racecourse above Kragujevatz and organized dispensaries to serve the civilian populations in numerous Serbian towns and rural areas.[40]

The fate of the Serbian volunteer units was a bleak one. Most arrived in the spring of 1915, at a time when military hospitals in Serbian bases were overrun with epidemics of typhus. During the hot summer, nurses protected themselves from the lice which transmitted the disease by caring for their patients in heavy overalls with taped sleeves, masks, heavy boots, and rubber gloves. Offering total nursing care to large numbers of sick and wounded soldiers—many of whom were utterly prostrate with typhus—in such heavy clothing was, no doubt, exhausting.

The work of the Serbian units was to be of short duration. That autumn, the German high command decided to launch a huge offensive, designed to knock Serbia out of the war. Austrian and German divisions attacked from the north, while their Bulgarian allies invaded from the east. The Serbian army was rapidly overwhelmed and driven into headlong retreat. The British hospital units serving it were forced to choose between the equally unattractive options of remaining where they were and awaiting capture or retreating just ahead of the army. Some units, notably those of Elsie Inglis and Lady Paget, chose the former course.[41] Others decided to escape, and most of these found themselves fleeing on foot across Serbia, Montenegro, and Albania to the Adriatic coast. The retreat of which they became a part was 'not that of an army but of a Country', as huge numbers of civilians fled the joint German and Bulgarian advance.[42]

When interviewed later by a correspondent of the *Nursing Times*, 'Miss Caldwell', the matron of a Red Cross unit based in Vrnjatchka Banja, described how she had called out, as the Austrians entered the town, 'Bring me a clean apron', explaining that 'for the honour of England I could not appear before the enemy in a dirty one!' She had tried to persuade her staff not to attempt to escape from Serbia and now believed that her decision had been correct: the Austrians treated the nurses of her unit well, although food was very scarce, and the journey from Serbia to Switzerland difficult and full of privations.[43]

The town of Krushevatz, where Elsie Inglis's unit was based, was overrun by the German army, and the unit's staff was placed under arrest. Their patients were transferred to a large Serbian military hospital, where Inglis's nurses were allowed to care for them under conditions of severe overcrowding. At one time, a hospital originally intended for 400 patients was housing 1,200 sick and wounded men. It was later reported in the *Nursing Times* that only the nurses' scrupulous attention to cleanliness and order had prevented a typhus epidemic. In February, the unit, along with others, was taken via Belgrade and Bludenz to Switzerland and freedom. Another unit of the Scottish Women's Hospitals, led by Alice Hutchinson, was also eventually freed after having been imprisoned for a time in Austria.[44]

## Flight from Serbia

In the summer of 1915, the First British Field Hospital had been posted first to Belgrade and then to Skoplje, where the majority of its patients were Austrian prisoners. In the late summer, in antici-pation of the attack that was to come, it had been moved to Pirot on Serbia's eastern frontier, to open a clearing hospital. On 14 October, staff were 'awakened at dawn by the "boom, boom" of heavy guns', to the news that 'the Bulgarians had become our en-emies'. For the next two weeks, the hospital took in huge numbers of Serbian wounded and the sound of artillery drew closer. Even-tually, shells could be seen bursting on the mountain sides within view of the hospital. On 28 October, the entire unit was evacuated by train in the direction of the British base Salonika. Severely wounded patients were given large injections of morphia, and settled as comfortably as possible in train carriages, but several died in the first few days. The next leg of the journey—to Mitrovitza— was made in ambulances along narrow, winding mountain roads. Eventually, having reached Ljoom-Kula, the staff were informed that the only way, now, to reach Salonika was to walk. The first stage of their march, of 100 miles through a narrow mountain pass to Debra, took seven days. The path was slippery with ice, over which a thick layer of snow was falling. Shelter was found in a variety of buildings: peasant huts, stables, lofts, and rest huts. Eventually, on reaching Monastir, the staff were able to board a train for the British base of Salonika.[45]

The hardships endured by the First British Field Hospital were considerable; but they seemed nothing when later compared with the suffering of those units forced to make their retreat across the Albanian Alps to the Adriatic. Several units arrived in England just before Christmas, and their stories provided ample fuel for a national press keen to feed the appetites of a public hungry for tales of heroism. The nursing press, too, chose to recount their experiences as a series of 'exploits' or 'adventures'. An edition of the *Nursing Times*, issued on New Year's Day 1916, began:

> We are thankful to hear of the safe arrival in this country of some of our heroic nurses from Serbia and glad to know that about 75 of them, including 22 members of the Scottish Women's Hospital and 33 of Mrs Stobart's party, arrived in time to spend Christmas at home. The party…walked 200 miles through Serbia, Montenegro and Albania (a daily 16 mile tramp) under the most awful conditions possible through knee-deep snow over high mountains.[46]

In similar style, the *Daily Telegraph* lauded the 'extraordinary courage and heroism of these British women'.[47] Mabel St Clair Stobart, who led her unit through the Albanian Alps on horseback, was celebrated as a national heroine: 'The Lady of the Black Horse'.[48]

As nurses' and doctors' stories emerged, it became clear that their long trek westwards from Serbia to the Adriatic had been both gruelling and terrifying. For most, even the first stage of their journeys from their postings in Serbia to Ipek had been difficult: some had travelled in motor cars, others on bullock wagons. All had been issued with a small daily ration of bread, and they considered themselves lucky. Serbian soldiers had no such rations, and each time a horse died by the roadside, it would be seized upon by groups of starving soldiers and cut up for meat. But both bread and meat soon froze 'as hard as iron'. As the journey continued, the roadside corpses of starved Serbians—both soldiers and civilians—became a common sight. At nights the units slept wherever they could find shelter, sometimes in stables, 'with snow blowing in through the roof and sides',[49] sometimes in shelters where the air was fetid and the floor was crowded with the bodies of refugees.

As the units continued their journey west, all found themselves in the town of Ipek, where roads stopped and narrow mountain-tracks provided the only means to cross the Alps. Wagons and cars were swapped for pack-ponies, and a long single-file column of refugees made its way on a five-day trek across the frozen mountains. This was the most testing part of the journey, but, having reached lower ground once more, the units met again at Podgoritza, then Scutari. After a brief rest, the final leg of the journey— a further two-day trek—took them to San Giovanni di Medua, where all were eventually able to obtain passage across the Adriatic to Italy.

One of the clearest narratives of the journey was offered to the *Nursing Times* reporter by Janet Middleton, a nurse with a Scottish Women's Hospital unit evacuated from Milanovacs on 12 October. On their journey across the Albanian Alps, staff had been obliged to sleep wherever they could find hospitality: in stables, lofts, and kitchens; sometimes on hay, sometimes on bare floors. Occasionally they had camped in the open air in sub-zero temperatures. Middleton described how they had climbed mountain passes to a

height of 7,500 feet above sea level, adding: 'I had to lead a pony
for six days over mountain tracks slippery with ice. We came down
a mountain side by candle-light over a path that I am sure we
would not have dared to attempt in the daytime. We had to cross
broken bridges and wade through rivers that were icy cold.' The
party had survived on half a loaf of bread per day, and had gath-
ered sticks for their evening fire as they walked. Sometimes, the
bread froze in their pockets. Some unfortunate nurses, whose boots
wore out or fell to pieces, suffered frostbitten toes. At times the
snow was knee-deep and the party would often lie down to sleep at
night in wet clothing.[50]

Middleton's story was typical of the experiences of the Serbian
units. Another nurse, Elizabeth Atkinson, described how she had
trekked over the Alps in a 'terrific blizzard' and had, with a small
group of friends, lost sight of the rest of her party. They were
helped by an Austrian prisoner they had nursed in Serbia, who
found them shelter in a ruined hut, built a fire, and attended to her
frostbitten feet. She commented: 'I would like to say that all the
Austrians we came into contact with were most kind and good to
us. Those we had nursed would do anything for us.' Descending
the other side of the mountains, this nurse found herself on a path
that was slippery, 'like glass', and her party lost most of its luggage
when their horses fell: 'In many places the mountain track was
barely a foot wide along the edge of the precipices, and we saw
both men and animals fall over. The ponies were so weak from
want of food that a slight collision between their loads and the
jagged points of the rock was sufficient to hurl them over.'[51]

The *Nursing Times* eagerly recounted narratives from a number
of national and local newspapers in a way that reveals the hunger
for heroic narratives of war nurses. The *Manchester Guardian* had
offered a rather whimsical piece describing how 'London shoppers
in the gay west-end shops were a little startled at the sight of groups
of very ragged, dishevelled women and girls, their clothes not only
travel-stained but begrimed, the most poverty-stricken shoppers

those splendid stores had ever seen'.[52] These were, of course, returning nurses and doctors, passing through London on their final
journey home. The decision of the *Guardian*'s reporting and editorial teams to juxtapose the squalor and filth of the women's dress
against the splendour of London's West End was undoubtedly
fuelled by a desire to depict the women's behaviour as both stirring
and aberrant. Such extreme behaviour could hardly be viewed as
the norm and was, thus, portrayed as both rather wonderful and
essentially ridiculous. The *Guardian*'s column went on to describe
the journey which had so disarranged the attire of the heroine-
nurses: during their climb to a height of over 7,000 feet, braving
blizzards and wading through knee-deep snow drifts,

> the track was so indistinguishable that often they only knew they
> were on the right way when they looked upwards and saw the thin
> black line of refugees winding up the mountain side far above them.
> Often they could only find their way by following the course of some
> stream, and often when the bridge was broken they waded knee
> deep in water to the other side. But the sun shone and the scenery, if
> terrifying, was magnificent…But on that mountain trek it was
> everyone for herself, and she helped best who kept going and did not
> block the way for others.

Again, the juxtaposition of intense suffering with 'magnificence' is
incongruous, as is the claim that 'the sun shone', when the nurses'
narratives refer explicitly to heavy rains on lower grounds, and blizzards in the mountains. At the end of 1915, the British perspective on
the war was, clearly, still heavily influenced by heroic narrative tropes,
which assumed that the British could always conquer hardship.
Danger and deprivation was seen as a fitting challenge for daughters
of the British Empire. It was, furthermore, taken for granted that
those daughters would, having conquered some of the most daunting
terrains in Europe, return to safe domesticity on the home front.

The romance theme was taken further, becoming epic in its
beauty and intensity, in a description given by Mrs W. Aldridge, a

member of Mabel St Clair Stobart's 'Women's Sick and Wounded Convoy Corps', and published in the *Daily News*:

> On the road from Prizrend to Ipek we outspanned one beautiful moonlight night by the road-side and made a jolly fire. Then one of the Serbian orderlies who were with us brought out some sort of rude bagpipes and played a strange melancholy music, while the others, linked together, swayed backwards and forwards in a slow rhythmic dance. And some of the nurses from Ireland sang sad Irish songs. Then we inspanned and by-and-bye [*sic*] came out by a pass upon a wonderful prospect of the Montenegrin mountains. Everything was drenched with the clearest silver moonlight. And as we stood there one of the girls said: 'It seems like being in eternity—no time or space'. That was how one felt after going through the Valley of the Shadow in Serbia.[53]

In the recounting of the nurses' stories, the use of classic techniques of epic-romantic writing, such as the recounting of the sad music of Serbian orderlies and Irish nurses, and the use of the biblical phrase 'Valley of the Shadow', are set alongside the grim realities of frostbite and the witnessing of death from starvation of a large part of the Serbian army. The strange incongruity thus created seems to have been a feature of the nurses' lives as willing participants in what they still viewed as a heroic struggle, but were increasingly beginning to recognize as a squalid waste.

The nurses' stories became legendary, and are found often recounted in the diaries and letters of their colleagues. Katherine Hodges told, in her diary, the story of one British nurse, 'with the courage of a lion', who, after having worked under bombardment in Antwerp in 1914, had gone to Serbia, only to join the retreat. She had been shot through the lung during a fight for food, and her unit had left her by the roadside. Her friend had remained with her until the Central Powers had overtaken them, and both had been taken prisoner. She recovered and was repatriated, only to volunteer for the Galician Front the following year. Another of Hodges's Russian acquaintances told of a dramatic accident, in which a motor car carrying a group of nurses had toppled off a mountain road over a cliff, killing one nurse instantly and wounding others. Hodges's acquaintance had sustained a mild head injury, but believed that her life had been saved by two heavy, thick braids of hair, wound around her head, which had cushioned her fall from the vehicle.[54]

## Conclusion

On the Eastern and Serbian Fronts, the First World War was a mobile conflict, requiring a highly-responsive medical and nursing service. In Russia, nurses served in 'letuchka' or flying columns, where they packed their patients' wounds with salt or iodoform and wrapped them tightly in bandages before placing them on ambulance trains bound for base hospitals in major cities. On their arrival, other nurses literally tore these dressings away, exposing newly raw wounds that were surgically treated and carefully monitored. At the Anglo-Russian Hospital in Petrograd, an international unit of nurses offered care to such patients. British and Dominion nurses, such as Dorothy Cotton, commented on the differences between Russian and British nursing practices. Whilst the former were scrupulously aseptic, the latter appeared to them to encompass a more patient-centred approach, and could, perhaps, be seen as less technical and more artistic. British and Dominion nurses also commented on how their lives and those of their Russian colleagues seemed to be imbued by an emotional and spiritual intensity, which allowed their experiences to take on a quality of epic romance.

In Serbia, the squalor of caring for typhus patients in ill-equipped and crowded hospitals soon gave way to a more immediate threat, as the German and Bulgarian armies advanced, forcing hospital units to join crowds of civilians fleeing for their lives. A highly ingenious, and often unconsciously propagandist, press celebrated their trials, transforming them into 'heroic exploits'—a tendency that was often encouraged by the nurses themselves.

# 4

# The Eastern Mediterranean and Beyond

## April 1915–December 1917

### Introduction: the wounded of Gallipoli

The ill-fated Gallipoli campaign, which lasted from late April to December 1915 and took the lives of so many Allied troops, was planned as part of a strategy for breaking the deadlock on the Western Front. Devised by Winston Churchill—at that time First Lord of the Admiralty—it involved the capture of Constantinople by a fleet of warships, which would open up the Eastern Front to Allied troops and cut off supplies to the Central Powers.[1] Fighting in France and Belgium had stagnated to the point at which two deeply entrenched armies stared at each other across the lethal territory of 'no-man's-land'. Any attempt to break the deadlock—and most of those attempts came from the Allied side—resulted in tens of thousands of deaths in exchange for a few yards of devastated territory. It could not have been foreseen that the campaign in the Dardanelles would turn out to be just one more such costly, destructive—and ultimately worthless—attempt at 'breakthrough'.

Following the failure of an initial naval campaign, the Mediterranean Expeditionary Force was sent from Egypt to the Gallipoli peninsula. Hundreds of thousands of troops, many of them members of the legendary Australian and New Zealand Army Corps

(ANZAC) brigades, were cut down by machine-gun barrage and shellfire on the steep and craggy slopes above Anzac Cove and Cape Hellas, in territory where no casualty clearing station could be safely established. Many of the most severe injuries were incurred in the first nine days after the landings. Following hasty first-aid treatment at brigade posts on the beaches, patients were loaded into 'lighters': shallow barges which conveyed them to waiting hospital ships for transport to Egypt. For much of the campaign, these so-called 'hospital ships' were really only converted transport vessels, which quickly became crowded with casualties. Once in Egypt, the sick and wounded were transferred to base hospitals, which were obliged to expand rapidly as they became overwhelmed with casualties. As on the Western Front, the 'rushes' of casualties spread outwards from the Gallipoli peninsula like ripples on a pond.

In 1919, Elizabeth Oram, Matron-in-Chief of the Egyptian Expeditionary Force,[2] wrote of the difficulties she had encountered in working to put together a nursing service to care for the wounded. Because both politicians and military commanders had expected Allied military action in the Dardanelles to be short and decisive, detailed plans for a lengthy campaign had not been drawn up; nor had arrangements for the care of the hundreds of thousands of wounded who streamed from the Gallipoli peninsula for eight months from the end of April to mid-December 1915. Medical historian Mark Harrison has commented that the Gallipoli campaign, along with those in Salonika, East Africa, and Mesopotamia, 'produced medical catastrophes reminiscent of those in South Africa and the Crimea'.[3] A failure to involve medical officers in military planning, coupled with inadequate transport services, meant that many died simply because they could not be evacuated quickly enough.[4]

Matron-in-Chief Oram arrived in Port Said on 10 May, two weeks after the first landings at Cape Hellas and Anzac Cove, to find that 'a handful of nurses' were coping with tens of thousands of casualties, with the help of only a few local trained nurses and several willing volunteers.[5] Over 16,000 had been distributed among several makeshift hospitals within ten days of the first land-ings. Reinforcements were hastily requested to staff not only the military hospitals in Egypt but also the ships and trains that formed the evacuation line from the distant Turkish peninsula. At the end of July, it was possible to despatch some nurses to Mudros Bay on the Island of Lemnos, and from September, five months into the campaign, a number of fully equipped hospital ships began to ar-rive to supplement the few provided in April.[6] In the high summer, however, the numbers of casualties once again began to mount, during the devastating 'Battle of Sari Bair' (6–21 August). In the winter, new problems emerged: the cold and unhygienic conditions in the trenches gave rise to epidemics of typhus fever and huge numbers of cases of frostbite and trench foot. Troops were success-fully evacuated from Anzac Cove, Suvla Bay, and Cape Hellas during December 1915 and January 1916, but, by its conclusion, the Gallipoli campaign had claimed about 44,000 Allied lives, among a total casualty list of approximately 141,000.[7]

## ANZAC nurses in Egypt

If the nurses of the First World War were engaged in a multi-layered battle, one of its most significant layers was the fight for political and professional recognition. Nurses, as professional women, had, since the late nineteenth century, been involved in two significant campaigns: for professional recognition through state registration, and for political rights through female suffrage. Remarkably, New Zealand nurses had already won both battles. In 1893, New Zea-land women had secured the right to vote, and a professional register for nurses had passed into law in 1901. Australian nurses were campaigning vigorously for their own register through their influential professional bodies, the Australian Trained Nurses' Asso-ciation and the Victorian Trained Nurses' Association.[8] And yet the wartime service of 'ANZAC' nurses was fraught with the difficulties that came with female work in a military environment. The structural weaknesses of their nascent military nursing services left them vulnerable to exploitation, neglect, and abuse. Australian and New Zealand military nurses appear to have experienced the consequences of these weaknesses more acutely than their counterparts from other countries.

Unlike Britain or the USA, neither Australia nor New Zealand had a formal military nursing service prior to the First World War, although both had military nursing 'Reserves'. The war proved to be a catalyst for the rapid growth of the Army Nursing Services in both Dominions, but these were assembled somewhat hastily, and without close attention to issues of status, pay, and conditions of service. Their somewhat 'informal' status was to lead to difficulties, when both Australian and New Zealand—but particularly New Zealand—nurses were exposed to poor working conditions and harassment by a small minority of medical officers.[9]

The first seven Australian nurses to serve overseas joined the SS *Grantala*, bound for Rabaul, part of German New Guinea on 13 September 1914. Their stay was short-lived, as the Germans surrendered the island shortly after their arrival. In November twenty-five nurses sailed for Egypt with the first convoy of the Australian Imperial Force, with Ellen (Nellie) Gould as their principal matron. Gould had been born in Exeter, England, spent much of her childhood in Portugal, and then, after working as a governess for several years in Germany, emigrated to Australia, where she trained as a nurse at the Prince Alfred Hospital in Sydney. After nursing British troops during the Second Anglo-Boer War, she had returned to Australia to found a private hospital, but had remained active in the development of military nursing, helping to establish the New South Wales Army Nursing Reserve. This first small group of nurses to arrive in Egypt began by assisting British nurses already stationed there, but went on to form the core nursing staffs of the first two Australian General Hospitals (AGHs). Gould was appointed matron to No. 2 AGH.[10] A second and much larger group of 161 Australian nurses left Australia in December on the SS *Kyarra*.

Australian nurses found themselves assigned to some of the most unusual military hospitals of the First World War. The Heliopolis House Hotel was chosen as the home of No. 1 AGH. A building of great grandeur and beauty, situated on the edge of Cairo, the hotel proved a difficult place to work. Patients were housed in small rooms on many floors, requiring nurses to run up and down marble staircases several times a day. The building lacked the waste-disposal facilities required by a hospital and the difficulties and hazards presented by heat, dust, and thousands of flies caused great anxieties for the nurses, one of whose primary duties was to protect their patients from infection and other environmental hazards. Soon after the arrival of No. 1 AGH there was an increase in the level of sickness among troops stationed in the Egyptian base and the hospital became severely overcrowded. The nurses staffing No. 1 AGH appear to have coped with the workload by viewing themselves as 'pioneers', breaking new ground and forging a path for the future development of the military nursing service.[11]

In order to alleviate some of these problems, No. 1 AGH took over a nearby fairground, Luna Park, on 6 April 1915, just weeks before the first landings on the Gallipoli peninsula. In a somewhat bizarre melding of a surreal environment with a horrific wartime reality, hospital personnel transformed the Park's ticket office into an operating theatre and its skating rink, bandstand, scenic railway, laughter and skeleton houses into hospital wards (see Figure 15).[12] The premises were highly unsuitable for the care of patients, who were crowded into its spaces on uncomfortable wicker beds.[13]

Several of the first Australian nurses to arrive in December 1914 had joined a skeleton staff of British nurses in another converted luxury hotel: Mena House, a former royal hunting lodge. No. 2 AGH was established here in January 1915. After the Gallipoli landing, its staff were given twenty-four hours' notice to prepare 1,500 beds, and the hospital was obliged to find additional premises—taking over the Ghezireh Palace Hotel, a building of great splendour on an island in the River Nile.[14] At Mena House, Sister

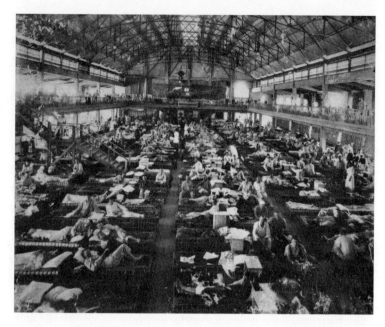

FIGURE 15 Heliopolis, Egypt, 1915. The interior of No. 1 Australian Auxiliary Hospital, formerly the Luna Park Skating Rink. Casualties from Gallipoli occupy beds of palm-wood, known as angeribs (photograph reproduced by permission of the Australian War Memorial, Canberra, Australia)

Nellie Morrice was ordered to prepare for large numbers of surgical cases just after the first Gallipoli landings. She found it almost impossible to obtain sterile dressings, having been told to apply to the matron at 8 p.m. (the wounded arrived at 6 p.m.). Eventually, she was able to obtain a large supply from the theatre sister. Nurses had to use their own personal supplies of surgical instruments, and there were insufficient pyjamas for the patients, who had to be put into thick grey flannel shirts. The sisters' living conditions were also 'rough', with cracked mugs and tin plates in their mess. When they complained, they were told it was 'active service' and they must 'put up' with the conditions.[15]

The operation of Nos. 1 and 2 AGHs expanded dramatically during the spring and early summer of 1915, as casualties from

Gallipoli exceeded all expectations. No. 1 AGH took over a casino, an atelier, and the sporting club pavilion in Heliopolis, along with part of the Abassia barracks. It also established an infectious diseases hospital at Choubra and a convalescent hospital at the Grand Hotel, Helouan. No. 2 AGH was working with a ratio of one nursing sister (assisted by orderlies) to 150 patients. Matron Nellie Gould commented that they 'succeeded where one could not have blamed them had they failed'. 'Local ladies' also assisted the work of the nurses, by preparing invalid foods and feeding helpless patients. Gould herself spent from 8 a.m. to 2 p.m. at Mena House and from 2 p.m. to 8 p.m. at Ghezireh Palace, super-vising the work of each institution in turn, before relinquishing control to two of her most senior sisters.[16]

Some Australian nurses were detailed to work with the British nursing services; none were happy with this arrangement, which meant that they had to accept the lower pay given to British nurses, and were less likely to nurse Australian patients. Eveline Vickers-Foote commented on her disappointment and resentment on finding that, although enlisting with the Australian Army Nursing Service, she had been made a part of the QAIMNS at the level of a staff nurse. She did, however, have great respect for the Matron-in-Chief, Miss Oram:

> She used to visit the hospitals and I liked her very much. I think she was the most impartial person I have ever met. The Australians were welcomed, and we all liked very much being with the British. The feeling was delightful towards us. The English girls could not do enough for us…They were told by the Matron, 'These Australians have come many thousands of miles from home, make them at home with you'.[17]

At the outbreak of war the New Zealand Army Nursing Service (NZANS) consisted of only one member of staff: the Matron-in-Chief, Hester Maclean, who was also president of the New Zea-land Trained Nurses Association and editor of the journal *Kai*

*Tiaki*. It was developed into a full service only with great difficulty and in the face of opposition from senior military medical figures, who were clearly opposed to the idea of women working close to the front lines in wartime.[18] But the precedents for a national nursing response to the First World War were multiplying. The British Queen Alexandra's Imperial Military Nursing Service had responded immediately to the outbreak of war and New Zealand's close neighbour Australia had sent nurses on active service to Egypt at the end of 1914. In January 1915 permission was granted for the recruitment of nurses to the NZANS, and the first fifty embarked for Egypt on the *Rotorua*, on 8 April 1915.[19] Unfortunately, Hester Maclean, probably feeling that the battle for a military nursing service had been won, did not argue for officer status for her nurses, and agreed that they might travel 'second class', even though medical officers typically travelled 'first class'. This led to a difficult voyage in airless lower-deck cabins, and snobbery from medical staff. In October 1915, Maclean wrote to General Henderson, Director General of the New Zealand Army Medical Services, requesting permission for nurses to wear badges of rank; this was not forthcoming, and it was only in 1941 that New Zealand's military nurses attained officer status.[20] These first contingents of nurses worked in British military hospitals throughout the Gallipoli campaign.[21] Rona Commons was placed in the Citadel Hospital, Cairo, and wrote home enthusiastically of how she had never thought she would live in 'such a magnificent palace'. She was later moved to the Heliopolis House Hotel, which she described—along with other Australian General Hospital sites—as 'simply Colonies from the Antipodes'.[22] Although they had a remarkable grandeur, the base hospitals in Egypt were far from healthy environments. In one of her letters home, Commons wrote:

> Did I tell you Sister Wilkie is off duty with dysentery? Sister Low is the same now; Sister Harris (Christchurch) has been off for a couple of days but is better now. Really I do think I am fortunate to keep so

well. Up at the Citadel some of the girls had most frightfully swollen legs from mosquito bites, and their faces bitten too, whereas I have hardly had anything worth calling a bite.[23]

In August 1915 a new series of assaults was launched against the Turks on the Gallipoli peninsula. Fanny Speedy, a sister with the New Zealand Army Nursing Service, believed that, had more staff been available, fewer lives would have been lost:

> Quite early in August convoys of wounded started coming in, such very ill cases too with dreadful wounds, some quite hopeless from the first; throughout the month, the Hospital, like all other hospitals, seemed unable almost to cope with the work, though each one did his level best, but we were still short-handed; this as one can imagine was remedied when the hardest of the work was over, one only regrets it because possibly one or two lives might have been saved, it is very hard to say, at least the sick and suffering might have had more attention.[24]

In addition to a shortage of trained staff, Australian and New Zealand nurses found themselves working with large numbers of orderlies, upon whom they relied to help with much of the time-consuming, 'caring' work of washing, feeding, and toileting patients. Many of these were drawn from the local Egyptian population and had no training at all, apart from what could be offered 'on the job' by nurses. Louisa Higginson, a New Zealand nurse based in a Red Cross hospital in Egypt, commented that the difficulties posed by working with untrained 'native' orderlies who could understand no English made her want to 'run away'.[25]

## Nursing on Lemnos

The experiences of nurses serving with No. 3 AGH were even more trying and extraordinary than those of nurses belonging to Nos. 1 and 2. Having left Sydney on the SS *Mooltan* in May 1915, they reached Britain in June and then travelled to Lemnos, an island in the northern Aegean Sea, within relatively easy reach of Gallipoli.

Hospitals were established on Lemnos in order to avoid the long sea voyage to Egypt, allowing casualties to reach a stable environment more quickly and with less risk. Alongside No. 3 AGH were Nos. 15, 16, and 18 British Stationary Hospitals, and No. 27 British General Hospital.[26]

Unfortunately, Lemnos was not only a hostile and inhospitable environment; its administration as a military base exhibited all of the worst features of the badly-handled Gallipoli campaign. Understaffed, and very poorly supplied with food and fresh water, No. 3 AGH in Mudros Bay was a challenging place in which to nurse the desperately sick and wounded men returning from the peninsula. Australian nurses arrived there in August 1915, and had to wait two weeks for equipment and supplies. Fortunately, most nurses travelled with their own equipment and were thus able to perform their work effectively.[27] Sister M. E. Webster, serving with the British nursing services on the hospital ship *Gloucester Castle* commented that, although from a distance Lemnos appeared to be a beautiful island 'of green hills, with bare stony summits and quaint windmills', in reality the area around Mudros Bay was 'a wilderness of drought', where human existence was poisoned by dust and flies, which contaminated food and water, infested wounds, and made sleep 'impossible'.[28] Sister I. Lovell commented on how, on first arriving at Lemnos, the nurses of No. 3 AGH had nursed patients under makeshift awnings, cutting up their own underwear to make bandages. 'Our lavatory and bathroom were the sea', she commented, adding that their food consisted of 'bully beef and biscuits'.[29] After three weeks, bores were sunk and fresh water was obtained for the first time; and, at about the same time, marquees and equipment for the hospital arrived.

No. 3 AGH cared for both sick and wounded. By the end of the summer, the sick came to far outnumber the injured, as typhoid and dysentery became prevalent among the overcrowded and malnourished troops pinned down in their shallow trenches on the peninsula. As winter set in, gastrointestinal diseases gave way to the problems of exposure, as the sub-zero temperatures and blizzard conditions attacked the emaciated bodies of malnourished troops whose winter uniforms failed to arrive before the first snows. Trench foot was rife, and nurses observed that the patients arriving at the Lemnos hospitals were dreadfully weak and emaciated. Lemnos itself could not offer much better weather conditions, and nurses worked hard to provide warmth and comfort for their patients in tented hospitals on the bleak hillsides above Mudros Bay, putting them into beds warmed with hot water bottles under multiple layers of blankets.

Soon large numbers of the nursing and medical staff of No. 3 AGH themselves became ill as a result of the inadequate shelter provided by their tents (which frequently blew down); malnutrition; and the hygiene problems associated with their very meagre water supplies (see Figure 16). Nurses spent their own money on visits to the hot springs at Therma, for baths, and it was reported that far fewer nurses than medical officers became sick.[30]

Working and living conditions for the nurses at No. 3 AGH were made even worse by a chauvinistic and harsh medical director, Colonel Fiaschi, who encouraged his medical officers to ignore the nurses' claims to seniority over orderlies in the care of patients. He was also slow to respond to their requests for equipment and supplies. Such deliberate obstruction from the officer-in-charge of the hospital could make life very difficult for nurses, who had no formal rank of seniority over orderlies, but were accustomed to 'taking charge' in their own wards. Indeed, many Australian nurses had spent much of their voyages out to the Eastern Mediterranean training orderlies in correct nursing practice, and were accustomed to being viewed as both the experts and the supervisors of such practice. Fiaschi appears to have deliberately undermined their authority. Fortunately, Grace Wilson proved an excellent leader and was very popular amongst her nursing staff. It was later acknowledged that she had performed an impressive feat in holding a nursing service together in trying circumstances. Wilson was,

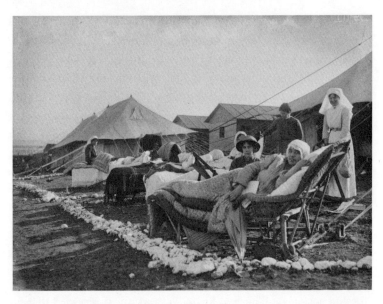

FIGURE 16 Sick sisters of the Australian Army Nursing Service convalescing in the tent lines of No. 3 Australian General Hospital, West Mudros (photograph reproduced by permission of the Australian War Memorial, Canberra, Australia)

perhaps, one of the most successful military matrons of the First World War. The way in which she overcame the problems associated with the almost impossible working conditions on Lemnos, and the obstruction of her work by a senior professional colleague, stands as an example of the resoluteness with which some senior nurses fought the battle for professional recognition alongside the struggle to save the lives of their compatriots. She was made temporary Matron-in-Chief of the AANS in September 1917, was twice mentioned in despatches, and was later to receive the Royal Red Cross (First Class) and the Order of the British Empire (Third Class). Wilson and her staff withstood enormous personal and professional pressures on Lemnos.[31] In January 1916, the last patients left the island and the hospital was packed up. Following a wait of more than twenty-four hours for their transport vessel—much of it spent on a cold rainswept pier—the nurses of No. 3 AGH left Lemnos for Egypt on 14 January 1916.

Winifred Lea, a trained British nurse based on Lemnos with No. 18 Stationary Hospital, commented in a letter to her father on hearing that the Gallipoli campaign was over: 'a nice old hash it has been—with a grand "halo" round it all the same—there must be a curious sort of atmosphere round certain parts of the Peninsular [*sic*] for those who could feel it—intense suffering—and Hell—and such courage and bravery as never was'.[32]

## Hospital ships in the Eastern Mediterranean

When planning for the Gallipoli campaign, General Sir Ian Hamilton had allowed for 11,000 casualties. At first, only three hospital ships and seven transport vessels were supplied for the evacuation of sick and wounded men from the peninsula.[33] Military commanders had assumed that the Allied forces would be able to push inland, and could then be supported by stationary hospitals; but Allied troops never made it beyond tiny beachheads, where their makeshift medical aid posts were pounded by artillery. Casualties were loaded into large flat-bottomed vessels known as 'lighters', and taken, still under fire, to hospital ships where they were winched to safety. Many were desperately ill, due to unsanitary conditions and lack of water on the beachheads. The earliest transport vessels were overcrowded, and medical orderlies struggled to provide the conditions of cleanliness and comfort that would allow their patients to recover. By the time the decision was taken to appoint female nursing staff to all vessels transporting wounded from Gallipoli, the medical services were in a state of crisis.[34] It is highly likely that the work undertaken by the earliest nurses on board hospital ships improved patients' chances of survival. Not only did nurses provide expert assistance to surgeons operating on urgent cases, and implement life-saving technical treatments, they also offered fundamental nursing care, washing, feeding, and hydrating men who were often louse-infested and weak from malnutrition and dehydration.

Sister M. E. Webster, nursing onboard the British hospital ship *Gloucester Castle*, wrote in her diary for the first week in August 1915:

> We are about a mile out from the shore at Gaba Tepe—now known as Anzac beach, in honour of the Australian and New Zealand Army Corps. There is only one narrow strip of beach, backed by bold red-coloured bluffs, deeply scarred and furrowed in their formation, and reaching a height of nearly 1000ft.... In the early morning and at sundown, this strange forbidding coast takes on a beauty of its own. The gullies are deeply blue and sea and sky glow with wonderful tints. Then, as darkness falls, lights spring out up and down the hill-side, like busy fireflies. The insistent tapping of machine guns destroys the silence of the night and the sharp reports of the snipers...sometimes we find stray bullets embedded in the wood-work on board.[35]

Nurses on board hospital ships in Gallipoli Bay probably came closer to the fighting than any other female participants in the First World War. But they had little time for passive watching. When they received patients, their first tasks were to overcome the damage that had been done, not just by exposure to combat, but also by the appalling conditions in which combatants had been forced to live. British nurse Mary Ann Brown recounted one journey on the *Devanha*, during which she was nursing men who were injured, ill, 'broken down', and exhausted. She described how ninety-five men were disembarked: 'They look the better for the rest they had here. One poor man said they would all be better dead than living the life they lived in the trenches.'[36]

Members of the New Zealand Army Nursing Service served on two hospital ships: the *Maheno*, which left Wellington in July 1915, and the *Marama*, which sailed in December of the same year.[37] New Zealand nurse Charlotte Le Gallais was on board the *Maheno*, which took wounded from Gallipoli to Lemnos and Alexandria. She described in her letters home how the ship would anchor about half a mile from the firing line, 'guns going off all around us, shaking the ship and startling the life out of me each time they begin'. She added: 'It's a dreadful place, Gallipoli. Dreadful and awful.'[38] She added that, for nurses, hospital ships were the most difficult postings. They received the wounded with the mud, 'flies and creepers' of the peninsula still on their bodies and uniforms. The work of 'cleaning them up', feeding and hydrating them was undertaken alongside the more technical work of treating shock and dressing complex wounds. In mid-September, she wrote: 'To my dying day I will never forget this last six weeks...It is much harder than I ever thought it could be.' On the first day at Gallipoli, the ship had begun taking on wounded at 4 p.m., and had continued through the night. The nurses continued caring for their patients throughout the next day, and then got two hours' rest before 'unloading' them at Lemnos. After this, the work of cleaning up the ship 'for the next lot' commenced. That night, she got to bed at midnight, but she was able to take a rest the next day, while the ship was returning to the peninsula. This pattern repeated multiple times, until she felt as thought she could 'sleep for a week'. She was suffering from the 'fleas and crawlers', observing that she was unable to stop scratching her skin which was 'nearly raw'.[39]

Eveline Vickers-Foote was assigned to the hospital ship *Assaye*, taking wounded from Gallipoli to Lemnos and Alexandria. Lighters transferring wounded men from shore to ship were shelled, killing some of the wounded. The ship itself was also shelled as it attempted to transfer lightly-wounded onto another vessel. Vickers-Foote commented: 'I do really think the Turks could have hit us if they liked, but it seemed as if they wanted to warn us to behave as a Hospital Ship.'[40] One of her worst wartime experiences was of overcrowding on the earliest voyages from Suvla Bay. Most of her patients had both wounds and dysentery. On 9 August, the ship—which had only six nurses—took on over 800 wounded men. Although the orderlies were 'pretty good', they had neither the skill nor the knowledge to care for badly-shocked and wounded patients with concurrent infections. Vickers-Foote and her colleagues experienced 'great anxiety' at the risks that were taken on those early voyages. Many of their patients were lying on deck, where 'they died like flies'. Her opinion of the medical officers was not good; she considered the officer-in-command 'about the weakest thing I have run across in the way of men'.[41]

Six members of No. 3 AGH had been given ten minutes' notice to join a French hospital ship, the *Formosa*, on their arrival into Mudros harbour in August 1915. Like Vickers-Foote, they received some of the first wounded from Suvla Bay. Sister I. Lovell commented on what 'terrible wounds they were—the majority of them were ten days old, flyblown and septic'.[42] The surgical team worked throughout the journey to Lemnos, amputating limbs that might have been saved had the patients only been embarked sooner. The ship made three journeys in three days from Suvla to Lemnos, delivering its patient-loads to No. 3 AGH. The following year, the *Formosa* was still plying Mediterranean waters, this time taking wounded and sick soldiers from Salonika to Malta and Egypt. Winifred Lea, who had been with No. 18 British Stationary Hospital on Lemnos, was transferred to the ship in the spring of 1916. She had heard that her mother had died, and was anxious to return home, but the War Office had refused to accept her resignation. Her transfer to the *Formosa* had been made in the hope that the ship would sail for England, but its orders were cancelled and Lea—who was not a good sailor—spent months sailing the Mediterranean, nursing in hot stuffy wards, suffering bouts of seasickness. Eventually the ship's matron arranged an exchange, and Lea was able to disembark at Malta—still a long way from home. This was where her letters ended, and it is not known how or when she reached home.[43]

On 24 November 1915, Sister Jentie Paterson of the QAIMNSR reported for duty at the busy East India Dock in London.[44] She was to serve on the SS *Braemar Castle*, a 'fine ship' fitted with beds for 300 patients, and with 'beautiful cabins' for the nursing staff.

Paterson's journey to the Mediterranean offered rest and tranquillity after her trying time earlier that year in an understaffed base hospital at Le Tréport. On 1 December, she saw the Sierra Nevada, 'towering into the snow line and tipped pink by the rising sun', and over the next two days, she revelled in the sight of Algiers and Tunis.[45]

On Tuesday 7 December, Paterson got up at 6 o'clock and went up on deck. She could see nothing but the 'bleak, dark and v cold' Mediterranean. At 8 o'clock the *Braemar Castle* entered the gulf of Salonika, and, as the sun rose, she enjoyed her first view of the old walled city, which sloped up the hill behind the harbour, its mosques and monuments standing high above its other buildings. The hills behind it were alternately white with tents and grey with huts. 'Truly the army have encamped', she exclaimed.

Three days later, Paterson was granted shore leave and began to explore the 'medley of East and West' that was the city of Salonika. Her diary is full of descriptions of 'Greek soldiers...Eastern veiled women...Men who outheralded [*sic*] any villain...Villanous looking faces with long knives stuck in their belts.'[46] It is also full of gossip, telling, for example, the story of two British privates imprisoned for brawling in the street with a Greek officer. The nationalistic—even jingoistic—quality of the writings is unmistakable. Both Paterson's patriotism and her prejudice resonate through the pages of her diary.

The *Braemar Castle* was taking on wounded from the failed Allied campaign in Serbia. The joint forces of Germany and Bulgaria had pushed the Allies south and west, and were forcing the Serbian army into its perilous retreat over the Albanian Alps. British forces were pushed back to Salonika, where wounded were treated in base hospitals, or embarked on hospital ships and taken to Egypt or Malta. The mountainous terrain of the Balkans, along with the mobile nature of warfare on the Serbian Front, meant that it was impossible to establish effective evacuation lines. Casualties arrived at the base filthy, malnourished, dehydrated, often with infectious diseases such as malaria and enteric fever, and with only a first field dressing covering their wounds. Nurses such as Paterson were often the first to hear their stories of defeat and suffering, and Paterson's diary stands as a remarkable record of their experiences. On 10 December, after a visit to the triumphal arch of Alexander, on which were 'wonderful carvings like the Egyptian stuff in Br. Museum', she helped load 100 patients. They were brought to the ship in three huge lighters drawn by a single tug. Down the centre of each of the wide, shallow boats were two rows of stretchers, and seated around them were less severely wounded men. A large wooden cage was lowered from the ship and the wounded were lifted into it before being hoisted onto the ship and directly down an opening in the deck to the wards in the hold. The process, which was highly efficient, was used to load wounded onto hospital ships throughout the Mediterranean. Paterson commented on her 'load' of wounded:

> I took on 10 officers filthy with mud some with lice. Men downstairs are alive. Frostbites, some awful ones. Private will lose 2 feet. Cold had been awful. They say we have lost 2000 frozen to death. One private was found frozen dead leaning on his rifle! One officer sadly told me the British line was broken we could do nothing sister against thousands on half rations!!! Terrible! I have one Capt with Enteric bad. 3 bad malarial fevers. 2 bad feet frost bitten. 1 gunshot thigh. 1 nerves, complete wreck... Hear more tomorrow. Got off duty 10.30 all comf asleep.[47]

Paterson did indeed 'hear more' the next day, when her patients were 'so much better'. One showed her a map of Serbia and Bulgaria, which had been made in Germany. The men had extraordinary stories to tell: of how 8,000 Allies were pitted against 15,000 enemy troops; men were surviving on a quarter of the normal rations; one small platoon was holding 26 miles of high mountain territory, and many fell to their deaths; and 500 men were frozen to death. Actual figures for amounts of supplies and death rates varied from one day to the next, but all were agreed that the campaign had been appalling. Paterson's recounting of the personal testimonies of her soldier-patients in her tiny pocket diary has an extraordinary—raw, yet almost unreal—quality. Part brisk relation of fact, part awe-struck recounting of an epic tale, her narratives are, perhaps, one way in which the reality of a generation passes into the legend of its time.

The next day, Paterson was getting down to the business of healing her patient's wounds. Some of her frostbite patients were experiencing intense pain. One man's toes had fallen off into his first dressing. Limbs were massaged, and patients were lifted onto the sunlit deck. Unfortunately, within three days, the weather had undergone a dramatic change and the ship had begun to 'roll and pitch most awfully'. Paterson's ward work was interrupted by frequent bouts of vomiting and she confided to her diary that she 'really felt I was doing something for my country this time'. As the storm passed, the ship was soon enjoying 'calm sailing all among the Grecian Isles again', but now there were mosquitoes in the cabins, and Paterson was finding lice among her clothes. As the *Braemar Castle* approached Valletta, Paterson exclaimed: 'I've got a *most* delightful set of officers. My typhoid is doing awfully well. So is Letchworth with shrapnel in his lung. Will get him up on deck tomorrow he was dying when he came on board.'[48]

In Valletta the wounded were unloaded and that evening Paterson was able to find time to explore the remarkable hospital of the Knights of St John, with its quarter-mile-long ward; and to stand in the Barracca Gardens looking at the 'twinkling' lights of military hospitals 'as far as the eye could reach'. On 21 December, she received a message to say that her patient, Letchworth, was dying, and resolved to find him. She was relieved to discover that the report which had reached her had been exaggerated. Letchworth was, in fact, much better, but all of her former patients were asking to be taken back onto the boat. Paterson's mood was undoubtedly lifted by her patients' obvious attachment to her; as she walked back to the harbour, she found that a 'glorious moon' was lighting up the island of Malta.

In November 1916 the *Braemar Castle* was torpedoed and sunk in the Aegean Sea. Paterson was, by this time safe at home in Glasgow, but the news of the destruction of her former home and workplace does not appear to have escaped her. A carefully excised piece from the *Daily Sketch*, containing a photograph of 'the brave nurses who faced death with a discipline worthy of our bravest fighting men' has found its way into her file at the Imperial War Museum, London.[49] In the margin, someone has drawn three exclamation marks.

Like Jentie Paterson on board the *Braemar Castle*, Mary Ann Brown used fresh air when she could, to help heal wounds. She reported how, having left Lemnos at 6.30 p.m. on 22 June, the hospital ship *Devanha* was soon 'passing quite near lots of peaceful looking islands', and that the patients were 'enjoying the nice breeze'.[50]

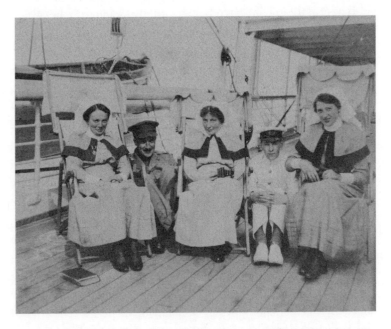

FIGURE 17 Nurses on board the hospital ship *Dongola* (photograph reproduced by kind permission of the Wellcome Library, London, UK)

Patients on board the *Kanowna*, being moved from Suez to Australia, do not appear to have experienced many 'nice breezes'. Sister Ruth Taylor commented in her 'narrative' that the heat on board was 'very trying'. Many patients were very seriously wounded and had to be nursed below decks where there was 'very little air', a shortage of electric fans, and an inadequate supply of ice.[51] Eleanor Jeffries was also having a very difficult time on board the hospital ship *Dunluce Castle*, taking Serbian soldiers on a four-day voyage from Valona to Tunis. The patients were suffering from a mysterious form of relapsing fever which, the medical officers concluded, must have been typhus. Forty died on the voyage, and Jeffries commented that she had never nursed such seriously ill men in her life. After 'unloading' them, the ship was quarantined for four days. Soon after this, it took 700 convalescent patients to Southampton, where Jeffries was forced to report sick and spend ten days in hospital.[52]

Barbara Mildred Tilly wrote to her mother from the *Marama*, on 29 January 1916, of how her ship was carrying some of the last troops to be evacuated from the Gallipoli peninsula. Her view of the English wounded on board was somewhat pitying: 'The English men are nothing in comparison with our NZ and Australian boys. They are such a weakly looking unkempt dirty toothed lot and yet one cannot help but feel sorry for the poor fellows. Some are eyeless, some legless and others have most ghastly wounds. The condition of the frost bite ones is also appalling.'[53]

**Tragedy at sea: the sinking of the *Marquette***

One of the most tragic maritime disasters of the First World War was the torpedoing and sinking of the SS *Marquette* in the Aegean Sea on 23 October 1915. As a rule, the Allied military authorities only moved hospital personnel from base to base on carefully marked hospital ships. But on this occasion several nurses of No. 1 New Zealand Stationary Hospital were being transported from Alexandria to Salonika on board a troopship.[54]

A report, published in the New Zealand nursing journal *Kai Tiaki* and reprinted in the *British Journal of Nursing*, offered a heroic narrative of the courage and self-sacrifice of the nurses. The ship was reported to have sunk very rapidly—in less than fifteen minutes. The thirty-six nurses on board calmly presented themselves at muster stations, and boarded their lifeboats. It was then that their real problems began. Major Wylie, of the New Zealand Medical Corps, told, in his official report of how the lowering of the boats was 'bungled': 'on the port side one boat descended heavily on top of one already in the water, and thereby so seriously injured several of the nurses as to kill them outright, or...make their subsequent existence in the water impossible'. Meanwhile, on the starboard side, another boat 'assumed a perpendicular position and emptied [the nurses] into the water'. A third boat became waterlogged and sank. Wylie expressed his admiration for the bravery of the surviving nurses, who spent seven hours in the water, clinging to the ship's debris: 'At no time did I see any signs of panic or any signs of fear on the part of anyone, and I cannot find words adequately to express my appreciation of the magnificent way in which the nurses behaved not only in the vessel but afterwards in the water.'[55]

Almost seventy years after the sinking of the *Marquette*, one of the nurses who had been on board that day spoke to an interviewer of her ordeal. The ship had seemed to 'go down inside of 10 minutes' and Emily Hodges had found herself falling into the sea: 'I thought that was the end of all things. I couldn't believe it when I came to the surface and I was alive.'[56] But relief was to turn to pain and exhaustion, as the nurses were to spend many hours in the cold water waiting for rescue. Some would not survive.

One nurse described her experiences later to a *Kai Tiaki* correspondent: she was one of a dozen survivors who clung to a raft, which was occupied by three men. She watched as one after another of the survivors—many of them 'strong men'—died and sank into the water; some 'went raving mad'. Three of the nurses clinging to this raft died of hypothermia and exhaustion. One of these, Nona Hildyard, was said to have been 'merry and bright' singing 'Tipperary' and 'Are We Downhearted', before suffering heart failure and drowning.[57] One anonymous nurse told a *Marlborough Express* reporter of how some of the lifeboats had been both damaged and overcrowded. These continuously overturned, pitching their occupants into the water: 'We were swamped again and again until we were exhausted. It was pitiful to see nurses and soldiers tiring in frantic struggles, finally releasing their grasp on the gunwale, floating for a few seconds, and then slowly sinking without a murmur.'[58]

The destruction of the *Marquette*, like all such stories, became a rich source of myth and propaganda. It was reported in the international press that the heroic nurses had called to the crew of the French destroyer who rescued them: 'Take the fighting men first!' It seems that the story had emerged as a result of the concern of some nurses for one of their colleagues: they had been keeping an exhausted orderly afloat. The wave from the rescue ship pulled him out of their grip and one of them asked the sailors to 'pick up that man first'.[59] Other strange myths formed around the behaviour of the nurses. One survivor, Mabel Wright, wrote an indignant refutation of some of these. It was not true, she said, that nurses had stood on the deck of the *Marquette* and cheered as men escaped the wreck in lifeboats.[60] Nor was the claim of some medical officers that they remained on board until all the nurses were safely in the lifeboats. The reality of the behaviour of those on board the *Marquette* was—as might be expected—a mixture of self-sacrifice and self-interest. Some medical officers were reported to have helped nurses onto rafts of floating debris. Others focused only on their own survival. Some nurses were said to have missed their opportunity to get into a lifeboat because they were helping wounded orderlies and had jumped into the water just before the ship sank. Others found themselves able only to watch as their friends died before their eyes.

Ten nurses died. One of these, Margaret Rogers, had written to her family before boarding the *Marquette*: 'There is no romance about war. It spells suffering, hunger, filth. How thankful I am every day that I came to do what I could to help and relieve our brave boys.'[61] Rogers is commemorated, along with her two Christchurch Hospital colleagues Nona Hildyard and Lorna Rattray, at the Nurses' Memorial Chapel, a small building near to the hospital at which they trained, which was funded by public donations and opened in 1927.[62]

## Challenging scenarios: Palestine, East Africa, and Mesopotamia

Some nurses—many of them from Australia and New Zealand—who had cared for the wounded of the failed Gallipoli campaign remained in Egypt to nurse those injured during the Palestine campaign,[63] where the system of casualty evacuation which had evolved on the Western Front was used with some success. Long lines of evacuation back to Egyptian base hospitals required careful planning.[64] In 1917 several hospitals moved north and east through Palestine to El Arish, Gaza, and Belah. No. 36 Stationary Hospital had already moved from Suez to Mehemediah on the North Sinai coast. After the First and Second Battles of Gaza in the spring of that year, hospitals were said to be 'overflowing' with casualties.[65]

New Zealand nurse Winifred Spencer was moved 'up the line' from her posting in Egypt to join No. 24 Stationary Hospital, consisting of approximately 1,000 beds under canvas, where she spent the last two years of the war. Each time a convoy arrived, the hospital would receive almost 1,000 new cases to treat and these would be operated upon, stabilized, and then moved 'down the line' as rapidly as possible, to prepare for the next 1,000. The work was 'terrific'. She later commented that her feet had been 'ruined...from tramping through the sand'. The weather was 'blazing in the day' and 'freezing' at night.[66]

Some hospital units followed the successful Allied advance deep into Palestine, and after General Allenby's successful capture of Jerusalem in December 1917, nurses were sent there to establish a casualty clearing station (CCS) in a partly built Italian hospital. They were said to have had 'a heartbreaking time', as their CCS was so poorly equipped. At first, they had to nurse patients on stretchers or mattresses laid on the floor. It was only with the help of the British and Australian Red Cross Societies that they were able to properly equip the hospital and make their patients comfortable.[67]

Nos. 15 and 16 British Stationary Hospitals were moved directly from one highly challenging environment on Lemnos to another: German East Africa, where their staffs encountered the hazards of extreme heat and parasitic infections.[68] Malaria was a huge problem in East Africa. The two best-known measures for protecting troops against this debilitating and life-threatening disease were mosquito-eradication and quinine prophylaxis. Neither was implemented successfully, resulting in tens of thousands of patients arriving in stationary hospitals in desperately-ill and sometimes moribund states.[69]

In Mesopotamia, the Allied campaign was hampered by increasingly stretched supply lines, which extended from the Persian Gulf along a vulnerable route to Baghdad. Medical provision was inadequate: wounded and sick men, many suffering from diarrhoeal diseases such as dysentery, were being transported on the decks of crowded riverboats to the coast, with no facilities. It was said that the foul smell emanating from these vessels reached those standing on the riverbank some distance away. On reaching the coast, those who had survived the journey were embarked on hospital ships for India.[70]

Thousands of men died during the siege of Kut in April 1916. Some nurses were moved from Egypt to base hospitals in India, which took patients from Mesopotamia. Heat in these scenarios was often a serious problem. Sister A. J. Low, based in India, was nursing sick soldiers just arrived from Mesopotamia, including some who had just been through the siege of Kut. They were said to be in a 'very emaciated condition' and 'it was only after weeks of care and good nourishment that they were able to be sent by hospital ships to England'. The journey to base hospitals in India was itself 'trying': patients were taken from Baghdad to Basra by ambulance boat, then to Bombay by ship. The final leg of the journey by train to the large new 1,200-bedded base hospital in the hills at Poona, 'in terrific heat', meant that even with the best possible care on board, patients arrived debilitated and dehydrated.[71]

Following the appointment of a Central Sanitary Committee and a Medical Advisory Committee in the spring and early summer of 1916, evacuation lines in Mesopotamia were improved, and female nurses were appointed to both field hospitals and river steamers. Survival rates appear to have improved dramatically.[72] Nurses were asked to volunteer to travel 'up the line' to care for patients in these dangerous settings. In an oral history interview conducted almost seventy years after the end of the war Winifred Lemere-Goff spoke of a quest for adventure, which took her to Mesopotamia, where wards were all 'out in the open' and conditions 'a bit primitive', yet 'quite enjoyable'.[73] Although they were immunized against plague, nurses were not well protected against the vast range of diseases which could be contracted in Mesopotamia. Lemere-Goff herself was hospitalized with malaria and had to be invalided home to India.

Nursing in India could be fraught with social and professional as well as clinical challenges. Historian Ruth Rae has examined a particular incident at the 34th Welsh General Hospital at Deolali, in which a Turkish interpreter accused five Australian nurses of sexual impropriety with their patients. The accusation was taken seriously by the medical officer commanding the hospital, and it was some time before the nurses were cleared of any misconduct by the Director General of the Medical Services in Australia, Major General R. H. J. Fetherston.[74]

## Nursing at Salonika

In September 1915, an agreement between the Allied states and the Greek prime minister, Eleftherios Venizelos, permitted the landing of Allied troops at Salonika, where an extensive base was created to support troops joining the Serbian campaign. The entry of Bulgaria into the war, and a decision on the part of the Central Powers to focus their attention on crushing Serbia in the winter of 1915, meant that the Allies were pushed back to a narrow enclave around Salonika, where they remained pinned down for much of the remainder of the war. As troops from the failed Gallipoli campaign were sent to Salonika, hospital units accompanied them. Conditions around the city and in the valleys of the Struma and Vardar, where troops were encamped, were unhygienic, and the whole region was infested with mosquitoes. Despite efforts to eradicate these, and to protect troops with quinine prophylaxis, malaria became so rife that it came to be seen as an almost inevitable consequence of a posting in Salonika.[75]

Salonika was a difficult workplace. Winifred Seymour, a British VAD, commented in her diary on the feeling that her time was being wasted on mundane work. Still, she found her patients themselves a consolation. One in particular, Boyer Collin, who appears to have been suffering from some form of relapsing fever—probably typhus—entertained both staff and fellow patients: 'When his temperature is high he is tucked under the bedclothes—directly he is better he is keeping the whole ward in fits of laughter.'[76] Another VAD referred to Salonika as a 'wild, rough place'.[77] Most hospitals consisted of huge encampments with 'rows and rows of wooden huts, and a good number of tents', often with around 2,000 beds. Water was scarce and nurses had to apply for a weekly bath by adding their names to a list.[78] Some nurses enjoyed the experience of 'camp life'. Sister K. E. Maloney of the Australian Army Nursing Service found the life 'appealing', 'simply loved' her work, and enjoyed the picnics and concerts which were organized for convalescent patients.[79] British VAD Mary Rumney, in contrast, was depressed by the constant sight of 'flies in the tea' and 'terrible dried up meat'. She described how patients often suffered from so-called 'Balkan tap': 'a form of depression due to not knowing what was to happen, having no news of the war, and being very bored'.[80]

The greatest threat to the health of both patients and staff in Salonika was malaria. British nurse R. Osborne described the precautions that had to be taken by those on night duty during the malarial season: 'the nursing staff went on duty wearing mosquito veils over their hats, mosquito gloves and thick puttees. The difficulties of nursing with these additions to the uniform can better be imagined than described.'[81] Australian Nurse Wray described how 'practically everyone, including soldiers had malaria in Salonique. Even the children have large malarial spleens.'[82]

Staff Nurse C. E. Strom was posted to No. 66 British General Hospital in 1917. In her first letter home she described how 'the evenings and mornings are beautiful but the nights are surprisingly cold; at least so it seemed to us last night!' On the day of their arrival, she and her colleagues had been supplied with tents, mosquito nets with collapsible frames, collapsible lanterns, ground sheets, macintoshes, and candles. That night they slept on the ground inside their tents:

> each girl laid her stock of blankets on the top of her ground sheet, heaped everything else available on top, and crawled in amongst it all. At first thoughts one would say, 'And a very cosy bed too'! but alas, it was nothing of the sort. The ground of Greece is astonishingly hard and stony, there are prickles and knobbly bits of roots there are clumps of clay. One girl even included a tortoise as part of her share of the earth! And cold! It was freezing...I think tomorrow we shall hie us forth and make the beds, and reduce the chaos a trifle. There are patients arriving tomorrow; so they say.[83]

Strom had several days in which to put her ward—which consisted of two adjoining marquees—in order. Its furniture had a strangely lopsided look, as the floor consisted only of a tarpaulin and was nowhere flat. Between the marquees was a 'wonderful pantry' which her orderly had been able to stock with a wide variety of foodstuffs. Strom's orderly, in fact, proved to be a 'gem' with 'friends in high places – i.e. the cookhouse'. He seemed able to procure goods such as tins of cocoa and soup without the usual 'fussation' and Strom was careful never to ask how this was achieved.

Nurses on day duty at No. 66 British General Hospital woke at 5 a.m. and walked to the bathrooms. Breakfast was at 6.30 a.m. and ward duty began at 7 a.m. Half of the day staff worked until 7.30 p.m., with a rest period between 1.30 and 5 p.m.; the remainder worked through until 5 p.m. Dinner began at 7 p.m., and 'lights out' was at 9 p.m., which meant that nurses had very little time to themselves. Strom was hoping that once the hospital was settled, she and her fellow nurses would get one half-day's leave per week, and a full day once a month.[84]

In September, Strom was placed on night duty. The work was onerous, each nurse caring for the patients of five wards, each of which contained twenty-nine patients; she was assisted in each ward by only one orderly. The first part of the night was spent making patients comfortable for sleep, but the process of waking them again began early in the morning so that beds could be made and the wards would be 'shipshape' before the day staff arrived. For the rest of the night, her time was spent checking on her patients' conditions and supporting those who were ill or in pain. Although the work was hard and the hours were long, Strom appears to have enjoyed night duty. She viewed her patients as 'great kids—such boys most of them', enjoyed their banter, and appreciated the help the convalescent 'up-patients' gave her with her morning duties. She also found the night-time atmosphere of the hospital soothing:

> There is something wonderfully peaceful about the moonlit, sleeping camp, with its long lines of marquees. The very tents seem asleep.

I often stand and look at them—and wonder. Somehow over all of
them, on these moonlit nights, there seems to hang an atmosphere
of serene hopefulness, and quiet peace; it is the atmosphere of per-
petual benediction. Alas! That the daylight blinds the eye![85]

In November 1917, Strom was transferred to a dysentery hospital
on a site about 3 miles from Salonika with 'splendid' views of the
harbour, but in the midst of other hospitals, depots, and camps.
Inhabitants of the 'foggy, muddy, bedraggled' hospital were obliged
to 'slog about in the mud', and the nurses shortened their skirts to
just above their gumboots. The site was infested with flies and the
work was challenging; great care had to be taken over patients'
diets to ensure good nutrition without damaging the lining of the
gut. Fortunately, Strom's two orderlies were 'splendid chaps' who
soon had the ward cleared of mud, in good order, and well supplied, and her medical officer was a 'joy to work for'.

Strom remained in Salonika throughout the winter of 1917/18
and into the last summer of the war. She found it a 'miserable hole'—
full of mud and slush in winter, and even worse in summer, when
it was full of 'flies and dust, and mosquitoes, and heat and smells
ad nauseam'. As summer progressed the flies seemed to get 'dreadfuller and dreadfuller...Nowadays we wear panamas to, and on,
duty, except in the evenings. The sun is scorching and the winds so
dry and hot.'[86]

One of the most interesting observations in Strom's account of
her experience at Salonika relates to the position of Australian staff
nurses vis-à-vis their own more senior colleagues—the sisters of
the Australian Army Nursing Service, and the so-called British
'Imperials'. Strom felt that she and her fellow nurses were badly
misunderstood. In one of her letters she explains how much she
would have loved to have formed friendships with the British nurses
some of whom seemed 'bonza', but they did not understand her—
nor she them. Her relations with Australian charge-sisters were,
however, even more distressing, and she and her fellow staff nurses

formed a union to offer each other mutual support and ensure that the vote at mess meetings would not go against them. The invidious position of an Australian army staff nurse is illustrated in the following passage in one of Strom's letters, which is couched in carefully light and witty terms:

> If we talk to the heads but sparingly, and that when we are addressed, we are cool, over-independent, and even impudent, and courtesy costs nothing.
> If we are cheerfully conversational, we are out to get an RRC.
> If we spend money on the Tommies, we are fools; the boys don't appreciate it, and, after all, it's only bribery on our part. Perhaps we can't keep them in order without promise of reward.
> If we don't spend it, we are mean. Look at the poor old things, without a cigarette to smoke except the issue with no matches, with nothing to read, and nothing to write home on. And us will all our screw!! Well, Well.
> If we are friendly with our orderly, we are familiar and lacking in dignity, and should be suppressed.
> If we are addicted to the 'Orderly' habit, we are stuck up and regimental, and ought to be ashamed of ourselves.
> If we converse amicably with the MOs, we are flirtatious creatures, and old enough to know better.
> If we leave all the conversing for the other sister to do, we are unnecessarily aloof.
> If we laugh with our Tommies, we are forgetting the dignity of our position. If they joke with us, and talk to us of their homes, they have been encouraged to be friendly, and should be pushed back…into their places. If we scowl at them, and our wards are of an atmosphere of gloom and despair, we are forgetting our duty to the community. Have we not any interest in our patients?[87]

Strom remained in Salonika until the late summer of 1918. The Vardar winds were one of her greatest trials. When they were at their most 'ferocious' they caused a 'bellying of the tent walls', knocking over lockers and screens and causing electric lights to dance up and down'. They also terrified the shell-shocked patients. Even worse than the winds and mud, however, were the mosquitoes. By the summer of 1918, malaria had come to be viewed as an occupational hazard, and in August Strom herself contracted the disease, taking several weeks' sick leave before returning to duty on a night shift because she found it difficult to endure the heat of the sun.

## Conclusion

An 'ANZAC legend' has formed around the courage and endurance of those Australian and New Zealand soldiers who faced the guns of their enemies on the Gallipoli peninsula. Many died on the cliffs above Anzac Cove, or in hastily-erected aid posts on the beach. Huge numbers of casualties were loaded onto transport vessels for transfer to base hospitals in Egypt. Long before anyone at home knew of their suffering, nurses at the base were listening to their stories, healing their wounds, and restoring their emaciated bodies to health. For those who made it as far as Egypt alive but were too badly damaged or severely infected to survive, nurses stayed with them, ensuring that they were as comfortable and pain-free as possible in their last hours.

The campaign was already several months old before new and fully-equipped hospital ships began to be supplied and, even then, nurses sometimes faced severe overcrowding and a lack of trained help in the often-stifling wards below deck. The Eastern Mediterranean could be a dangerous scenario in which to work. Designated hospital ships, clearly marked with Red Crosses, were rarely attacked (though they were still vulnerable to the indiscriminate destruction caused by sea mines), but transport vessels were considered legitimate targets for submarine attack, and when nurses were transported on a troopship, the *Marquette*, they were as vulnerable as their male compatriots. Following the successful withdrawal of troops from Gallipoli, many hospital units in Egypt and Lemnos—including Nos. 1, 2, and 3 AGHs—were transferred to the Western Front. Others provided services along hazardous evacuation lines in Palestine and Mesopotamia, and a few were posted to East Africa or sent to support nursing services already operating in India. In these scenarios, infectious diseases such as typhoid and malaria posed serious threats, and nurses found themselves nursing large numbers of very sick patients, and, at times, succumbing to infection themselves. Some nurses wrote narratives of their experiences after the Armistice. It is clear from these writings that they viewed themselves as an integral part of the war effort. By allowing themselves to be posted to dangerous scenarios and performing work which they saw as vital, they believed they were playing a significant supporting role in what they saw as the heroic effort of their soldier-comrades.

# 5

# New Challenges on the Western Front

## 1916

### Forces of destruction: Verdun and the Somme

By 1916, it was becoming clear that neither the Allies nor the Central Powers were able to muster sufficient force to break through their enemy's lines on the Western Front. Both sides began to consider 'raising the stakes' of warfare, by risking even greater numbers of casualties in the hope that they could overwhelm their opponents. The 'Great War' was becoming a war of attrition, in which the winning side would be the one which lost the fewest men—the aim of its commanders to kill and disable as many opposing troops as possible.[1] For nurses in casualty clearing stations, trains, ships, and base hospitals, this translated into overwhelming 'rushes' of tens of thousands of men, arriving en masse at each successive point down an overstretched evacuation line. Already worn down by eighteen months of overwork and emotional stress, they now experienced an intensification of pressure. Faced with impossible workloads, they pushed themselves to their limits, working sixteen-hour shifts or longer, and taking breaks only to eat and sleep; but, still, they faced the grief and frustration of what they saw as potentially avoidable deaths.

As the year began, both Allied and German high commands had been making plans for devastating large-scale attacks on the Western

Front designed to drain manpower from their opponents. Erich von Falkenhayn was planning an attack at Verdun. He had reasoned that the French could be relied upon to defend what was not only an important border stronghold but also a symbol of national pride. Verdun, with its twenty forts, had been the last fortified city to surrender at the end of the Franco-Prussian War in 1871, and was viewed as impregnable. He reasoned that, if it were lost, French morale would crumble. Falkenhayn's plan was to pour troops and artillery into the region and wear down French resistance to the point where France would run out of resources and be knocked out of the war.[2]

Douglas Haig had been planning for a similar 'push' from the Allied side, in the Somme sector, since December 1915, but the opening attack at Verdun on 21 February pre-empted and distorted his plans. The Allied campaign had been planned as a joint British and French attack, but, with the French pinned down at Verdun, the burden of the assault fell upon the British army. At the same time, the British found themselves under pressure from their French allies to use decisive force to relieve pressure on Verdun.[3]

By the beginning of 1916, the British forces were composed of what was left of the regular army (many of whose officers had been wiped out during the first eighteen months of the war); Lord Kitchener's 'New Army', composed of volunteers who had enlisted since the outbreak of war; and the first of the conscripts, drafted into service following the implementation of the Military Service Act on 27 January. In practice, those troops who faced the German army alongside the River Somme in the summer of 1916 were mostly the willing volunteers of 1914 and 1915 who, although they had undergone several months of rigorous training, lacked military experience. Nothing in the quiet civilian lives of the teachers, bankers, factory-workers, and farm-labourers who went 'over the top' into no-man's-land on 1 July 1916 could have prepared them for the carnage that would follow. Witnesses later described how tens of thousands of British troops 'marched in formation', directly into a hail of machine-gun fire.[4]

The disaster that was the 'Battle of the Somme' has passed into legend. Although it was a joint British and French assault, it was in its British sections that things went terribly wrong. It was a peculiarly British disaster, creating a peculiarly British legend. The myths that surround it are manifold: the heroism of the ordinary British soldiers who went 'over the top' that day; the crassness of the senior military commanders who sent them to almost-certain destruction; the revelation of the horror of large-scale industrial warfare as colossal lists of the dead and missing reached the home front. The British strategy was to have been, essentially, no different from that which had been employed with occasional, limited success during 1915; but its planned force was to have been much greater. An initial bombardment, designed to wipe out enemy troops and artillery in the front-line trenches and break the German wire, was to have been followed by an attack, protected by a 'creeping barrage' just ahead of the advancing troops. In fact, the success of the entire strategy depended upon the success of the initial bombardment, which, unfortunately for the Allies, had not taken into account the depth or resilience of the deep German bunkers, some of which were located 40 feet below ground. If the heroism of the British was to become legendary, then so too were the courage and endurance of the Germans who survived the ferocious seven-day bombardment.[5]

The advance, when it took place, was mistimed, permitting the German defenders to ascend from their defensive bunkers, reach their front-line positions, and fire their machine guns into a mass of slowly advancing men. Other elements of the strategy also failed: the battle was prefaced by the detonation of 20 tons of explosives in deep tunnels below the German trenches, but the craters and gashes in the landscape created by these enormous explosions impeded the British advance, making its troops even more vulnerable, breaking communication lines, and creating confusion. The date, 1 July 1916, has been called 'the bloodiest day in the history of the British Army',[6] resulting in 57,470 casualties, of which 19,240 were deaths.[7] Many of those who managed to find their way back to their own trenches, or who survived long enough to be carried off the battlefield by stretcher-bearers, were maimed and debilitated by deep, mutilating wounds.[8]

The so-called 'Battle of the Somme' lasted until 18 November, resulting in only moderate territorial gains for the Allies, with the loss of 146,000 lives.[9] Its horror is symbolized by the vast memorial at Thiepval, which commemorates tens of thousands of men who have no known grave. Some of the bodies of those killed were so pulverized or so deeply buried in the churned-up clay of the Somme fields that they were never recovered.[10] In recent years, historical scholarship has offered a number of revisions to the interpretation of the Somme battle as a waste of lives—a conflict in which 'Lions' were led by 'Donkeys'.[11] Its apparent futility has been questioned by those who have pointed out that military innovation (in particular, the invention of the 'tank') and the heavy casualties inflicted on the German forces were significant in securing an eventual Allied victory.[12]

On 1 July 1916, as the first Allied troops mounted the parapet and began their desperate advance into no-man's-land, nurses in military hospitals throughout northern France and England were preparing thousands of extra beds. Everyone knew that a 'push' was planned on the Western Front and that it would yield thousands of casualties. No one anticipated that those casualty figures would escalate into hundreds of thousands over a period of just a few months. Meanwhile, nurses behind the lines close to Verdun had been experiencing overwhelming pressure since mid-February. French nurses, many of whom had little formal training, were becoming experienced in hospital work as they worked alongside members of the British French Flag Nursing Corps and fully trained American nurses.

## Nursing the poilus of Verdun

In the second decade of the twentieth century, nursing services in France were in a state of flux. A process of social reform, which had removed many nuns from hospital service in the late nineteenth century, had left something of a vacuum, in which most nursing work was undertaken by uneducated women with very little training. When the war began, it was regarded as natural that their services would be supplemented by the work of 'Red Cross ladies'. A few schools for professional nursing had been founded, but these were not able to recruit sufficient numbers of students to supply the needs of French hospitals, even in peacetime. The crisis of war had exposed the inadequacy of nursing provision, revealing the difficulties under which a small cadre of professional nurses and a few remaining, highly-experienced nuns were labouring.

After the Battle of The Marne in 1914, Grace Ellison, a British woman living in France, offered to create a corps of fully trained British nurses for service in French field hospitals. She realized from the start that offering such support would be a delicate diplomatic mission. Rather than establishing entire British units in the French war zones, she wanted to offer the services of individual nurses, who would assimilate themselves into French hospitals, offering nursing care of the highest quality, without disrupting the work or routines of the hospitals.[13] The fact that she was able, with the help of her honorary treasurer, Ethel Gordon Fenwick, to recruit large numbers of British nurses for such difficult and trying work, illustrates the initial failure of the British medical services to harness the willingness—indeed, the anxiety—of fully trained British nurses to participate in the war effort.

Ellison's corps was given the name 'French Flag Nursing Corps' (FFNC). By the middle of May 1916, when the Battle of Verdun had been raging for three months, Ellison spoke at a meeting in London of how this 'little corps of splendid nurses, recruited not only in the United Kingdom, but in Canada, Australia and New Zealand', had already taken care of over 27,000 wounded men.[14] She commented on the diplomacy of the nurses, who had been obliged to work, at times, under conditions they considered inadequate or inappropriate. Language differences could cause difficulties: 'For instance, a Frenchman might call his wife a cat or a little cabbage, as a term of endearment; an Englishwoman by no means regarded these terms as compliments.' Similarly, nurses learned that they must not make requests to French orderlies by using the familiar 'je veux', but must, rather, always remember the respectful 'je voudrais'.[15]

Even allowing for the somewhat propagandist reports published in Fenwick's *British Journal of Nursing*, the FFNC appears to have been highly successful in carrying out its mission of bringing expert nursing care into French field hospitals. Many FFNC nurses wrote articles and letters to the journal, expressing their delight in the appreciation they received from the French wounded—particularly the 'poilu': the ordinary French soldier and equivalent of the famous British 'Tommy'. Some patients corresponded with their nurses long after they had recovered from their wounds and returned to the front lines; their nurses, in return, sent them small presents such as cigarettes and soap. One nurse recounted a story of how she believed one day that she had lost her autograph album:

> There seemed to be some mysterious amusement among the wounded when I asked about it: 'peut-être quelqu'un va le remettre en place bientôt Madelle,' was all the answer I got. At last it was 'found'—and what a thrill it gave me! As I turned over the leaves, I found each patient had contributed some expressions of their gratitude, with etchings, verse, portraits, and in a small packet trinkets and rings made from bits of shell out of their wounds.[16]

The collection of macabre souvenirs appears to have been a peculiar interest of both nurses and soldiers. One nurse at the 'Urgency Cases Hospital' in Révigny wrote to the *British Journal of Nursing* of witnessing the shooting-down of a German Zeppelin close to her hospital, adding: 'some of us went to see the wreck next morning. It was a terrible sight—the remains of dead and half-burnt Germans amongst the ruins. The Zep seems to have been made entirely of aluminium, with a sort of canvas covering. I have got a bit of the aluminium.'[17]

Not all relationships between British nurses and their French colleagues were as good as those so frequently recounted in the *British Journal of Nursing*, nor were all British nurses and volunteers as diplomatic as Grace Ellison would have liked to believe. In 1915 a wealthy volunteer-nurse, Dorothy Cator, published a book in which she regaled her readership with tales of conflict with doctors, nurses, and orderlies in a French field hospital.[18] Just before the opening of the Verdun offensive, the editor of the *Nursing Times* had offered a scathing review of Cator's book, commenting: 'Our sympathies are with the unfortunate *médecin chef,* who if he had not been the courteous Frenchman he evidently was would assuredly have refused to be bothered with these Englishwomen.'[19]

The sensitivity felt by trained nurses when untrained, wealthy, and influential volunteers risked causing offence within a military medical service with which they were attempting to establish a rapport was understandable. So, too, was the tendency for journals such as the *British Journal of Nursing* to colour their tales of British professional nursing with tints of heroism. At Bergues, for example, it was reported that a group of FFNC had taken over 'a hospital filled with delirious typhoid patients' with no water and very little equipment. No sooner had they transformed it into a 'model fever hospital' than it was shelled by the Germans and the nurses were obliged to carry their patients to the cellars and nurse them there.[20] The corps received remarkable support from the home front, and this may in part have been the result of the campaigning zeal of its supporters. One letter to the *British Journal of Nursing* spoke of the 'grey flannel bed jackets with scarlet collars' which had been supplied by 'the dear old ladies at the Barnet Workhouse'.[21] In reality, French field hospitals were desperately poorly equipped and nurses were heavily dependent on their relatives and friends at home to send basic items such as pillows, blankets, and pyjamas. One nurse wrote of patients struggling to drink from condensed-milk tins and having only canvas-covered straw for pillows.[22]

The nursing care offered to the 'heroes' of Verdun was reported in the *British Journal of Nursing* with great eagerness and, sometimes, in quite emotional terms. One correspondent wrote of how slowly the news of the German attacks had reached French field hospitals: 'almost before one realised that the gigantic struggle had actually commenced wounded were pouring in, and all wounds of the severest type, the lighter cases being sent direct into the interior'.[23] French evacuation lines were completely overwhelmed by the crisis, and nurses found that patients were arriving in their hospitals in similar conditions to those who had been evacuated to British base hospitals from the Battles of the Marne and Ypres in 1914. Often transported on straw in goods carriages, a first field dressing wrapped around their wounded limbs, with only one thin blanket, and without food or drink, these patients arrived in emaciated states and with severe infections. Many of their wounds were compound fractures, in which the damaged bone protruded through muscle and skin, causing extensive soft-tissue damage. These wounds were often gangrenous, and many patients' conditions were either dangerous or clearly hopeless. For many, amputation was the only course of action that could offer any chance of survival, and nurses found themselves assisting in operating theatres in ways they could not have dreamed of in civilian life. One nurse wrote later of her horror at being 'pushed into giving anaesthetics'. Initially, she was 'terrified', but 'soon became quite courageous when I could hear the pandemonium of noises hailing from the countless stretchers which crowded the floor in the adjoining room'.[24] Another wrote: 'as long as I live I think I shall hear the cries of pain, and often the sobbing of these brave men, when they are dressed'.[25]

At Verdun, the German forces adopted military techniques designed to overwhelm their enemies into rapid submission. One of their strategies was to follow a bombardment with an attack protected by a creeping barrage, in which front-line storm troops were armed with flame-throwers. As a consequence, nurses saw large numbers of severe burns: 'practically every part of the body being involved, the burns of the head and face usually being of the 4<sup>th</sup> or 5<sup>th</sup> degree'. They dressed the deepest and most severe burns with picric acid, in the hope of avoiding infection, but many patients died of shock before their wounds could even begin to heal. Wet saline dressings were applied to less severe burns, and these often healed well, with a minimum of scarring. One correspondent of the *British Journal of Nursing* wrote, in emotional language, of her involvement in this work:

> Never, never can we forget the horror of these days on the one hand and on the other the joy and thankfulness that one feels in the possession of the precious right as a trained nurse, to have a real and responsible share in the magnificent methods in surgery of dealing with suffering humanity in connection with these brave patient heroes. We feel as never before that our presence and work here behind the French line is amply justified, and the work itself 'worth while' beyond all telling.[26]

In late September 1916, trained nurse Mabel Jeffery, now working for the French Flag Nursing Corps, moved to Hôpital Complémentaire No. 32, Ambulance 1/69, Château Thierry, close to the French lines (see Figure 18). When she went home on leave in October, two of her patients, Paul Leleux and 'Pasturel', wrote poignant letters thanking her for her care. Leleux wrote of how

> Your departure has been so quick that I have not had the time to say you how I am thankful for all the cares you gave me, for all the trouble I was the cause to you. I thank you very much for them and I will remember a long time your kindness towards me…It's not so difficult to see you are gone away. Tables are not washed every day, nor the beds made! and I am obliged to ask it twenty times at the least, to have hot drinks or a dry shirt. Bah! We don't die for that. And Pasturel is now my 'nurse', and a very clever and good one.[27]

Pasturel himself sent similar thanks, in French, ending with an English postscript: 'I am always a notty boy.'[28] The tendency for

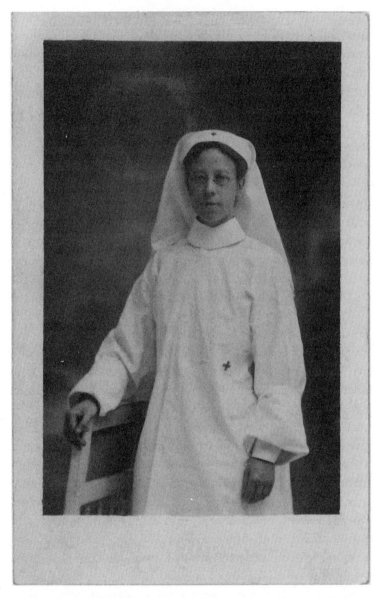

FIGURE 18 Portrait of Mabel Jeffery in French Red Cross uniform (image from Marian Wenzel and John Cornish, *Auntie Mabel's War* (London: Allen Lane, 1980), reproduced with the kind assistance of the Department of Documents, Imperial War Museum, London, UK)

nurses to view their patients as 'boys' was clearly encouraged—at least in some cases—by the 'boys' themselves. Another of Jeffery's patients thanked her not only for her 'bravery and devotion', but also for looking after him and his fellow patients 'as if you were our mother'.[29] This imitation of highly personal, familial relationships was typical of the ways in which nurses in military hospitals related to their patients. It aroused mixed emotions within governments and army commands. The tendency for female nurses to adopt 'mothering' roles (whilst still deftly combining those roles with scientific acumen and technical proficiency) was welcomed as an indication that women 'knew their place' within the military hierarchy. Yet, at the same time, their behaviour aroused fears that their kindness and nurturance would 'soften' the soldiers who came under their influence, rendering them unfit for military service.

## British nursing services on the Somme Front

Even before the 'Somme push', nursing services on the Western Front were operating under severe pressure. Jentie Paterson, based at No. 26 General Hospital, Étaples, commented in her diary, on 31 March, of having gone into her ward to find a 'man (regular been out since Mons) been admitted last night and never cleaned up! Shot through bridge of nose and left eye and cheek. Low condition. I tackled him at once, shaved and went ahead. He is on the list. Will be a squeak.' Paterson's hasty account reads almost like a coded message. 'On the list', undoubtedly referred to the fact that this patient was entered into the 'dangerously ill' (DI) list for the ward. His survival would be a matter of both good nursing care and chance. In 1960, Paterson added a marginal note to her diary, perhaps before depositing the document in the Imperial War Museum: 'Yes was, but we nursed him back to life in France. I begged him to be left sunny weather verandah and I do his dressing. He finished up with only loss 1 eye!' Of another patient, she also commented in her later 1960 notes: 'He got *well*: deaf one ear. 1 glass eye! He and wife so grateful wrote me for years. Always p.c. [postcard] on day he got well.' On 8 April, Paterson wrote of one of her worst cases: 'An American who is with Canadians fighting for us. Shot through both eyes...when they advanced to hold the crater...24 hours became a target for shrapnel. Is a mass of wounds,' adding immediately afterwards: 'My other eye man is round the corner had his bed lifted out in the sun today.'[30] On 24 April, Paterson's diary records that her father died at 8 p.m. She was granted seven days' emergency leave, but was, once again, obliged to resign from service with the QAIMNSR because her mother was ill and 'absolutely alone and unable to attend to a host of business affairs'.[31]

Elizabeth Haldane reported that, at the beginning of 1916, there were twenty-four General Hospitals, three isolation hospitals, thirteen stationary hospitals, twenty-nine casualty clearing stations, twenty-two hospital trains, and twelve hospital barges operating as the British medical services in France.[32] Yet, even before the Battle of the Somme, the provision was inadequate, and nurses were operating under intense pressure. On 13 March, at No. 1 British General Hospital at Étretat on the coast of northern France, Sister Edith Appleton wrote of a particularly sad death on her ward:

My poor little boy Kerr died yesterday, he had been in 15 days suffering from gas-pneumonia, bronchitis & had been extremely & dangerously ill at the time, but only the day before yesterday he realized that he was not going to get well. I am glad to say we never left him night or day & he was fond of us all. Yesterday was a difficult day to be 'Sister'—He kept whispering all sorts of messages for home & his fiancée—then he would call 'Sister' & when I bent down to hear—'I do love you' 'when I am gone will you kiss me?'—& all the time heads would be popping in 'Sister—20 No—so & so—to . . .' 'The S. Sgt wants to know if you can lend him a couple of men to . . .' this & that—but in spite of all—I did kiss the boy first for his Mother & then for myself—which pleased him—then he whispered 'but you

still will when I'm gone' The night before he asked me what dying
would be like—& said it seemed so unsatisfactory—he felt too young
to die—& not even wounded—only of bronchitis. Then another
time he said, 'They wouldn't let me go sick every time they said it
was rheumatism & would wear off—& marching with full pack &
dodging the shells was dreadful.' Thank Goodness—what I told him
dying would be like happened—exactly—a clear gift of Providence.
I told him it would be—that little by little his breathing would get
easier—& he would feel tired & like going to sleep—& then he
would just sleep—& with no morphia—that is exactly what did
happen—without a struggle.[33]

In 1916, the staff of Nos. 1 and 2 Australian General Hospitals
arrived in northern France, to be informed that their units must—
in the short term—be broken up and their nurses sent to assist
various British units in the area. The news caused much disappointment, yet Australian nurses were also keen to find out about
the working practices of their 'imperial' colleagues. Ellen Cuthbert
was sent to the officers' surgical wards at No. 3 British General
Hospital at Le Tréport, situated close to another British and two
Canadian hospitals in 'very beautiful' surroundings on the cliffs
above the town. The wards were housed in a large hotel with small
rooms and long flights of stairs—highly unsuitable for the nursing
of severely wounded men.[34] Gertrude Doherty spent three months
nursing at a British General Hospital on the quay at Le Havre. She
worked with a minimal staff of orderlies on night duty on the so-
called 'bath ward' where badly wounded limbs were kept sub-
merged in baths of sterile water, saline, or mild antiseptic. Three
of her patients had had both legs amputated and were nursed on
specially constructed 'Carters' beds, which permitted them to be
lifted into the air whilst the bed was changed.[35]

On 10 June, Ellen Cuthbert and three other Australian nurses had
been posted to No. 6 British Stationary Hospital, which had taken
over premises vacated by No. 42 Casualty Clearing Station. The hospital was right beside a railhead, within walking distance of the

trenches behind the Arras sector of the front, well north of the Somme. It was the first receiving hospital behind the field ambulance, and Cuthbert remarked on the poignancy of watching the smiling and waving troops marching past the hospital en route to the trenches and then receiving them into her ward as wounded men days later, desperately ill and yet still displaying the same 'wonderful spirit of cheerfulness and endurance—grateful for any care they received'. Here she experienced for the first time the use of Thomas Splints for fractures and Carrel-Dakin treatment for wounds.[36]

By mid-1916, the Allied medical services on the Western Front were treating more casualties in France than ever before. The experiences of 1915 had taught senior medical staff that treatment as close as possible to the battle lines was both more economical and more likely to yield success than the rapid evacuation of wounded back to Britain. The chaos following the Battle of Loos, in which some CCSs had been overwhelmed whilst others were left empty, led to the development of a new system of 'pairing' CCSs, so that one would 'take in' cases until full, when it would hand over to its neighbour. Eventually, this system was to evolve into one in which three CCSs would be located in close proximity to each other, each 'taking its turn' to admit casualties, while the other two focused on performing essential operations and evacuating patients onto hospital trains. On the eve of the Battle of the Somme, the system of 'pairing' CCSs was in place, and plans were being drawn up to bring into the area a sufficient number of ambulance trains to evacuate 10,000 wounded men per day—clearly an underestimate.[37]

In the days following 1 July, staff in CCSs and on trains found themselves under intense pressure. A 'specification tally' was always attached to a patient's uniform at the regimental aid post before he was put into a motor ambulance for transfer to the CCS. This contained information on his wounds, his prognosis, and whether he had received morphine and anti-tetanus injections. Upon arrival at the 'reception hut' of a CCS, the patient would undergo further 'triage': the process which would enable a rapid decision to be taken about treatment. Depending on their conditions, patients would be declared to be: 'moribund' (without hope of survival); in need of immediate emergency treatment for shock, in which case they would be transferred to the resuscitation ward; requiring urgent surgery; able to await surgery; or fit to travel immediately (either as a 'lying' or as a 'sitting' case).[38] Sister Blair, based at a CCS in France, described the systematic efficiency with which the now highly-experienced staff in her CCS worked during the Somme 'push':

> On the morning of attack by 9am the ambulances began to roll up and we would receive 300 wounded in an hour, when we switched off, and another CCS would take in, we worked in pairs. When they had received 300, we again took in, and so on till all were dealt with. The walking wounded arrived first, often travelling down in London buses, and passed through the dressing tent, then on to a Marquee on the railway siding, for a hot meal and smokes, thence onto the hospital train for the base. Another train immediately took its place and waited for the first load of operated-on cases. Meantime all the stretcher cases were examined and dressed and labelled as to which ward they would go into. The resuscitation ward received those very collapsed cases which had to be revived before being fit for oper-ation. In the operating theatre we had 3 tables going at one time, continuously day and night, until all the wounded had passed through once. To each table was appointed a surgeon, anaesthetist, sister and orderly ... When the last train-load for the time being, had departed we settled down to nurse those too ill for evacuation, all head wounds with fracture of the skull and laceration of the brain, abdominal wounds, chest wounds and multiple wounds were kept for a few weeks at the CCS before being sent to the base.[39]

Blair's description resonates with a sense of mastery and com-posure. Yet, not all nurses experienced such apparent calmness during their work in CCSs, many of which were rapidly over-whelmed by the sheer numbers of casualties during the first few days of the Battle of the Somme.

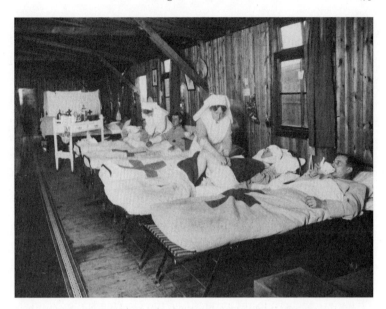

FIGURE 19 An Australian Casualty Clearing Station on the Western Front (photograph reproduced by permission of the Imperial War Museum, London, UK)

Elsie Dobson was posted to No. 10 Ambulance Train in early 1916. By this time, even adapted passenger-trains were much better equipped than those on which the earliest transport nurses had struggled to care for patients. Dobson's train had 'spring stretchers and every convenience'. At normal times it would carry about 750 patients, but during a 'push' this could increase to almost 850 'and there would be stretchers everywhere—on the floor, in corridors, one walked on the edges of stretchers'. Footboard-walking was still a feature of train work and Dobson later described how it was achieved:

> Short full skirts and sensible shoes were necessary for this perform-
> ance for the coaches were separated by a gap of 3 or 4 ft wide—but
> there was always an orderly with a guiding hand to help one over the
> chasm! On another train an orderly fell and had both legs cut off.
> We were then told we must not walk the footboards, but I for my

part did not obey that instruction—it was quite impossible to do so and still carry out one's duties…A necessary supply of stimulants, drugs etc. was carried in a bag on my belt, and a bag of cigarettes and matches was also on my belt. The orderlies in each coach would report on loading any severe cases and in due course each coach would be visited by me.[40]

During the Battle of the Somme, the train took on huge number of patients from overcrowded CCSs. Dobson recalled making five trips in three days, resting on the return journeys. On one occasion, the train arrived at a completely full CCS; severe stretcher cases had been placed 'in a field of beautiful maize'. Well over twice the usual number of cases was loaded onto the train and Dobson 'just did the best [she] could for the very bad cases'.[41] Sister Leila Smith, also working on an ambulance train, witnessed distressing scenes at the CCS at 'Germaincourt'. Patients were 'lying everywhere in the grounds of the clearing station' and the walking wounded had to be held back by a guard as they fought to get onto the train.[42] Down the line in bases such as Boulogne, hospitals were coping with massive influxes of patients. Matron Nellie Gould commented on how, when the 'rush' of casualties was at its height, 'the wards would fill and empty again into the hospital ships at Boulogne two or three times in [each] twenty-four hours'.[43]

## Coping with crisis: July–November 1916

On 3 July, Edith Appleton wrote in her diary of the 'much-longed-for advance'.[44] Her writing bears witness to the British peoples' hope that the Somme 'push' would be the breakthrough that would end the war—hopes that were cruelly dashed. The next day, Edith wrote of the arrival of 'hundreds upon hundreds' of wounded at Étretat.[45] Their injuries were horrific, some infested with maggots, others clearly gangrenous. Staff in CCSs and hospital trains had not had time to wash and feed them all, so the work of making them clean and comfortable fell to the base hospital staff. The work was often heartbreaking, as it became clear that many of the wounded had no chance of survival. Several patients died within hours of reaching the hospital, and Edith wrote of 'one poor lad' with 'both eyes shot through and there they were, all smashed and mixed up with the eyelashes. He was quite calm, and very tired. He said, "Shall I need an operation? I can't see anything". Poor boy, he never will.'[46] Two days later, Edith had given up trying to put into words the crisis at Étretat: 'it beats me', she wrote. The system whereby base hospital staff were warned in advance of an approaching hospital train had completely broken down as overloaded train after overloaded train arrived without notice. The hospital had expanded into a restaurant, a garage, part of a casino, and some of its own staff's quarters to accommodate patients.

Among Appleton's most poignant diary-entries are those relating to a young soldier named Lennox, who had been brought into No. 1 General Hospital on 13 July, with a piece of lead lodged in a lung. For forty-one days, she noted his condition in her diary. On 16 July he was 'holding his own', but she feared that he would have died next time she came on duty. 'My poor little chest boy is dying', she wrote the next day, adding that he was in an 'agony of pain'. By 28 July he was coughing up pus from a number of abscesses and by the 31st had a 'generally poisoned condition'. On 8 August, Appleton wrote that her 'boy' Lennox seemed unable to die, although he could never recover.[47] She was offering him mental as well as physical relief, by sitting at his bedside composing comforting letters to both his mother and his fiancée. Finally, on 23 August, she wrote:

> Lennox died soon after 8 o'clock last night. Never have I seen such a slow, painful death. It was as if the boy was chained to Earth for punishment. Towards the end it was agony for him to draw his little gasping breaths and I felt I must clap my hand over his nose and mouth and quench the flickering flame. I am very glad for the boy to be away.[48]

Appleton's next two diary entries are dated 28 August and 8 September, and explain that she has written very little because she had been ill and 'miserable' with an ear infection.[49] Perhaps the strain of caring for this and other hopeless patients was beginning to tell.

During the heaviest rushes of casualties, CCSs and base hospitals in France became so overwhelmed that many patients were moved more rapidly down the line to Britain than would normally have been the case. Claire Tisdall, a volunteer 'ambulance nurse' in London, described her shock upon seeing one desperately wounded patient lying on a stretcher on a London railway platform. Thinking, at first, that the lower part of his face was covered by a black cloth, she realized, as she got nearer, that 'the whole lower half of his face had been completely blown off and what had appeared to be a black cloth was a huge gaping hole'.[50] The wounds created by the sometimes indiscriminate shelling of opposing forces were rarely clean or simple, and, because shells burst upwards, facial injuries were common. Patients with jaw injuries required particularly intricate care. Often finding it almost impossible to eat, they had to be fed through rubber tubes, inserted through excruciatingly painful open wounds. Great care had to be taken that feeding tubes were passed into the stomach, not the lungs, before milk, beef-tea, and carefully liquidized foods were poured into them. Once this messy and painful process had been accomplished, the wounds were irrigated with antiseptic to remove any germ-harbouring food substances, before being re-dressed. Since the only really effective analgesia at this time was morphia, which had to be used with care because of its toxic and addictive properties, the feeding of facially injured patients was a tortuous time for both patients and nurses.[51]

On 17 April 1916, No. 1 Australian General Hospital (AGH) took over the premises of No. 12 British Stationary Hospital, on the racecourse at Rouen. Meanwhile, in the same month, No. 2 AGH arrived in Marseilles and established a temporary infectious diseases hospital in the south of France, before moving to Wimereux,

near Boulogne, where it opened a specialist unit for the treatment
of fractures. The new 'Sinclair's swing bed', which allowed patients
to be cared for without the need for the painful dismantling of
splints, enabled nurses to save time and conserve energy.[52] Later
that year No. 3 AGH took over the Kitchener War Hospital in
Brighton on the south coast of England, where it remained until
May 1917, when it was relocated to a site near Abbeville behind the
Somme sector.[53]

## At the front

American-trained nurse Alice Fitzgerald was 'donated' to the British
nursing services on the Western Front by a committee of philanthropists in Boston, Massachusetts, USA. Inspired by Edith Cavell's
'sacrifice' and anxious to show their support for the British, the
'Edith Cavell Committee' funded the salary, travel, and expenses of
the 'Edith Cavell Nurse from Massachusetts'.[54] When they began to
recruit for the position, they knew that they would require someone
who was both an expert clinician and a consummate diplomat.
Fitzgerald, who had trained at the Johns Hopkins University Hospital in Baltimore and then pursued a successful career before becoming Superintendent of Nurses at the Robert W. Long Hospital,
Indianapolis, easily met their criteria: she was a 'gentlewoman' by
birth, from a wealthy family which had travelled extensively through
Europe during her childhood and youth.[55] Her command of several
European languages was enhanced by her excellent communication
skills. Fitzgerald worked alongside QAIMNS and other British
nurses, first at a base hospital in Boulogne, then at a CCS at
Méaulte, situated between Bray and Albert on the British sector of
the Somme Front. Her experiences on the Somme were so harrowing that, on her arrival in London on leave in December 1916,
she was diagnosed by a doctor as suffering from 'shell-shock'.[56]

In her unpublished diary, Fitzgerald wrote that hers was considered to be the nearest CCS to the front lines, adding that the

shelling was 'thunderous and continuous'. Situated on raised ground, it offered a view across several Allied rest camps. Forty observation balloons were tethered nearby and floated, seemingly, directly above the heads of the CCS staff. She felt that she was 'all but in the firing line'. On days off, she walked close to the CCS, picking up pieces of shell, or was taken by army officers on visits to see captured German trenches—marvelling at their depth and complexity—or to view British tanks. Her accommodation was a small bell tent, in which she could only stand upright at the very centre. Nurses' accommodation was not floored, and when the rains began in the late summer her home turned into a quagmire, and she was obliged to spend all her time in gumboots, with her dress pinned up 'as far as I dare'.

Fitzgerald's patients were laid on stretchers on the ground, and she was obliged to kneel in the mud to nurse them. Her diary documents her anxiety at not being able to give them the care they really needed: 'What is nursing here? There is not time even to undress the patients except a few who are to be operated upon and even they often go to the operating room in khaki. If the cases are serious they are then taken to the tent which has beds but if only a sight operation has been performed they are not undressed and come to us for evacuation in the same khaki.'[57] Coping with the mud inside the hospital tent offered her, she felt, an insight into the horrors facing the men in their trenches, and although she had to 'slip and slop around in great style', she could be glad for those of her patients who were likely to survive that they had (at least temporarily) escaped the horrors of the trenches. Among her wounded were German prisoners, whose letters she helped to censor. One prisoner-patient had written to his mother, explaining how happy he was: the sister in his ward spoke German, and he felt as though he were on holiday, having escaped from the fighting. Fitzgerald felt that her job was made more difficult by the attitude of the CCS's commanding officer. He was 'overbearing and antagonistic toward the nurses', making it plain that he did not want them in his unit. She added: 'Well, at least, the patients like to have us and that is more important than his personal prejudices.'[58]

In 1916, Sir Anthony Bowlby had been made Consultant Surgeon to the British Expeditionary Force. He took a special interest in CCSs, arguing that they needed to be enlarged, better staffed, and placed much nearer to the fighting lines. His recommendations had been taken into consideration during planning for the Somme offensive.[59] Hence, nurses such as Fitzgerald found themselves not only within sight and sound of shellfire, but, on more than one occasion, actually under fire themselves. On 24 September 1916, Fitzgerald wrote in her diary of a 'terrifying night' during which a high explosive shell was dropped just outside the camp. She likened the noise to 'the sudden collapse of a thousand buildings with the crumbling of stone and the shattering of glass and metal'. This incident was followed by the worst 'rush' of casualties she had ever experienced. Many of her patients had chest or abdominal injuries and she felt she had 'never worked harder nor more hopelessly in my life'. Most patients were covered in blood and the air was thick with flies. Gas shells were being dropped on Bray, and Fitzgerald was afraid that the prevailing wind might carry the poison into her compound.

On 11 October, she experienced another 'night of terror', when moonlight brought a series of fierce air raids. A nearby French anti-aircraft gun boomed, and shells 'whizzed and whistled by'. The next day a new batch of wounded was brought in, many of them with severe wound infections. They had lain in no-man's-land for days waiting for rescue. On 13 October, Fitzgerald recorded in her diary that even worse cases were being admitted:

> Some of these men had been lying in no man's land for seven days without food or drink; they lived in shell holes through several bombardments, were eye witnesses of advances and retreats, afraid to make a sound because of enemy snipers, and yet are alive to tell the tale. One must marvel at human endurance for the wounds, after such a long time without any care, are dreadful beyond description.[60]

After a further air raid, during which 'our tents shook as if they had been blades of grass in a breeze' and 'shells just whizzed like bumble bees around us', she felt so physically and emotionally exhausted that she was unable to raise her limbs from the bed. She was also numb with cold, as the mud had turned to frost and she was able to keep warm in bed only with several blankets and coats. She commented: 'It is impossible to describe the concussion felt after an explosion, even at a distance, nor the horrible sinking feeling that grips you as you wait for the next jolt which you know is bound to come.' Fearing facial injury more than anything else, eventually, on 10 November, she borrowed a steel helmet from a sergeant, padded it with a piece of blanket, and placed it over her face when lying down at night. From then until her leave in December, she slept marginally better.[61]

It was not only British and Dominion nursing services that saw 'action' behind the Somme sector in the summer of 1916. Mary Borden, already the 'directrice' of a highly successful French field hospital in Rousbrugge, Belgium, petitioned the French military services to permit her to form a second, much larger hospital to support the French wounded of the Somme campaign. Her huge, 1,400-bed field hospital, 'l'Hôpital d'Evacuation', approximately 3 miles behind the front-line trenches, at Bray-sur-Somme was just a few miles from Alice Fitzgerald's posting at Méaulte. The size of the hospital and its extreme proximity to the front lines meant that its nurses worked under intense pressure. Not only were they frequently inundated by 'rushes' of severely damaged men, they were also within sight and sound of shellfire—their nights, like those of Fitzgerald, frequently disturbed by the booming of heavy artillery. Borden wrote in her extraordinary book *The Forbidden Zone* of how she—a volunteer nurse, tutored by some of the most highly-trained professional nurses in the world—worked in the reception hut of her own field hospital 'triaging' patients, deciding who could survive, performing shock therapy, and rushing the most urgent cases to the operating theatre. She described her life-saving work as a process of dragging men back from the brink of a vast ocean; of creating 'the flow against the ebb...like a tug of war with the tide'.[62]

## The development and extension of nursing work

The Battle of the Somme produced hundreds of thousands of casualties. Many were wounded during the first attack on 1 July, when troops marching across no-man's-land were met by a barrage of machine-gun fire and shell-blast. The wounded streamed into casualty clearing stations along a large sector of the Western Front, almost overwhelming these small field hospitals and resulting in practices that would only ever have been permitted in an emergency. Operating theatres found themselves running up to eight complex operations at the same time, and some nurses were obliged to assist more than one surgeon. Many casualties had multiple wounds and the team could work much more quickly if the nurse attending the surgeon undertook some of the minor surgery, while the doctor concentrated on the more complex wounds. Some nurses found themselves removing shrapnel and other debris from smaller wound-beds, and closing and suturing even the largest wounds, whilst the surgeon moved on to the next case. Sister Kit McNaughton, a trained Australian nurse from Little River, Victoria, found herself crossing such boundaries of professional practice, when she removed a bullet from a patient's back.[63]

Gas shells were used for the first time during the Somme offensive.[64] These released asphyxiating gases such as chlorine, bromine, and phosgene directly into Allied trenches, suffocating their victims, and causing severe eye irritation. For those who survived, it might be several days before their eyes could be opened. Nurses in both CCSs and base hospitals became adept at positioning their patients to allow them to breathe as easily as possible, administering oxygen and stimulants and bathing eyes with sodium bicarbonate.[65] Often a damp compress was left over the eyes until the pain and photo-phobia (shrinking from light) began to be relieved. Most patients regained their eyesight, although some were blinded by the toxins in the chemical weapons. Although the majority of patients who made it as far as CCSs survived the destructive effects of gases on the lungs, many were left with chronic lung damage, which would predispose them to tuberculosis and other lung infections later in life.[66]

As nurses took on more medical and surgical work, they were obliged to delegate more of their fundamental care work to order-lies. This could cause difficulties. In French field hospitals, British and American nurses commented, with both amusement and exas-peration, on the vagaries of French orderlies. One corporal with Ambulance 1/69 in Château Thierry wrote to thank Sister Mabel Jeffery, confessing: 'I was always in a temper, but please believe me it was not because of you…I hope that when I work with a lady nurse again, it will be with one like yourself.'[67]

### In 'Blighty'

The Battle of the Somme created overwhelming pressure for CCSs close to the front lines, and for base hospitals in northern France. The pressures encountered by these units were pushed outwards like ripples on a pond. As far away as northern England a huge 'rush' of work was being experienced. Janet Miller, a VAD at the Second Western General Hospital in Manchester (see Figure 20), described how her leave, which had been planned for July 1916, had to be cancelled because all staff were urgently required. She recalled how 'miserable' that summer was for nurses working at the hospital, because, no matter how hard one worked, it was impos-sible to offer the care that was really needed: 'one had no time to do more than the barest necessities for the men. Their wounds did not get anything like the proper attention.' She later recalled one 'Irish boy, Hussey', who 'lingered between life and death for several

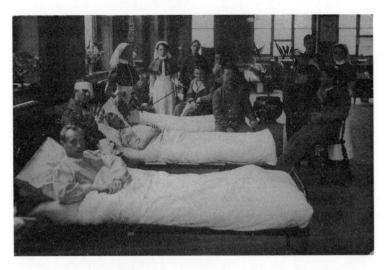

FIGURE 20 Second Western General Hospital, Manchester (photograph reproduced by kind permission of Sue Light)

days, but died eventually'. The weather was hot and their bulky dressings and bandages made the patients uncomfortable: 'the poor Tommies felt it so, but with very rare exceptions, they behaved wonderfully well and were marvellously patient and anxious not to give trouble'.[68]

Yet, once the first 'rushes' of patients were over, many base hospitals in Britain were able to establish more relaxed routines, and create environments in which healing could take place. In the summer of 1916, the No. 1 New Zealand General Hospital moved from Abasseye in Egypt to Brockenhurst in the southern English county of Hampshire. Nurses wrote of their pleasure at finding themselves transferred from the Egyptian desert to the beautiful ancient woodland of the so-called 'New Forest', not far from where they had disembarked at Southampton.[69] Their hospital took over several sites which had been established by philanthropist Lady Hardinge for nursing Indian troops in 1915. Forest Park Hotel became an 'officers' hospital, with a tented convalescent hospital on meadowland opposite; the Balmer Lawn Hotel was reserved mainly for 'medical' and 'neurological' cases; the Morant Hall was converted into a convalescent hospital for patients who were recovering prior to their return to active service or repatriation.[70] A large hutted hospital was also constructed on a site close to the village church, and several private houses became small wards. Modern visitors to the ancient churchyard of Brockenhurst can stand beneath the serene canopy of its ancient trees and view the cenotaph erected in 1927 in the middle of the ninety-five carved granite monuments to those whose lives could not be saved.

About 300 nurses were based at Brockenhurst, some billeted in private homes, others on the top floor of the Balmer Lawn Hotel.[71] The presence of large numbers of recovering and convalescing patients in the village created a lively social atmosphere. Patients, dressed in their 'convalescent blue' uniforms, attended 'cinematographic pictures', dances, concerts, cricket matches, and picnics. Wealthy local residents drove small groups to patriotic concerts on the coast in nearby Bournemouth. Convalescent patients were also able to engage in a number of vocational classes, including metalwork, carpentry, leatherwork, sign writing, and bee-keeping, and to attend lectures on a range of subjects. One patient with a below-knee amputation wrote home:

> I do hope you won't worry over me because we are treated like lords here. You would probably imagine the ward as a place of wailing and gnashing of teeth whereas you would not find a more cheerful crowd in the hospital. We get great treatment here. The nurses are real good sorts and you would be astounded at the fun that goes on. No one is allowed to be gloomy in this place.[72]

The No. 2 New Zealand General Hospital was also relocated to a beautiful site at Walton-on-Thames. By April 1917, New Zealand nurse May Chalmers, the sister-in-charge of its auxiliary hospital, was referring to it as 'a truly lovely place'.[73]

## Conclusion

The wounded of the Somme endured a long, hazardous, and often tedious journey before they arrived at convalescent hospitals in places such as Brockenhurst. The transformative process by which a man sent 'over the top' into the death-zone of the Somme could feel himself treated 'like a lord' in a picturesque New Forest village was a complex one, involving nursing and medical staff in many treatment scenarios: field dressing stations, casualty clearing stations, hospital trains and ships, and base hospitals. In addition to assisting in operative procedures and giving medically prescribed treatments, nurses spent much time at their patients' bedsides, offering food and fluids to restore strength, and a combination of bracing humour and gentle sympathy to provide reassurance.

Behind the lines at Verdun, French and other Allied nurses offered total patient care to men who had somehow lived through massive bombardment and held defensive positions against storm-troop tactics. Many nurses' writings reveal a viewpoint in which the poilus were 'heroes' and they themselves were performing a vital service to the 'motherland'. But the Somme and Verdun were turning points in the consciousness of Allied citizens. No longer could the lengthening casualty lists be ignored or put to one side. It was becoming clear that the First World War involved a horrific loss of life and, while nurses still saw the Allied cause as a 'just' one, they could no longer avoid the realization that they were watching suffering on a scale that had never been witnessed before.

# 6

# War of Attrition on All Fronts
## August 1916–March 1918

**Transformation on Western and Eastern Fronts**

The year 1916 ended in a mood of resignation for Allied nations.[1] The failure of the push at the Battle of the Somme had convinced many that the two forces engaged in the Great War were so evenly matched that the conflict might last for decades. But, for Allied nurses, anxieties about an uncertain future were offset by a new sense of clarity and purpose about their work and its achievements. The care of patients with battlefield wounds so horrific that their cases seemed hopeless was becoming commonplace, and ways were being found to save them. Nurses were drawing confidence from their successes. At the same time, the once-strained relationships between trained nurses and their now-experienced volunteer assistants was solidifying into something resembling close and respectful cooperation.

In August 1916 a new ally—Romania—entered the war: but its support proved fragile. Its initial military campaign was disastrous and the country was rapidly overrun by advancing German and Bulgarian armies. Its high command managed, with Russian support, to hold the region of Moldavia, where—in the ancient city of Jassy—it established its base. British-born Queen Marie of Romania became an important symbol of patriotism as, dressed in a spotless white Red Cross nurse's uniform, she toured military hospitals, distributing gifts to the wounded.[2]

Although it had promised continuing stagnation, 1917 proved to be an unexpectedly eventful year. Its first major upheaval came in March, when the initial phase of what has come to be known as the 'Russian Revolution' resulted in the abdication of the Tsar and the formation of the Provisional Government. The Revolution had been preceded by military and humanitarian catastrophe on a vast scale: the Russian army had sustained over 2.5 million casualties, and huge numbers of civilians had been forced from their homes and condemned to live as refugees in squalid 'barracks' in cities such as Petrograd and Moscow. There were fears among the Allies that the Provisional Government would pull Russia out of the war, but these were unfounded. The government did, however, issue its famous 'Order Number One' allowing army units to form soviets and become self-governing. The short-term consequence of this well-intentioned, egalitarian policy was a general breakdown of military discipline. In April, the Germans secretly assisted the prominent anti-war revolutionary 'Lenin' to return to Russia from exile in Switzerland. As leader of the Bolsheviks, he declared himself against the war and won widespread support. During the October Revolution, the Bolsheviks took power, and on 15 December they signed an armistice with Germany at Brest-Litovsk. Their conflict was now to become a civil war in which Russian turned on Russian; it would last until 1921.[3]

Russian nurses found themselves in the midst of civil and military upheaval from the late spring onwards. As military discipline began to break down, many were forced to make their own way—often with great difficulty and across hazardous terrains—back to their home cities. Many foreign nurses (including those from Britain and the Dominions) remained at their posts until the autumn, when widespread disorder and the descent into civil war made their existence, even in cities such as Petrograd and Moscow, precarious.

Eventually, they were forced to return home, some via Finland and Sweden, others making long, arduous train journeys across Siberia to Vladivostock and the Pacific Ocean.

Long before Russia's withdrawal from the war had become inevitable, another great power had entered the conflict on the Allied side. Many citizens of the United States of America had expressed sympathy for the Allied cause since the beginning of the war—and this sympathy had been heightened by the sinking of the *Lusitania* by a German submarine on 7 May 1915. The American president, Woodrow Wilson—'a man of peace to the core of his being'—had argued for neutrality,[4] yet American munitions and loans were already helping sustain the Allied cause. So were thousands of American volunteers, some of them fully trained nurses, most working under the auspices of the American Red Cross, some serving directly with the French Service de Santé.[5] Following a German policy of unrestricted submarine warfare, and the release of the 'Zimmermann Telegram' promising Mexico three southern US states (New Mexico, Texas, and Arizona) should it support the Central Powers, the United States Congress declared war against Germany on 6 April 1917. Hundreds of thousands of volunteers and conscripts joined the American Expeditionary Force, and large numbers of trained nurses—some of whom were already members of the Army Nurse Corps—prepared themselves to travel to Europe to care for their countrymen. American troops first fought on the Western Front in October 1917.[6] By this time, large numbers of American nurses, working in US 'base hospitals', had already been caring for their British and Dominion allies for about six months.

On the Western Front, Allied commanders attempted new and audacious breakthroughs. The 'Nivelle Offensive', which began in early April, pitched French troops against defensive positions close to the 'Chemin des Dames' ridge; it resulted in well over 100,000 casualties within four days.[7] British troops, under Haig's command, launched a diversion close to Arras in the same month. In a close imitation of their unsuccessful strategy at the Somme, the British bombarded Vimy Ridge for three weeks prior to the attack, then advanced, taking the ridge on 12 April. In June, the British launched a further offensive, this time prefacing their advance by detonating thousands of tons of explosives in tunnels beneath Messines Ridge, killing approximately 10,000 German soldiers.[8]

Nivelle's failed offensive led to a widespread breakdown in military discipline among the French forces, with soldiers refusing point-blank to obey their officers, and fraternizing with German troops, in a mirroring of the widespread fraternization which was taking place on the Eastern Front. The French mutinies were brought under control with mass courts martial. Five hundred death sentences were passed, although there were only forty-nine executions. Following an improvement in the conditions and leave entitlements of French troops, morale improved. Its collapse had not been replicated among the British forces, although the writings of nurses attest to the widespread despair and anger among their patients. The sense in which the Great War could no longer be seen as anything but a 'war of attrition' was heightened by the bloody Third Battle of Ypres, which lasted from 31 July to 10 November, and was popularly named the Battle of Passchendaele after the village which formed the Allies' primary objective. Among its troops were large numbers of Australian, New Zealand, and Canadian divisions. Allied casualties numbered well over a quarter of a million, in exchange for the capture of Passchendaele, partial control of the ridge on which it was located, and an advance of approximately 5 miles.[9] An attack at Cambrai, at which tanks were used successfully for the first time, enjoyed moderate success, but in the same autumn the Italians endured a crushing defeat at Caporetto, in which they lost half their army.

## Lines of evacuation on the Western Front

The system for the evacuation of casualties from the battlefields of the Western Front underwent a remarkable evolution between

early 1915 and the end of 1917. The transformation was brought
about partly through the intervention of Douglas Haig, who, in
1915, had witnessed poor coordination between CCSs, such that
some had been overwhelmed with rushes of dangerously injured
casualties, whilst others remained idle. By the time the military
medical services faced the challenges posed by the Battle of the
Somme, these problems had, largely, been overcome and CCSs were
working in pairs—or sometimes groups of three. One hospital
would 'take in' patients until full, at which time it would close and
focus on operating upon and evacuating its existing casualties.
Meanwhile its 'partner' CCS would begin its own 'take-in'. This
system appears to have been working smoothly by 1917,[10] but it was
to be severely tested by the Battle of Arras, which began on 9 April
that year. CCSs were already under pressure due to the burden of
sickness in the Arras sector—particularly from trench foot—which
had resulted from a period of cold, wet weather. Arras was said to
have had the highest average daily death rate of any battle fought
by the British during the First World War,[11] yet CCSs and ambulance trains appear to have functioned smoothly, evacuating men
quickly and efficiently to bases.

Some CCSs behind Arras came under shellfire and had to be
moved. By this time, base hospitals on the French coast were also,
at times, coming under severe bombardment. Later that year, Julia
Ashbourne Herbert was awarded the Military Medal, 'for con-
spicuous devotion to duty, when after being wounded in the head
by an aerial bomb, she came on duty in the operating theatre, and
continued to work there the whole night and all the next day'.[12]
Nurses were acutely aware of the danger they faced during such
fierce offensives, but were, perhaps, unaware of the ways in which
their experiences were used to fuel the Allied propaganda machine.
Maud McCarthy, Matron-in-Chief of the British Expeditionary
Force, was regularly asked to forward stories of heroism to the War
Office for use by its Propaganda Committee.[13] Following Arras,
careful instructions were issued to directors of medical services

that CCSs must be located far enough behind enemy lines to avoid shelling.

In March 1917, Australian nurse Gertrude Doherty was posted to No. 3 Australian Casualty Clearing Station, which moved 'up the line' to Bapaume on 8 April. The weather was cold and wet and the ground was saturated with snow and slush. The nurses went on duty in their gumboots. All duckboards had been commandeered for the front, so there was no flooring to the hospital tents:

> I was put in the theatre where operations commenced before every-thing was unpacked. There were no beds mattresses or pillows etc, only stretchers and blankets so as soon as a patient was operated on and put back on the stretcher it gradually sank in the mud. There was no time to remove the men's clothes or boots. When we were just about full a hospital train came in and relieved the pressure. The stretcher bearers had a fearful time wading through the mud carry-ing the men to the carriages.[14]

During the battle for Bullecourt in May the CCS had a 'fearful number of casualties', but this time it was aided by the arrival of two more CCSs. Casualties were arriving within two hours of being wounded, and four surgical teams were operating around the clock. Upon arrival, casualties were labelled 'A', 'B', 'C', or 'D' ac-cording to the severity of their illnesses. If there were too many 'A' and 'B' cases, 'C' and 'D' cases had to be loaded onto trains without having been operated upon.[15]

Another Australian nurse, Sister A. Smith of the AANS, was posted to No. 2 Australian CCS at Trois Arbres in January 1917. She was amused by the stories of her patients, who spoke con-stantly of 'taking' Messines Ridge: 'We heard of that ridge so often, and the time it was going to be taken,' she commented, 'that we only laughed when they spoke of it and decided the day had not yet dawned for "that ridge".'[16] But months later as she lay in her bell tent one early morning in June, she felt the 'concussion of the earth' as the mines beneath the ridge were detonated. From that morning onwards for the next several weeks, wounded men poured into her CCS: 'strong healthy men . . . dead, dying, unconscious and moaning'. Many arrived with limbs 'blown off'. A large marquee was erected to act as a reception tent, where the wounded were sorted and sent to the resuscitation ward, X-ray, the theatre, the pre-op ward, or the moribund or 'dying ward'. Staff worked well beyond their shifts, realizing that their colleagues on the next shift could not cope without help. They took only as much rest and sleep as they felt was necessary to allow them to continue with their work. Sleep was, in any case, almost impossible, with 'shells bursting overhead, anti air craft and machine guns going continually with the noise of general bombardment and the screech of shells overhead'.[17] The colonel of the CCS received a commendation after the battle for treating 2,300 cases in nineteen hours, many of whom were operated upon. For several days, Smith was put in charge of the moribund ward, where only hopeless cases were placed. The work was emotionally testing:

> It was a hopeless, heartbreaking place. Rows of dying men mostly Australians and New Zealanders, nearly all headcases and unconscious, semi conscious or else raving in delirium, and pulling their bandages off. None likely to live more than a few hours, and pronounced hopeless by the doctors. Each on a mattress on a stretcher, mostly in their khaki. They were the only cases not undressed in the admitting tent. Every hour or so, someone dying and being taken out, only to be followed by someone else in an hour or so. All we could do was try and get them to take nourishment, give injections to deaden pain, undress them and make them comfortable.[18]

Smith's unit, like many CCSs, was placed close to an observation balloon and experienced particularly fierce bombardment, as the German artillery attempted to destroy the balloon:

> On the afternoon of this same day, the Germans had been shelling the balloon pretty frequently and pieces were falling in different parts

of the camp. One large piece came down and buried itself in a tent between two patients, who were side by side on stretchers. It missed both and one of the patients was an elderly man, and was very much terrified, and practically suffered from shellshock all afternoon. His luck was further out however, as he was one of the patients killed by the bomb that night.[19]

The Third Battle of Ypres, like the Battle of the Somme, has entered the psyche of the British nation. The suffering of its troops has been immortalized by the writings of war poets such as Siegfried Sassoon and Wilfred Owen.[20] Even before the assault, CCSs and base hospitals were already under pressure, because the cold, wet conditions, which had turned the entire zone of the armies into a quagmire, had caused a great deal of sickness—particularly trench foot, which was reaching almost epidemic proportions. During the 'push' it became difficult to collect the wounded from the battlefield: six or eight men were sometimes needed to carry a single stretcher, and their progress would be slow as they waded through several feet of mud.[21] As a result, the incidence of anaerobic wound infections began, once more, to rise, along with the need for amputation of limbs. Many infections were so intractable that death was already inevitable when the patient arrived at the CCS. All that could be done was to place him in the moribund ward, offer him rest, nourishment, and emotional support, and wait for death. The Third Battle of Ypres was also characterized by an escalation in the use of chemical weapons, and by November CCSs and base hospitals were overflowing with patients, some suffering from multiple concurrent problems: wounds, gas poisoning, and illness.

At this time, a greater degree of specialization was brought into the system of casualty evacuation, with particular CCSs focusing on, for example, abdominal or chest wounds, in a way that would not have been possible without the logistical efficiency with which casualties were now labelled, sorted, and moved 'down the line'. At Brandhoek, just south of Poperinge, Kate Luard, as Sister-in-Charge

of No. 32 CCS, an Advanced Abdominal Centre, was supervising
well over thirty nurses. Abdominal surgery had undergone dramatic
improvement since the beginning of the war. In March 1915, a
number of innovative surgeons had begun to experiment with new
approaches in CCSs. Patients who faced certain death because of
the extent of their injuries underwent radical—and often quite
heroic—surgery.[22] At first, these patients' survival seemed almost
miraculous. Later, it became clear that their lives had been saved for
three reasons: the rapidity with which radical surgery had removed
infectious matter from their bodies; the skill of the specialist surgeons who treated them; and the expertise of the nurses who cared
for them pre- and post-operatively and assisted in their surgical operations. By the end of 1916, No. 32 CCS was viewed as one of the
most significant specialist emergency-treatment centres for such
cases, and Luard's position as its Head Sister was one of the most
responsible of the war. It was also one of the most dangerous: the
unit had been located to an area of Brandhoek between Poperinge
and Vlamertinge in late July 1917, to serve the 'push' that was to
become known as the 'Battle of Passchendaele' (see Figure 21).
Soon after arrival, its staff found that shells were flying over their
heads 'both ways'. American neurosurgeon Harvey Cushing commented in his diary that, 'if the coming push does not result in an
advance in the first few hours, they [the CCSs] will be heavily
bombarded'.[23]

No. 32 CCS was almost overwhelmed with patients during the
earliest days of the battle. Thirteen tables were operating, and
Luard had responsibility for a much larger number of staff than
was usual for a CCS. In early August, her unit nursed Noel Chavasse, a military surgeon and the only man to win two Victoria
Crosses during the First World War. Sadly, Chavasse died of his
injuries on 4 August. The nurse who cared for him during his final
hours was Ida Leedam, who had worked as a nurse at the Royal
Southern Hospital when he had been a registrar there. After his
death, she wrote a letter of condolence to his father:

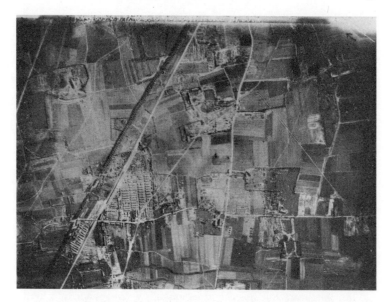

FIGURE 21 Aerial photograph of Brandhoek, taken in summer 1917 (photograph reproduced by kind permission of Talbot House, Poperinge, Belgium)

He was sitting up in bed...delighted at finding a Southern nurse for his night sister. The first night (August 2ⁿᵈ) he was with us, he passed a very comfortable night, sleeping off and on, talking now and then of the Southern days. The next day (August 3ʳᵈ) was also another comfortable day, sleeping off and on, worried a little about his men and servant (Rudd) who was very badly wounded (since dead)... I came on at night...At 11pm he became restless, pulse poor and asked me not to leave him...At 3am (August 4ᵗʰ) pulse much worse, still more restless but cheerful. At 4am became worse...These were his last words he ever spoke to me, 'Sister, write that letter for me', which I did and sent to Miss G. Chavasse. 'Give her my love, tell her Duty called and called me to obey'.[24]

The part of Brandhoek in which Nos. 32 and 44 British CCSs and No. 3 Australian CCS were located was close to an area known as 'Remy Siding'.[25] Because of its proximity to a munitions dump and a strategically important railhead, it was subjected to severe bombardment. On 21 August, 1917, the shells began to fall close to the units. Luard describes the terrible events that followed:

> The business began about 10am. Two came pretty close after each other and both just cleared us and No. 44. The third crashed between Sister E.'s ward in our lines and the Sisters' Quarters of No. 44. Bits came over everywhere, pitching at one's feet as we rushed to the scene of the action, and one just missed one of my Night Sisters getting into bed in our Compound. I knew by the crash where it must have gone and found Sister E. as white as paper but smiling happily and comforting the terrified patients. Bits tore through her Ward but hurt no one. Having to be thoroughly jovial to the patients on these occasions helps us considerably ourselves. Then I came on to the shell-hole and the wrecked tents in the Sisters' Quarters at 44. A group of stricken M.O.s were standing about and in one tent the Sister was dying. The piece went through her from back to front near her heart. She was only conscious a few minutes and only lived 20 minutes. She was in bed asleep. The Sister who shared her tent had been sent down the day before because she couldn't stand the noise and the day and night conditions. The Sister who should have been in the tent which was nearest was out for a walk or she would have been blown to bits; everything in her tent was; so it was in my empty Ward next to Sister E. It all made one feel sick.[26]

Nellie Spindler, the nurse who died, was a 26-year-old fully-trained nurse from Wakefield, Yorkshire. She was taken to nearby 'Remy Siding' and was buried in the military cemetery at Lijssenthoek. Many years later, the Commonwealth War Graves Commission erected a white marble headstone above her grave, referring to her as 'A Noble Type of Good Heroic Womanhood'. At the beginning of the twenty-first century, museums both at Lijssenthoek Cemetery and Talbot House, Poperinge were still celebrating her in terms of heroism and sacrifice, displaying faded images of propagandist newspaper clippings, which refer to the 'huns' barbarous conduct'. Visitors today can view her grave: 'the only woman in a silent white city of 11000 casualties'.[27]

Immediately after Spindler's death, an urgent meeting was held on the 'central duckboards' at No. 32 CCS, between Kate Luard, the commanding officers of Nos. 32 and 44, the Director of Medical Services, and the Quartermaster General. Luard urged total evacuation, but at first the general wanted No. 32 to remain. Fortuitously, a shell landed on the railway close by just as he was making his final decision. All patients and staff were evacuated from the area.

Harvey Cushing noted that three CCSs close to Remy Siding had been closed as 'untenable'.[28] Their loss created a huge gap in the surgical provision for severely wounded men who were still being moved 'down the line' from the Ypres Salient, and an attempt was made to reopen them: they remained active for several days, before their final closure in early September. With her work temporarily halted, Luard took a brief period of leave in Folkestone.

Australian nurse Gertrude Doherty was part of No. 3 Australian CCS, also based in Brandhoek. She was one of those who was evacuated and then returned days later to 'very heavy and strenuous work caused by the terrible hard fighting in front of Ypres'. British and American surgical teams joined the station and eight operating theatre tables were kept running day and night. Each team specialized in a different type of wound—one taking all head wounds, another all abdomen wounds, and so on.[29] In 1917, mustard gas was used for the first time. It caused severe chemical burns to the skin and mucous membranes, resulting in much greater damage to the airways than chlorine or phosgene. Mustard gas poisoning was difficult and laborious to treat. Burns had to be dressed using an aseptic technique and oxygen was needed to assist breathing.[30] During October, gas casualty figures were so high that a special unit for their treatment was established at Brandhoek.[31]

French field hospitals also established 'forward' units close to the front lines. The Scottish Women's Hospitals unit at Royaumont formed one at Villers-Cotterêts, which took wounded men directly from aid posts close to the trenches. The unit was overrun by the German advance in the summer of 1918, and had to be hastily evacuated.[32]


## Base hospitals

By 1917, the provision of nursing services on the Western Front was so complex that Maud McCarthy decided to hold a conference for all the 'overseas' Matrons-in-Chief. The meeting, at Abbeville, was attended by Margaret Macdonald (representing Canada), Grace Wilson (representing Australia), Mrs E. R. Creagh (representing South Africa), Mabel Thurston (representing New Zealand), and Bessie Bell (representing the USA).[33] Base hospitals continued to expand. Australian army nurse Elsie Tranter commented that the district of Camiers and Étaples was a 'regular city of huts and tents'. Her own hospital alone, 'No. 26', had 2,600 beds. She commented on how understaffed all hospitals were, observing that even if they could double their numbers, nurses would still be working under pressure.[34] During the Cambrai offensive, Elsie Dobson commented on the 'race' to get through her workload one night, when she was caring for large numbers of severely wounded men, many of them 'double amputations'. She and an orderly evacuated twenty-three 'acute surgical cases' from her ward, and were just clearing up the debris of 'soiled linen, ring cushions, splints, dressing buckets, carrell's tubes [*sic*], and such like' when they were informed that a new convoy was due to arrive in thirty minutes.[35] At such times nurses could only do what was possible and their focus was on the preservation of life.

Many nurses and VADs had experience of nursing German prisoners of war. One of the most vivid passages in Vera Brittain's *Testament of Youth* refers to her work in a 'German ward' at Étaples, where staff numbers were much reduced by comparison with the main wards, and where the sister-in-charge cared for her patients with a mixture of contempt and compassion.[36] The attitudes of nurses towards their prisoner-patients were often ambivalent. Australian nurse E. Steadman commented that 'Fritz made a good patient, but I am sure he had not the fine sensibilities of our own British boys. I have marvelled as I did amputation dressings, huge through and through gun shot wounds, penetrating chest wounds and Fritz never turned a hair.'[37] She added that nursing the Germans felt very different to nursing one's own wounded. The work was done with conscientious pride but 'without a vestige of sentiment'.[38]

The late summer and autumn of 1917 also saw an increase in enemy bombardments of bases in northern France. Prior to this, it had only really been nurses at CCSs who experienced severe bombardment. Now, nurses in base hospitals many miles from the front lines could be vulnerable to enemy attack from the air. One night, Australian nurse Ellen Cuthbert was awakened from a deep sleep by 'the noise of bursting shrapnel falling on the roofs of our quarters, which were shaking on their foundations, then everything began to fall on the floor photo frames and ink stands were two-stepping round the room and nose caps from anti-aircraft guns were also falling on the roofs'.[39] Cuthbert and her colleagues soon discovered that several bombs had fallen close to the railway line beside their billets. Such experiences were common for nurses in both British and French military hospitals, who soon learned to distinguish between the booming of their own anti-aircraft guns (often positioned very close to their quarters) and the explosion of the enemy's bombs.

Nurses were also working under difficult conditions at General Hospitals in Britain. Many seem to have appreciated the assistance of VADs, some of whom now had more than two years' experience in military hospitals. In 1917 US nurse Minnie Goodnow published a 'text-book for the auxiliary nurse'. Having served at the American Red Cross Hospital in Paris, Goodnow had considerable experience of supervising nursing assistants. She knew that such assistants lacked many of the advantages of trained nurses, whose years of experience as probationers had given them an understanding of how to 'handle' vulnerable patients. One of Goodnow's main concerns was to emphasize the ethic of caring inherent in such work:

> It must be borne in mind that the relationship between a sick man and his nurse is one which does not exist in ordinary life, and which must, therefore be governed by special rules. Nursing involves a certain amount of mothering, if you will, of handling the person, of a peculiar sort of intimacy new to both patient and nurse. There must be real friendliness without loss of respect, a fine balance between condescension and cordiality…The war nurse should, therefore, maintain a dignity and purity of life commensurate with the high purpose which everyone assumes her to possess.[40]

British nurse Violetta Thurstan devoted a whole section in her *Text Book of War Nursing* to 'The Probationer in a Military Hospital', including all inexperienced nurses in her readership. She acknowledged that the work was 'often arduous and monotonous', but added that 'the patients' health and comfort depend much on the services rendered by the junior nurse'.[41]

Even as professional nurses were coming to appreciate the needs of VADs for careful supervision and on-the-job training, VADs themselves were growing in confidence. Florence Egerton wrote to her mother on 26 August, of the patients at her hospital in Leicester:

> I want you to realise what the work is that calls and grips me. One boy of 20 has two fractured legs with gaping wounds and has had to be drugged till he's simple and is practically helpless. It takes 3 of us to make his bed. Another has a gash from the mouth, along the jaw (fractured), down the neck and on to shoulder. It is sewn up as far as the jaw and then all the length of the jaw is an open, dirty gash. It's the most gruesome thing I've seen. He also has a wound on one arm, on his ankle and his thigh and is as patient as a lamb. He never gets cross even over feeding which is just awful. Another has a shrapnel

wound in thigh and has also been gassed by the *new* gas. It's hellish—his body is literally scorched nearly black all over, while some parts, eg. legs and arms, face and neck are a mass of blister as from burns. His eyes are made up and his voice nearly gone. Yet he still smiles. Those are the worst, but the others each have more than one wound. In all, we have 24 patients for dressings in a morning—a few at night according to how they feel, and 27 beds, backs and washing of helpless patients in an evening.[42]

Egerton's reference to the *new* gas illustrates one of the new challenges facing nurses in 1917. On 13 July, the Germans had used dichlor-ethyl-sulphide, or 'mustard gas', for the first time. Its effects were to burn the skin and respiratory tract, and to violently inflame the eyes.[43] Its worst effects were on areas of skin which had been in contact with clothing, or where the victim had been sweating. These areas were affected by the 'mass of blisters' referred to by Egerton and were intensely painful. Patients affected by mustard gas were helpless and required both careful pain relief and total nursing care.

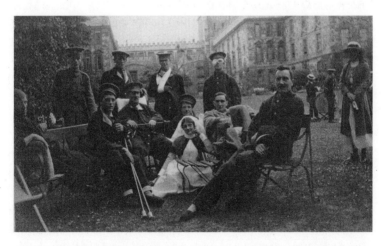

FIGURE 22 Sister Isabel Wace with convalescent patients at New College, Oxford, UK (photograph reproduced by kind permission of Judy Burge)

Throughout Britain, nurses were struggling to care for patients in a range of settings—some more suited to hospital work than others. Nellie Morrice was made a head sister at No. 3 AGH in Brighton. Space was scarce and one of her wards of 100 beds was placed underground. As many of the patients were suffering from nephritis, Morrice found the conditions highly unsuitable.[44] In England, at Cobham Hall, an officers' hospital, Australian Matron Nellie Gould was experiencing an acute shortage of staff, and was finding that orderlies who had been well trained by experienced nursing sisters could perform valuable work. In a later narrative, she remembered 'L.Cpl Browne, a Queenslander who was a gentleman, a true nurse and all that is best in a bona fide Australian. He was originally a gunner, but after over a year in France had bronchitis and had to be invalided to England, nothing daunted he faced the guns of orderly life and made a complete success of it. He had his 21st birthday while I was there.'[45]

## Romania's ordeal

Born Marie Alexandra Victoria on 29 October 1875, 'Queen Marie of Roumania' had impeccable royal credentials: she was a granddaughter of both Queen Victoria of Great Britain and Alexander II of Russia. Marie married Ferdinand of Romania on 10 January, 1893, at the age of only 17, and chose to become deeply involved in the nationalist sentiments of 'her' people—an ethnic group inhabiting not only the 'Kingdom of Roumania' but also many of the lands held by the Austro-Hungarian Empire. Her memoir, *Ordeal: The Story of My Life*, is one of the most interesting—though possibly distorted—accounts of Romania's involvement in the First World War.[46] The majority of Romanians were profoundly attached to the idea of the unification of their territories to create a 'Greater Roumania'. Marie, whose natural allegiance was to the allies of the Triple Entente, became a symbol of their patriotic hopes, and is said to have been instrumental in arguing for Romania's entry into the war on the Allied side. Her husband's more natural affinities were with the Central Powers, but he too recognized the huge groundswell of opinion in favour of the Allies and against the Autro-Hungarian Empire within his nation.

Marie's anxiety to be of use to her people infused her actions during the war, but her account of her involvement in Romania's war makes incongruous reading for a modern audience. She writes of how she longed to establish her own hospital in Romania's war-time capital, Jassy, but found herself to be more useful visiting hospitals and distributing small gifts to the wounded; of how difficult it was to live in a private railway carriage whilst her palatial residence at Jassy was being prepared; of how she was so busy on one particular day that she almost had no time to 'dress for dinner'; and of how she wore a snow-white dress, with a red cross emblazoned on the chest and a flowing veil as a symbol of her patriotism and service to the nation, but viewed with passive despair the legions of typhus-carrying lice which infested her country's field hospitals.

Marie believed that her greatest contribution to her country's war effort was her ability to raise the morale of its troops. Some might argue that she was, in fact, one of the most powerful propagandists of the conflict. She was clearly adored by her people—or, at least, her own memoir speaks eloquently of her sense that they loved her and believed she belonged to them. When she visited the wounded and asked about their suffering, the reply was often: ' "Yes, I am suffering, but never mind as long as you become Empress of all the Roumanians" '. She added, however, as an honest rider to this statement, that not all of the wounded expressed either love or joy:

> They keep looking at me when I enter a room as though all their eyes took possession of me; a strange weight to carry, the look of so many eyes—I never knew it would be so heavy. All those eyes, one after another, staring up at me, some with love, some with astonishment, some with sad indifference, some with joy which lights up their faces, some with mute pain, some as though calling for help, but one and all resigned, terribly resigned.[47]

Queen Marie of Romania appears to have genuinely wanted to do her duty and support the cause of her nation. She and the aristocratic ladies who assisted her, clearly acted with courage and energy, within the limits of what was considered appropriate for 'ladies'. She recounts how, on one occasion a man with a severe thigh injury was brought into a military hospital bleeding to death, and remarks on how 'her' ladies 'behaved admirably, everybody volunteering to help, even those least accustomed to such sights'.[48] One cannot help wondering how the surgeon coped with such an influx of genteel offers of support, whilst struggling to repair a torn artery. And yet, the symbolism of the 'queen-nurse' was clearly a potent one: 'they feel less forsaken, less in danger, less unprotected when I suddenly appear in their midst', she asserted.[49] And Marie's genuine compassion is revealed by her refusal to wear rubber gloves when visiting the wounded during Romania's great typhus epidemic in the winter of 1916/17, because 'the soldiers all kiss my hand, and I really cannot ask them to kiss India-rubber!'[50] On another occasion she expresses her fear and horror of the lice that infested the wards:

> I am not exaggerating when I say that they were covered from head to foot with lice! At first I could not understand what was that white sand or dust which lay in every fold of their clothes, and could hardly believe it when I was told that it was neither dust nor sand, but lice! And it was those lice, it seems, which carried the typhus infection! This was the first time I thoroughly understood how dangerous this was, because how could I defend myself against an insect no larger than a grain of sand?[51]

Romania's history of the war is a remarkable one, and Marie's own story is intimately entwined with it. That she chose to dress as a nurse and 'care' for the wounded illustrates how powerful the symbol of the 'warrior-nurse' was: it reassured, and gave an almost fanatical belief in the rightness of their cause to those who had entered into a contract with their state to fight against a powerful enemy, when their odds of survival were desperately poor.

## Nursing on the Eastern Front

Katherine Hodges, an ambulance-driver-turned-volunteer-nurse, had served with the Scottish Women's Hospitals on the Romanian Front before being evacuated to Petrograd. In the winter of 1916, she joined a Russian field hospital run by a female doctor on the Galician Front, finding herself placed in an epidemic hospital close to Zaleschiki, a 'terribly devastated' village on the banks of the River Dniester. Driving by sleigh to her posting, through the devastated zone close to the front, she reflected on 'the dreadfully sinister effect of a vast cemetery of soldiers' graves along the road, the black wooden crosses sticking out of the white snow in a tragic, desolate manner. Destroyed, splintered woods, barbed wire entanglements, huge shell holes, devastated villages, all the refuse of war exposed itself as mile after mile slowly unfurled before us.'[52]

Hodges—an untrained volunteer-nurse—appears to have found her experience in an epidemic hospital close to the front lines truly daunting, although the spirit of her diary is one of determination to view the experience as a 'great adventure'. Caring for patients with infectious fevers was one of the most intense and skilful types of nursing in an era before antibiotics and Hodges was clearly out of her depth. She encountered patients with diseases ranging from the louse-borne typhus fever, through severe skin infections such as erysipelas, to dangerous airborne diseases such as diphtheria, scarlet fever, and measles. But it was a local epidemic of the deadly 'black smallpox' that proved most frightening. Her doctor-friend had practised vaccination techniques on Hodges so many times that she felt sure that she was protected against the disease, but when she woke up one morning with a rash all over her face and body, she was terrified. Her complaint proved to be rheumatic fever, contracted during the long, cold journey to Zaleschiki.

Smallpox was not the only epidemic disease to wreak havoc on the Eastern Front. The macabre quality of Hodges's diary is heightened when she describes a night spent caring for one of the hospital's doctors, who was dying of influenza. The Russian general commanding their sector of the front insisted that the doctor should have a full military funeral, and her dead body was borne a mile and a half to the graveside, propped up in her coffin, with her mourners following behind: 'it was agonisingly cold and the dreadful macabre effect of poor Dr F's nodding head and shoulders, which moved as the coffin jolted as the officers marched, haunts me still'.[53]

During the summer of 1917, Hodges was moved to a surgical hospital near the front, where she encountered the dressing techniques used by Russian surgeons and nurses. Typically, and in contrast to the wet antiseptic dressings and irrigation techniques in use on the Western Front, wounds were tightly packed with dressings of iodine-soaked gauze, which were left in place for several days. Such techniques had become common practice out of necessity, because of the long train journeys between front-line flying columns and base hospitals in cities. A dressing was required which could be left in place and which would not shift and expose the wound if disturbed. British nurses commented on the suffering of patients when the dressings were, finally, removed. Typically, they stuck to the inner surfaces of wounds and had to be 'ripped away', taking much healthy tissue with them.[54]

Some of Katherine Hodges's most harrowing stories relate to patients whose suffering could not be controlled, because of the extent of their wounds and a shortage of morphia. In one 'appallingly dreadful' episode she witnessed the pain of a patient whose head wound was being dressed and whose piercingly shrill scream she described as 'the sound produced from a human being in a state of agony, which eliminated reason'. Hodges, the volunteer, was often delegated to hold the hands of patients whose painful dressings were being performed. She commented that her arms were severely bruised from the 'frenzied grips' of the suffering men. Because it was common for patients to have been left for several hours—sometimes days— on the battlefield, many wounds were severely infected, and some also infested with maggots. For many—particularly the gas gangrene cases—amputation was the only solution.[55]

## History in the making: witnessing the Russian Revolution

On 4 March 1917, Canadian nurse Dorothy Cotton, based with the Anglo-Russian Hospital in Petrograd, wrote home about the extraordinary events taking place in that city. The Russian imperial flag was being torn down and replaced with the red flag of the Revolution. Hospital staff were ordered by men 'with fixed bayonets' to remove the imperial insignia from their hospital.[56]

Days later, nurses on the Eastern Front began to hear news of the events taking place in Petrograd. At first there were rumours that the Tsar had abdicated; then soldiers began to hear news of 'revolution', and frequent spontaneous celebrations were common. By late March army discipline was beginning to break down. Well-organized army units were turning into 'straggling groups of soldiers'.[57] Katherine Hodges heard that desertions were due to the circulation of a rumour that every man could choose whatever land he wanted from within his own village; this led to a mass exodus from the army as each man 'tore off in the direction of home as fast as he could go to grab the best bit of land'. No one bought rail tickets any more; they simply boarded any train they could, resulting in overcrowding and, sometimes, violent scenes at railway stations.

The downfall of the tsarist government in March 1917 did not put an end to Russia's Great War. In spite of the early breakdown in discipline in some areas and widespread fear among officers that they would not be able to control their troops, fighting continued along the Eastern Front. During the period between the March and October Revolutions Katherine Hodges found herself moved from her epidemic hospital to a surgical hospital closer to the front lines. It was here that she began to encounter the wounds of war. Once again, she was 'terribly nervous and worried', despite the stalwart help and support of the 'very capable and experienced sister' under whom she worked, who was 'wonderfully good and patient with my stupidity'.[58] Hodges's narratives of the surgical hospital are, if anything, even more shocking than her descriptions of the epidemic hospital. One story, in particular, stands out both as witness-testimony to the horrors of war and as an illustration of the importance of skilled nursing care. One day, in the dressing room, after massive wounds to a patient's torso had been dressed, the sister asked Hodges to 'rub his back'—a euphemism for providing pressure area care to the buttocks—and return him to bed. As the two turned the patient, they discovered that his back was covered in dirty dressings. Hodges was instructed to soak these away, to reveal the patient's hidden wounds:

> I couldn't think what was wrong with it. One shoulder, part of the spine and one hip were nothing but large, open suppurating wounds and in the middle of them something gleamed that looked to me like mother of pearl. I called E. She came across, gave one look and said '*My God!*' The Mother of Pearl stuff was *bone*. These wounds were bedsores, and his hipbone, shoulder blade and several vertebrae were completely exposed. It was terrible. We couldn't think why he seemed so sensitive to pain right down in the groin of the uninjured leg. E. thought there must be something wrong somewhere of which we had no report, so she examined him thoroughly, found that he was septic and that the affected part was a bullet! He had been in the hospital about six weeks and Heaven knows how long the bullet had been there. We cleaned that up and at last got the poor soul back to bed. We fought and fought over him, but he died eventually, E. said as much from the bedsores as from his wounds.[59]

On 4 March 1917, Florence Farmborough, still based with a letuchka close to the front lines, heard the news of the Tsar's abdication with dismay. Although the Revolution appeared to be a bloodless coup, and although she recognized the patriotism of Kerensky and other revolutionaries, she shared the grief of her fellow nurses that their Tsar had been humiliated; as members of the elite, most were stalwart royalists. She also began to recognize that the Central Powers had 'embarked on an artful ruse to spread unrest among Russia's fighting men in the trenches'.[60] Soldiers being brought into the field hospitals were beginning to display an apathy not seen before; they seemed utterly war-weary, no longer caring about the conflict's outcome. While her unit was at Podgaytsy, she went to hear Kerensky, later acknowledging in her diary that he was a great orator: 'His sincerity was unquestionable; and his eloquence literally hypnotised us.'[61] But not even Kerensky's stirring patriotism could halt the slow and corrosive decline in morale which was infecting the Russian armies: a decline that would soon turn into a complete breakdown in military discipline. A new offensive was launched and the letuchka was once again overwhelmed with work. This time, though, for Farmborough, the suffering of the wounded seemed insupportable, and her work meaningless. Decades later, her evocative writing—drawing upon her original diary—was to capture this new sense of hopelessness:

> I went into the large tent where the heavily wounded were lying. Two torches provided a dim illumination and a lighted candle flickered on the small table in the middle of the tent. I sat at the little wooden table and tried not to be upset by the groans and cries of pain. There was a dreadful smell of pus and gangrene. Two men with smashed stomachs had just died…Not far [away] was a little stout man in a half-sitting position; the rattling noise in his throat was dreadful to hear. He had been shot through the right lung and his open wound was big enough to insert my fingers. The usual injection of morphia had little or no effect and his frightened eyes were gazing at me with a great pleading in them.[62]

Farmborough began to feel that there was no longer any real value in her work. Her disillusionment mirrored that of the troops her unit was serving. Some were refusing to return to the trenches after rest periods.

As army discipline broke down, hospital sanitars became disorderly and disobedient.[63] Katherine Hodges commented that 'a general discontent was slowly seeping through the troops around us', who were, increasingly, questioning the purpose of the fight. At the end of June, upon returning to the epidemic hospital at Zaleschiki, Hodges found that orderlies were 'lazy and indifferent'. A dispute with the new matron led her to resign from the hospital and return to Petrograd via Kiev, where she witnessed the beginnings of the Ukrainian uprising.[64] By now, all journeys were made in overcrowded, often rowdy, trains and it was difficult for foreigners to obtain the papers they needed. It was only with difficulty that Hodges managed to return to England, via Finland and Sweden. En route, she once again enjoyed the hospitality of the Anglo-Russian Hospital. While in Petrograd, she witnessed mass rallies and frequent unrest in the streets. Food was becoming scarce, and agitators were distributing guns and ammunition from lorries in the streets of the city—even to small boys, who 'popped them off' causing several deaths.[65] Dorothy Seymour, who had been placed at the Anglo-Russian Hospital in September 1916, managed to get onto a train leaving Petrograd for Finland, eventually reaching Aberdeen, after a rough and dangerous sea-crossing from Bergen.[66]

Farmborough's journey back to England was even more tortuous. It was not until March 1918 that she realized her work in Russia was at an end. The Treaty of Brest-Litovsk had been signed and Russia—no longer at war with the Central Powers—was about to tear itself apart in civil war. After struggling on crowded trains to reach Moscow, Farmborough boarded one of the last goods trains to take Westerners across Siberia to Vladivostock. Here, she embarked for the USA from where she eventually reached England.[67]

Few Western nurses remained in Russia until the signing of the armistice of Brest-Litovsk. Many left long before this, as it became obvious that Russia was descending into chaos. One rare individual—Margaret Barber—decided to offer her services to a Bolshevik relief agency. Barber was a professional nurse, who had travelled east to care for civilians in Armenia, but had been forced to leave as the Turks advanced into that country. After a short time at the Anglo-Russian Hospital, she had joined a 'Friends'' relief unit travelling to the village of Buzuluk in Samara. Her posting was extremely remote; the train journey took fifty-six hours, followed by a drive of 57 miles across the steppe. Barber, like many British nurses, was clearly captivated by the remarkable landscape of the Russian steppe and the extraordinary way of life of its people, and would later write of her experiences in romantic tones. En route to Samara Province, she sighted 'the Volga by moonlight, a broad, ample, stretch of water so majestic that one felt quite awed by it'.[68] The steppe itself, she found to be 'a vast plain looking just like the sea'. In winter, snowstorms known as 'burans' would blow up, and snow would drift across the one track across this bleak landscape: 'During a buran the church bells are tolled all night to act as a guide to those within earshot, but often the drivers can only leave it to the horses' instinct...Many cases which we could not decide were dead or alive were brought into our hospitals after these storms.'[69]

When news of revolution reached Buzuluk, its inhabitants reacted with 'mild apprehension and astonishment'. At first the local Cossacks' threat to resist the revolutionaries aroused great fear, because it was known that they 'spared no one when they fought', but eventually it was heard that the Cossacks had, for the time being, decided to accept the new regime. In the event: 'the Revolution affected us very little. We were simply told by the peasants one morning at our dispensary that there was no Tsar, and this was afterwards corroborated by the local paper. The returning soldiers held meetings on the market place, assuring us that the millennium had come, and that we were now all free.' On 16 May 1918, Barber's unit returned to Moscow, as local doctors and nurses began to come home from the war. In Moscow, food was scarce and it was now almost impossible to get back to Britain, as lines of communication had been broken. Yet, Barber appears to have experienced a strange sense of comfort amongst the Bolsheviks. In spite of having to live in poor quarters and queue for food, she enjoyed calling 'everyone, man or woman, high official or potato man "tavarish" or comrade'. She witnessed the procession of Red Guards and workers' unions in Moscow, which marked the anniversary of the Revolution. 'One felt', she commented, 'that Bolshevism had got a firm hold on the people when the huge crowds joined in singing the "International" as they dispersed.'[70] In August 1918, she left for Astrakhan, as part of a Bolshevik relief unit to Armenia. Here she nursed civilians during a typhus epidemic, until forced to leave. Her work for the Bolsheviks was arousing suspicion amongst the local 'Whites' and she was informed by the British that her situation was 'serious' and that she would not be allowed to return to Bolshevik Russia. She was escorted to Britain via Constantinople, where she was declared a 'sick sister' and placed in the military hospital at Woolwich, until able to convince the staff that she was neither a military nurse nor ill. At the end of her book, Barber listed the reported atrocities of the Russian Civil War, concluding that these had been committed on both sides, although she herself had not witnessed any. She added:

> It is sad to think of those banished Armenians in Astrakan still longing to return to their homes and wondering why I have not kept my promise to come back. This I am prevented from doing; nor can I send them any message. I fear their faith in the British must be shaken.[71]

The closing of Russia's borders was a traumatic event for many Western nurses who appear to have felt a genuine and deep love for their adopted country. Russia was to remain isolated for the remainder of their lifetimes, and none would ever return. For one nurse, Mary Britnieva, an Anglo-Russian born in Petrograd, Russia was actually her homeland. She had married the Russian head doctor of her letuchka just after the war. Britnieva tried to remain in Russia, struggling to safeguard the survival of a young family through Bolshevik rule, civil war, and famine. She was eventually forced by tuberculosis to travel—a refugee—to England, via Finland, where she and her children were able to build a new life with her

British relatives. Her autobiography, *One Woman's Story*, is tinged with grief and nostalgia. Written in 1934, it conveys her sense of a lost world. In 1930, her last link with Russia was broken when her husband was shot as a spy by the Stalinist regime.[72]

## With the doughboys in France: American base hospitals on the Western Front

For the first two and a half years of the Great War, US opinion had been divided over whether the country should join the Allied side. The official government line was that the conflict taking place across the channel was a 'European war', and was not the business of the USA. Nevertheless, the sympathies of the majority of US citizens were with the Allies—particularly the French, with whom they had felt a particular affinity since the American Revolution. By 1917, these sympathies had already been reflected in the movement of large numbers of volunteers across the Atlantic, many working under the auspices of the American Red Cross, as ambulance drivers, nurses, and hospital volunteers, some joining the Allied forces as combatants.[73]

As early as April 1916, George Crile, Professor of Surgery at Western Reserve University in Cleveland, Ohio, had suggested that American university hospitals should form units that would act as 'base hospitals' in the event of a US declaration of war. The idea was greeted with some enthusiasm and large hospitals began to organize along the lines proposed by Crile. When the long-awaited declaration came on 6 April 1917, very little work was required to bring several US military base hospitals to a state of readiness.[74] Typically, the unit's medical staff were drawn from the hospital itself, and a senior nurse (often the existing superintendent or matron) was invited to form a corps of nurses who would act under the joint auspices of the Army Nurse Corps and the American Red Cross.[75] These nurses were exclusively white and middle class; none of the 1,000 trained black nurses who had enrolled with the Red Cross were permitted to nurse overseas, although some cared for black patients in base hospitals in the US.[76] Hospital orderlies—known as 'corpsmen'—were recruited locally. Corpsmen were not officially under the command of nurses but, on 14 April 1918, a letter was circulated from the surgeon general's office to all base hospitals declaring that 'head nurses' were to be in command of their wards, with all staff deferring to them.[77]

In the spring of 1917 American nurse-leaders had begun to recognize the potentially very serious problem of a shortage of suitably trained nurses to staff US base hospitals. They began to debate the wisdom of hiring volunteer nurses similar to the British VADs. In March 1917, even before the US had entered the war, the idea had been put forward that the nursing workforce should be supplemented with bona fide student-nurses rather than with volunteers. This could be achieved, it was argued, by the establishment of an Army School of Nursing (ASN), whose probationers would act as untrained carers whilst obtaining an apprenticeship-style training in a number of military base hospitals.[78] The decision of US nurses to use students rather than VADs as assistant nurses is an intriguing one, which can be attributed in large part to the determination of nurse leaders such as Annie Warburton Goodrich (President of the American Nursing Association), Adelaide Nutting (Director of the Department of Nursing and Health at Teacher's College Columbia University), and Lillian Wald (Honorary President of the National Organization of Public Health Nurses). These and other influential nurses formed an emergency committee, which undertook a rapid survey of the nursing services available in the spring of 1917. They were able to deflect a Council of National Defense initiative to employ volunteer nurses in military hospitals by demonstrating that both volunteer nurses and enlisted men provided a substandard service in comparison to probationer nurses under the supervision of fully trained graduates. They also pointed out that the war had created an upsurge in enthusiasm for nursing among young women, which should be tapped in order to support a sustainable future for the US nursing services. Such a service would be in striking contrast to the British model, where the eventual departure of a temporary workforce would leave the profession bereft of experienced staff at the end of the war.[79]

At a conference attended by both influential nurses and senior members of the army medical services, the nurses' arguments proved convincing, and Surgeon General William Gorgas recommended to the Secretary of War that the need for a rapid expansion of the nursing workforce should be achieved by the formation of the ASN. The scheme was approved in late May 1918. It was recognized that the care of sick and wounded soldiers had suffered as a result of a lack of trained nurses during both the American Civil War (1861–5) and the Spanish-American War (1898). 'Enlisted men' had been used as nurses' aides, but the ratio of trained to untrained carers had clearly been inadequate. It was recognized that 'careful nursing' was a highly labour-intensive practice, which needed to be undertaken under close supervision. Typhoid patients, in particular, had died unnecessarily in their thousands because untrained carers were unaware of their patients' needs for special diets to protect their intestinal tracts from ulceration and perforation and for support with hygiene and toileting to avoid collapse.[80]

Annie Warburton Goodrich was appointed Head of the ANS, which was located in the office of the Surgeon General, but supported students in numerous base hospitals in the USA. Goodrich was later to acknowledge that the war had ended before it had been possible for nurses from the School to play much of a part in it. Nevertheless, by November 1918, it had a student body of 1,600, many of whom had given important nursing care to sick and injured soldiers in base hospitals at home. More importantly, the ASN did survive well into the 1930s as a nurse-training institution of high quality, providing nurses for both military and civilian practice.[81]

One of the medical units formed in the spring of 1917 was located at the University of Virginia, Charlottesville, which was, on

23 June 1917, given the official designation 'Base Hospital No. 41'. Its formation was driven by Dr William Goodwin; it ran entirely independently, and much of its funding was provided by a patriotic society calling itself the 'Benevolent and Protective order of the Elks of the US'. Margaret Cowling, who had travelled to Austria two years earlier as part of the Red Cross relief effort to Europe, had enjoyed a successful civilian career and was, by now, the University of Virginia Hospital's Superintendent of Nurses (see Figure 23). In an account written after the war, Cowling was to recount how

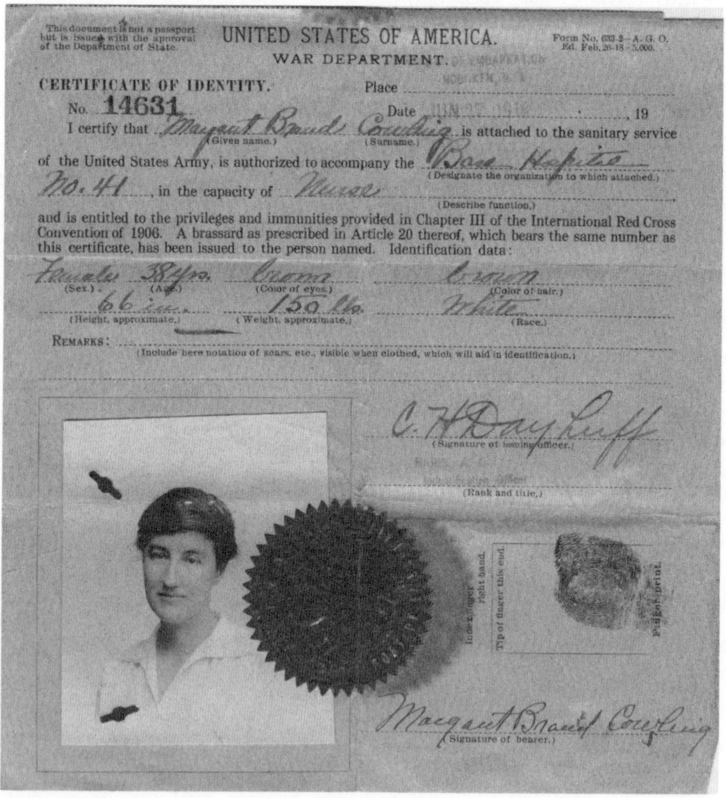

This document is not a passport but is issued with the approval of the Department of State.

UNITED STATES OF AMERICA.

Form No. 633-2—A. G. O. Ed. Feb. 26-18—5,000.

WAR DEPARTMENT.

CERTIFICATE OF IDENTITY.

Place

No. 14631

Date ..., 19

I certify that Margaret Brand Cowling (Given name.) (Surname.) is attached to the sanitary service of the United States Army, is authorized to accompany the Base Hospital No. 41 (Designate the organization to which attached.), in the capacity of Nurse (Describe function.) and is entitled to the privileges and immunities provided in Chapter III of the International Red Cross Convention of 1906. A brassard as prescribed in Article 20 thereof, which bears the same number as this certificate, has been issued to the person named. Identification data:

Female (Sex.) 38 yrs. (Age.) Brown (Color of eyes.) Brown (Color of hair.)

66 in. (Height, approximate.) 150 lbs. (Weight, approximate.) White (Race.)

REMARKS: (Include here notation of scars, etc., visible when clothed, which will aid in identification.)

C. H. Day Luff (Signature of issuing officer.)

(Rank and title.)

Index finger right hand. Tip of finger this end. Finger print.

Margaret Brand Cowling (Signature of bearer.)

FIGURE 23 Margaret Cowling's Certificate of Identity (image reproduced by kind permission of the Claude Moore Health Sciences Library, the University of Virginia, Charlottesville, VA, USA)

Dr Goodwin had invited her to act as 'Chief Nurse' to the rapidly forming base hospital. She agreed readily and created a nursing corps of 100 members, who underwent several months' preliminary experience in military hospitals in the US before travelling to New York on 20 June 1918 for mobilization.[82]

Margaret Cowling's motives for entering war service are not obvious, but seem to have had more to do with her love for her work than with patriotism. For someone with Cowling's experience, the invitation to lead a corps of military nurses to France was an opportunity to meet the challenges of a new and testing clinical leadership position. She was one of the few nurses—indeed one of the few individuals from any background—who provided practical support to both the Central Powers and the Allies during the course of the war. Whatever her motives, she clearly impressed her commanding officer with her apparent aptitude for military discipline. At the end of the war, Lieutenant Colonel Julian Cabell wrote to Stephen Watts, then Director of the University of Virginia Hospital, of 'the exceptionally efficient duty performed by Miss Margaret B. Cowling as Chief Nurse of the University of Virginia Base Hospital'. Cowling had apparently shown 'wonderfully good judgment' in staffing the hospital's wards, some of which were very large, housing almost 200 patients. Cabell's view was that Cowling

> deserves the very highest praise for the way she handled the nurses in general. As they were all graduate nurses, you can well understand how hard it was for them to appreciate the importance of military discipline and they naturally felt that they were being put back into a training school. Her service in this way was, however, most satisfactory...When it seemed impossible to look after more wounded in any sort of way with our personnel, which was estimated to be sufficient for 1000 beds only, we were ordered to expand rapidly up to nearly 3000 beds. Under these circumstances, when additional wards of from 300 to 400 beds were opened up, Miss Cowling always quietly complied with orders...I cannot begin to give Miss Cowling sufficient praise for the really wonderful results she accomplished

under the adverse condition of such rapid expansion in tent wards, which were pitched in muddy fields.[83]

A very different view of Cowling was offered by one of her own staff: Camilla Louise Wills (see Figure 24). A very young graduate of nursing, having just completed her diploma at the University of Virginia Hospital when Base Hospital No. 41 was formed, Wills was delighted to be chosen by her matron to join the war effort. She travelled with her unit's nurses, first to Camp Dix, New Jersey, to prepare for active service, then to New York for embarkation to Europe. She wrote numerous letters home to her aunt, one of which, written during the voyage to Europe, offered an ambivalent view of Margaret Cowling's leadership: 'Miss Cowling is not making herself very popular among the girls and I'm afraid we are going to have some trouble—but for Heaven's sake don't tell that. She has been very nice to me so far, so I'm trying to keep out of things.'[84]

Wills's perspective on wartime service appears to have been coloured by the optimism of youth and her own adventurous nature. Her diary and letters resonate with a sense of excitement. Although letters home to relatives often sanitized the less palatable aspects of wartime experience, Wills appears to have genuinely enjoyed 'roughing it' at Camp Dix, where she shared a dormitory with about forty other nurses and spent much of her time enduring 'red tape— physical examinations etc'.[85] The realities of war seem to have been far away in this large American base hospital. She enjoyed her stay in New York, awaiting embarkation for Europe, spending much of the time sightseeing, shopping, and visiting the theatre. Jennifer Casavant Telford has observed that the opportunity to become part of the American war effort was 'limited to those from upper-middle-class families with the means to support their endeavour'.[86] American nurses, such as Wills, were obliged to buy their own uniform and camp equipment and to take $50 dollars worth of gold with them overseas. Even Wills—clearly a young woman of some means—was obliged to borrow money from her aunt to fund all of this.[87]

After her arrival in France, Wills was to discover the real nature of wartime nursing and found herself part of a cadre of
trained staff each of whom cared for a ward full of desperately
wounded men with the help only of semi-trained orderlies. The
ultimate success of Base Hospital No. 41 is, in large part, a testament to the hard work and self-discipline of its staff. It seems
likely that Margaret Cowling's somewhat strict approach to discipline was a response to the understandable stresses of her position in charge of over 100 young women working in a foreign
country in dangerous circumstances. The need to follow orders,
even when it meant accepting inadequate staffing levels on wards
caring for the most seriously-injured and acutely-ill patients,
seems to have been accepted as part of 'active service'. Cowling
probably tolerated conditions which she might have found un-
acceptable in peacetime, because she saw herself fighting 'against
the odds' at a time of acute humanitarian crisis, when resources
simply were not available. In such times, it seems, poor conditions
and understaffing were simply seen as part of the 'great struggle
for civilization'. Julia Stimson, Matron of Base Hospital No. 21
(Washington University, St Louis) seems to have taken a similarly
positive approach to difficult work in trying circumstances. Writing
home to her family, she expressed satisfaction—even joy—at
finding herself at the heart of one of the greatest 'dramas' the
world had ever seen.[88] Stimson, like Cowling, enjoyed excellent
relationships with both medical officers and her own nursing
staff. She went on to become chief nurse of the American Red
Cross in France and then director of the nursing services for the
American Expeditionary Force.[89]

Not all American chief nurses enjoyed such harmony with their
medical colleagues. Historian Kimberley Jensen has argued that
their lack of officer status exposed some senior nurses to harassment and bullying.[90] 'I am sorry to say', wrote Camilla Louise
Wills, 'the officers of our unit are not as nice to the nurses as a
whole as they should be.' Wills and her colleagues socialized much

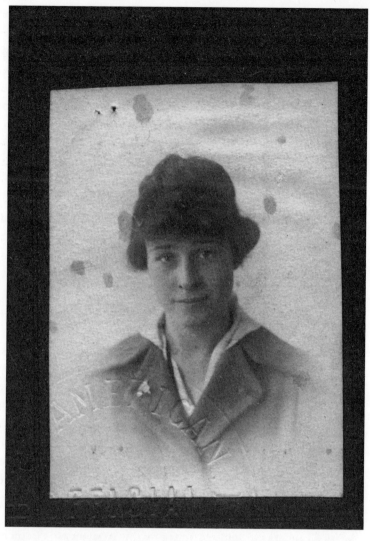

FIGURE 24 Photograph of Camilla Louise Wills, from her Certificate of Identity (photograph reproduced by kind permission of the Eleanor Crowder Bjoring Center for Nursing Historical Inquiry, the University of Virginia, Charlottesville, VA, USA)

more easily with the corpsmen of their unit, many of whom were
university students of a similar age and social background to themselves: 'Of course we are not allowed to go with the enlisted men
socially but I can certainly say that I have found some far superior
men among the privates since landing here than among the
officers.'[91]

Their position as important executors of treatment and care,
with no clear role or status, left nurses of all nationalities vulnerable to being at best ignored, at worst victimized, and although it
appears that relationships between nurses, orderlies, and medical
officers (particularly in US military hospitals) were, for the most
part, cordial, the obvious disadvantages of their weak status and
position drove many nurses to pursue better working conditions
and political recognition, through state registration and educational reform, after the war.

## In Italy

Military hospitals in Italy took casualties from highly destructive
campaigns such as that being fought on the Isonzo Front, where
repeated assaults led to multiple, severe casualties. There is very
little extant evidence in English about the work of nurses in Italian
military hospitals, and there appears to be a dearth of research
into the work of Italian nurses. Two British volunteer nurses have
left accounts of their work in northern Italy. Sybil Reeves had
joined a voluntary aid detachment in London in 1914. In 1915, she
had assisted in a mental nursing home in Bedford, at the West End
Hospital for Nerves and Shell-Shocked Soldiers, Bulstrode Street,
London, and in the soldiers' wards of the Westminster Hospital.
Eventually, in the spring of 1916, she was given a much-wanted
overseas posting at Villa Trento near Cormons in Italy, as part of
the First British Ambulance Unit. Vera Woodroffe, another VAD,
was posted to a mobile radiographic unit donated by the British
Red Cross Society to the Italian medical services in the same

sector. In a letter to her mother, Woodroffe referred to her work as 'killingly funny', and observed that she could really have 'done with much more work':[92]

> We rush about in Fiat ambulances the back of which is covered with apparatus...The roads are perilously precipitous and one dashes down a perpendicular hill round a corner at right angles and find the very narrow road thick with carriages or else a battalion of Alpini trampling along in marching kit most picturesque...we dash up to a large building built round a square immaculately white with pink oleanders growing up in the courtyard are met by various Italian MOs alternately looking like Nero or one of the Apostles with liver complaint who salute...insist on shaking hands all round very fatiguing...Our 2 orderlies with the help of some hospital pia-toni carry in the apparatus we get the circuit arranged and wired up while the orderlies leap about the room and nail up blankets...the coil is put through the window or door and Tordella runs the dy-namo from the car outside. We then get down to it and X ray Ital-ians of all shapes and sizes grades and wounds...When matters are over they invite us into their mess to drink coffee or ice cream and we chat politely...shake hands and dash off to the next where exactly the same proceedings take place.[93]

That autumn life became much less relaxed. In August 1917, Sybil Reeves was posted to a first line clearing and dressing station at Dolegna, 2 miles from Caporetto, and, following the overwhelming German victory that autumn, was forced to join the mass retreat as far as Vicenza, before boarding a train for Milan and safety.[94] Vera Woodroffe too, was experiencing a much busier time, although her letters remained upbeat: she was witnessing 'frightfully interesting and magnificent surgery against tremendous odds but it is mar-velous what is saved from the wreckage'.[95]

After the war, Sybil Reeves was one of the few VADs who en-rolled as a nurse probationer at St Thomas's Hospital, London. Unfortunately, she was forced to give up her training, following a severe attack of peritonitis and septicaemia.[96]

## Disaster at sea: the sinking of the *Mongolian*

In 1917, Eveline Vickers-Foote, an Australian who had been placed
with the QAIMNS, decided to return to Australia to attempt to
re-enlist with the Australian Army Nursing Service. She had volunteered to be part of the Australian Imperial Force (AIF) in 1915, but
had been placed with a British unit in Egypt, and then on the hospital ship *Assaye*. Although her experience of working with the
British had been a good one, she was anxious to nurse her own
countrymen. She had attempted to transfer services while in Egypt,
but permission had been denied, and she decided that the only way
to gain the transfer she desired was to resign and travel back to
Australia to re-enlist. She left Suez on board the transport ship
*Mongolian* in June along with two other Australian nurses.

As the ship neared Bombay it was mined and sank in less than
fifteen minutes. When she wrote later of her experiences, Vickers-
Foote marvelled at the way in which the ship's crew managed to get
all but thirty of the passengers into the lifeboats and away from the
sinking vessel in the middle of a monsoon. The passengers rowed
towards land for nine hours and eventually managed to make land-
fall on a rocky part of the Indian shore, where one of the boats
capsized, drowning two of its occupants and injuring several others.
The surviving 100 passengers 'camped in our life belts in tropical
rain, smashed up a couple of boats and made a fire'. They were on
the beach for three days. One of the passengers in the capsized
boat had contracted pneumonia, while another 'refractured an old
fracture'. The three nurses tore up their clothes for bandages and
splinted the limb. Yet another man had been badly burned when
the mine exploded; he died on the beach. After three days, a small
group of the shipwrecked passengers reached a neighbouring village, and stretchers were brought back for the wounded. The
nurses themselves walked for 12 miles with 'feet tied up with sail
cloth'. Eventually, they were evacuated by minesweeper from a
coastal village to Bombay, where they recovered at the Australian

'Victoria War Hospital'. Vickers-Foote's comment on the episode was: 'It was exciting all right.'[97] She returned to 'active service' in Europe later that year. In May 1918, she was placed with No. 3 Australian General Hospital. She found the work 'very hard, in the rushes, tremendous, but usually steady'.[98]

## Conclusion

From the last months of 1916 to the spring of 1918 nurses coped with crisis on many fronts. In Belgium, the Nivelle Offensive and the Third Battle of Ypres produced some of the most traumatic wounds of the war, made worse by an intensification of the use of chemical weaponry. On the Romanian and Russian Fronts, the efforts of nurses were hampered by the worsening political situation, as Russia descended into the chaos of Bolshevism and civil war. In April 1917, the United States of America entered the war on the Allied side. Some of its base hospitals were already in a state of readiness, and were able to travel to Europe that spring. By October they would be nursing their own compatriots. Nurses of all Allied nations were gaining confidence in their own expertise. Yet their vulnerability vis-à-vis their more powerful medical colleagues could, at times, cause tension. Nurse leaders in the USA were determined not to make the same mistakes as their British professional allies. Determining that assistant nurses in their hospitals should hold student status and be clearly placed under the supervision of fully qualified nurses, they formed the Army School of Nursing, an organization that went on to become one of the most highly-respected nurse-training institutions of the early twentieth century.

# 7
# Final Push
## March–November 1918

### Introduction: reversals of fortune

On 21 March 1918, the entrenched stalemate on the Western Front was suddenly broken by a dramatic series of German offensives. Drawing upon strategies they had perfected over the previous two years—'storm troops', hand grenades, and flame-throwers—the Germans hurled overwhelming numbers of men against four deliberately-chosen points: the Somme region, Ypres, the Aisne, and the Montdidier-Noyon sector.[1] It was well known among the Allies that Erich Ludendorff, the architect of the March breakthrough, had been planning a significant offensive since early winter, but the Allied forces, weakened by the failed Nivelle Offensive and the Third Battle of Ypres, were ill-prepared to counter any concerted attack, and were not, initially, able to withstand the scale and force of Ludendorff's offensives. Falling back along a wide swathe of the Somme sector, British and Dominion forces allowed the Germans to advance 30 miles in six days, and gave up all of the territories they had won at the Battle of the Somme. In April, the Germans launched the second phase of their campaign, recapturing Passchendaele Ridge and advancing on the ruined town of Ypres.

Allied evacuation lines were put under enormous pressure by the German advance. CCSs, within 5 or 6 miles of the front lines, were in immediate danger of being overrun. Staff, patients, and equipment were hastily evacuated, but at some CCSs a skeleton (male) staff was left behind to be taken prisoner, along with their helpless patients.

In May, the Germans launched the third phase of their attack, and succeeded in advancing as far as Château-Thierry, on the Marne. French field hospitals, like their British counterparts, were forced to retreat rapidly. It was only in July that Allied armies on all sectors of the front began to hold back the German advance, which was, in any case, losing momentum. The exhaustion and low morale of individual German soldiers was beginning to influence events; soldiers who had forced a breach in their enemy's lines now stopped to take food and wine they found in captured trenches and overrun villages.

At a conference at Doullens, on 26 March, the French general, Ferdinand Foch, had been given supreme command of the Allied forces, and this consolidation of command, along with the placing of American Expeditionary Force units with the British and French armies, gave new strength to the Allied forces. In late July and early August, they won decisive victories on the Marne and at Amiens. In both counter-offensives, the Allies broke with previous strategy and took the Germans by surprise, by dispensing with the usual pre-attack bombardment and simply advancing behind an effective 'creeping barrage'. In the autumn the American Expeditionary Force won a decisive victory at Meuse-Argonne, at the cost of 26,277 deaths and 95,786 serious injuries, making it 'the deadliest battle in all of American history'.[2]

In mid-September, the Allies launched a rapid and successful offensive out of Salonika, knocking Bulgaria out of the war and freeing Serbia. From June onwards, a series of Italian victories culminating with the Battle of Vittorio Veneto (24 October–2 November) completed the collapse of the Austro-Hungarian army.

On the Western Front, Allied forces—and the field hospitals serving them—began to advance. The campaign that followed, known as the 'Hundred Days Offensive', pushed the Germans back beyond the Hindenberg Line, the series of heavily fortified trenches from which they had launched their spring offensives. Because the Allied advance was achieved largely through infantry attack, casualty rates were enormous. The British Expeditionary Force alone lost approximately 314,000 men to death or injury.[3] And because the war was now highly mobile, CCSs were forced to find new ways of moving fast in order to place themselves in positions to receive the wounded.

Wounds sustained on the battlefield were only one of the ways in which troops could lose their lives during the Allied advance of 1918. The influenza virus which was to cause a global pandemic, killing more individuals than the war itself, is believed to have first appeared on 11 March 1918 at Fort Riley in Kansas. The movement of American troops to Europe probably began the spread of the disease, which was erroneously named 'Spanish flu', because the earliest accurate reports emerged from neutral Spain.[4] During the Hundred Days Offensive, the American Expeditionary Force alone reported approximately 360,000 cases of influenza. In CCSs and base hospitals, nurses fought to save the lives of men who were brought to them in collapsed states, unable to breathe, their faces and hands blue with cyanosis, some already in heart failure. Accustomed as they were to nursing people with severe infectious diseases, many commented that they had never seen anything like the 'Spanish flu'.

On 5 October 1918, Prince Max of Baden informed the Allies that Germany was willing to negotiate a peace settlement, and on 11 November the Armistice was signed in a railway carriage in the forest of Compiègne, sparking celebrations across Europe and beyond. But for those nurses who were still caring for the victims of war injury and influenza the war was not yet over. Many found that they had not the heart to join victory celebrations when grieving parents were sitting at the bedsides of dying young men.[5] And their own battles for political recognition—as both women and nurses—would outlast the First World War.


## Flight: March–July 1918

As the year 1918 opened, the routines of the Allied military nursing services seemed well established. Among the British, the QAIMNS and its Reserve continued to lead and direct the nursing work in most CCSs and base hospitals. By January 1918, there were approximately 5,000 members of the Territorial Force Nursing Service (TFNS), of whom about one-third were abroad. Indeed, fifteen of the British General Hospitals overseas were staffed entirely with TFNS staff.[6] Some Dominion nurses staffed general hospitals belonging to their own countries, whilst others worked alongside British staff. Most US nurses worked within base hospitals attached to their own units.

Medical historian Mark Harrison has observed that the military medical services on the Western Front were ill-prepared for the assault of March 1918: 'few expected an onslaught of the ferocity of the Ludendorff Offensive, or that it would overwhelm Allied defences so quickly'.[7] CCSs had been placed deliberately close to the front lines, to ensure that the wounded would be attended to quickly. Many had to be abandoned. Staff were forced to evacuate their patients onto already-overcrowded trains.

On 22 March, just one day after the beginning of the German offensive, Sister Ella Redman of the Australian Army Nursing Service was moved from No. 3 Australian General Hospital to a CCS at Méricourt. She was posted to the dressing station and found that the wounded were 'just pouring in'. Many severely wounded men—even some with abdominal and chest wounds—walked into the station and then collapsed as they reached safety. Those with severe wounds or poorly controlled haemorrhages were sent straight to the 'pre op ward'. The less seriously wounded were given hot drinks and tea in an overcrowded area outside the reception tent. After about thirty-six hours, the CCS ran out of splints, and food and dressings were becoming scarce:

> In many cases of broken limbs and in some cases where the limbs were just hanging on by muscle, all we could do was to bandage as firmly as possible, give an injection of Morphia and turn the case into the paddock with a couple of blankets...The men were splendid, not one of them complained, their only trouble was to get away before the Germans took them prisoners; in many cases as soon as they were dressed they started to walk hoping that some of the transport or an ambulance would pick them up.[8]

On the evening of 23 March, large numbers of retreating Allied troops and transports began to pass the CCS. Mingled with them were 'panic-stricken' civilians. In the early hours of the next morning, the colonel refused to take in any more wounded, as the station was now caring for 1,000 stretcher cases with no dressings, no food, and hardly any water. At around 4.30 a.m. the nurses were evacuated to Abbeville, each with one piece of hand baggage.

The next day, the nurses were posted to another CCS, this time at Corbie, arriving about 8 p.m. Conditions here were even worse than those at Méricourt. The Allied forces were retreating so rapidly that there was no time to establish any advanced dressing stations. Redman was called on duty at 3 a.m. to dress wounds tied up with puttees, handkerchiefs, and ties; all patients had to be given anti-tetanus serum and most also needed morphia: 'One case, a severe abd. case was carried in by four of his pals a distance of ten miles, the case was hopeless, we packed him with hot water bags, inj. Morphia; he died shortly after being admitted.'[9] At 5 p.m. on 26 March, with the German advance just 2 miles away and the bridges ahead of them ready to be destroyed by explosives, all cases were evacuated by train, and the nurses were taken by ambulance to Abbeville. They were allowed only two bags each, and Redman had to leave behind many of her prized possessions, including books, photographs, and souvenirs from all her previous postings. Redman's story is told as one of the 'Nurses' Narratives' collected by Colonel Arthur Butler to assist him in writing his official history of the Australian Army Medical Services during the war. One of her main concerns in writing her narrative seems to have been to explain how 'splendid' her matron, all of the CCS's medical officers, and the orderlies were. Indeed, the word 'splendid' appears repeatedly. She was anxious to convey a sense of how much the staff were willing to do for their wounded compatriots, emphasizing that many 'never rested day or night'.[10]

For Maud McCarthy, Matron-in-Chief of the BEF, the most stressful element of the spring retreat was an acute and worsening shortage of nurses. Workloads had increased dramatically—as had morbidity rates among her staff, which stood at 7.4 per cent in June.[11] Increasing numbers of nursing sisters and volunteers were being sent to 'sick sisters' hospitals' and in the six weeks from 21 March to the end of May no leave of any kind had been granted to those who remained at their posts. The work of repeatedly evacuating, packing up, moving, and then reopening field hospitals, on top of the stress of caring for those injured by 'storm-troop' tactics, was exhausting, and nurses' working hours were well in excess of the norm. If military hospitals behind the lines could be seen as, in Mary Borden's terms, the 'second battlefield' then this was a battlefield in which the casualty rates were steadily rising. But for McCarthy, a stalwart supporter of the British Empire, these trials served to highlight the heroism of her staff, and to prove that nurses, as well as soldiers, were vital components of the Allied struggle. In her report for the year 1918, she wrote of nurses 'in action' having to be supported by 'reinforcements' from heavily overworked bases.[12]

In May and June, requests were made for eleven surgical teams to be transferred from France to the beleaguered Italian Front, and McCarthy reluctantly moved seven nursing sisters and four 'lady anaesthetists'—who could hardly be spared—as part of these teams.

In spite of the pressures placed on them, the medical and nursing services on the Western Front continued the process of specialization which had begun the previous year. Expertise in particular conditions, or in particular areas of work, was considered desirable. Six 'dieticians' were appointed, one to each of the bases of Boulogne, Calais, Rouen, Étaples, Trouville, and Abbeville. Other specialist nurses were appointed to ophthalmics and aural divisions, to the specialist wards for fractured femur cases at No. 8 Stationary Hospital, and to the special 'Carrel-Dakin hut' that was attached to No. 26 British General Hospital. A number of nurses were sent to the 'Mental Division' of No. 8 Stationary Hospital— rare examples of general nurses being tasked with the specialist work of mental health care.[13] One particularly important nursing speciality, which had proved its worth during the war, was the 'Military Massage Corps'.[14] Nurse-masseuses performed much of the work that would later come to be understood under the label 'physiotherapy'. In addition to massaging damaged limbs in order to improve the supply of blood and lymph, masseuses also taught patients exercise regimes to help strengthen muscles and joints and improve mobility.[15]

The other highly significant development of summer 1918 was the formation of the Royal Air Force Nursing Service (RAFNS). On 1 April, the Royal Flying Corps and the Royal Naval Air Service had joined forces to create the British Royal Air Force. On 1 June a temporary nursing service, consisting of a matron-in-chief, four matrons, and forty sisters and staff nurses was recruited. Among its members was Joanna Margaret Cruikshank, who was, in November, to become acting matron-in-chief and would, in 1921, become the first permanent matron-in-chief of the Royal Air Force Nursing Service. She had been born in India and had trained at Guy's Hospital in the early years of the twentieth century, before becoming a sister with Lady Minto's Indian Nursing Association, and then enrolling for active service with QAIMNS. She had been invalided to Britain after contracting a particularly virulent form of malaria. The temporary RAFNS was to perform some important work during the last months of the war, but was not formalized until January 1921. On 14 June 1923, Princess Mary, daughter of George V became its president and it was renamed Princess Mary's Royal Air Force Nursing Service.[16]

Another important decision made during that uncertain summer of 1918 was that the service and expertise of VADs should be rewarded. The suspicion felt towards 'amateur nurses' at the outbreak of the war, which had at times shaded into open hostility, had by its closing months given way to grudging respect. Professional nurses could not forget the, at times outrageous, behaviour of some wealthy and influential 'lady-nurses', but they had had sufficient contact with enough hard-working and able volunteers to convince them that many—if not most—VADs were their genuine partners and allies in the provision of expert care. A decision was taken in June that 100 VADs should be promoted to the level of 'VAD Assistant Nurse'—perhaps a rather limited concession on the part of a nursing establishment which had been relying heavily on the VAD workforce for over three years. Many VADs had served continuously in military hospitals since the spring of 1915, and there were, by June 1918, 1,767 VAD members and special military probationers serving with the BEF in France.[17]

On the 'home front', some auxiliary hospitals were caring for increasingly acute cases. In May, at the Stamford War Hospital, Dunham Massey Hall, Cheshire, brain surgery was performed on Gordon Highlander, Private Johnstone. A small space at the foot of the grand staircase was converted into a temporary operating theatre, and the daughter of the house, VAD Lady Jane Grey, held a torch, directing light onto the operation site while Dr Percy Cooper performed the surgery. The following, somewhat harrowing, account was written later by Catherine Bennett, Sister-in-Charge of the hospital:

> Patient had one sinus in the head on admission, general health fairly good, complained of frequent headaches which increased gradually

in intensity, especially on the R. side. X-Ray Photo was taken in April, two pieces of shrapnel were discovered in the cerebrum, about ½ in. under the skull. Patient fell in a heap one a.m. after which pt. suffered very severely. Doctor Percy Cooper performed Trepan [*sic*] of the skull & extracted one piece of shrapnel; the other had sunk too low down. The following week patient was bright and suffered less. Suddenly, he developed symptoms of brain disturbance. Dr Cooper put him under Twilight Sleep, symptoms were subdued, for a time, but recurred with greater severity. Lady Stamford's Parlour was hastily prepared for a ward, where he was nursed alone. As the pain continued, the vitality became lower. All symptoms pointed to a cerebral abscess. He was transferred to the Royal Infirmary Manchester, for operation by a special Head Surgeon. He died in a violent fit before the operation took place.[18]

Such cases suggest that hospitals in Britain were severely overstretched during the spring and summer of 1918. The risks associated with performing major brain surgery in a non-clinical environment must have been recognized—and yet accepted—by the doctor involved. The patient was only transferred to the care of a specialist brain surgeon after his condition became critical.

By the early summer of 1918, large numbers of American nurses were arriving in Europe. Sara McCarron, one of the few who had the distinction of having served in both German and Allied military hospitals, arrived at the American Ambulance in Neuilly in July 1918.[19] She was moved, with five other nurses, to Jouy-sur-Morin at the end of the month. Her group arrived at a field hospital and were told that three of their number would have to go on night duty immediately. McCarron was one of those who went straight to the tented wards. That night they had to extinguish all lights as an air raid began. The wards had no flooring and the work was 'hard on the feet'. On 4 August eight gassed cases were brought into McCarron's ward, and she spent much of the day washing their eyes with sodium bicarbonate, and applying compresses. The hospital became very busy, and the situation was made worse by the fact that many wounds were very severe and had to be watched for haemorrhage—a very difficult task during the darkness of air raids. Some patients were so restless that they tore their dressings off. Others had wounds which bled so profusely that dressings had to be constantly reinforced. McCarron found herself too busy and anxious to eat or sleep, and at the end of the first week in August, she was forced to take a brief period of sick leave.[20]

Nurses in all parts of the Allied lines found themselves working long hours under great stress. On 3 June, Jane De Launoy, stationed at the Vinkem site of 'L'Hôpital de l'Océan' in Belgium, compared her role to that of an early modern 'Beguine': 'Not always easy, not always comfortable. Their role is to aid, to give the soldiers back to the country. They do that with all their will...No-one thanks them for suffering for strangers.'[21] The experience of Julia Stimson, Matron of No. 12 General Hospital, was altogether less bleak. In April 1918, she was appointed chief nurse to the American Red Cross. Then, in October, she was made director of nursing services to the American Expeditionary Force.[22] Meanwhile, Mabel Jeffery, who had recently been moved by the FFNC to Ambulance 12/14 at Vauxbin, near Soissons, at the request of its medical officer, found herself having to evacuate the hospital at a few hours' notice, and move back to a position much nearer to Paris at Pontoise.[23]

## Under bombardment

In the summer of 1918, German air raids on Allied bases increased in both frequency and severity. The worst of these, as far as the nursing services were concerned, took place on 19 May at Étaples, 29 May at Doullens, and 31 May—again at Étaples. In fact the Étaples nurses were having a particularly rough time. The raid on the 19th lasted three hours and caused damage to several hospitals. Maud McCarthy reported that, 'at No. 1 Canadian General Hospital, 1 sister was killed, and 2 so severely wounded that they died shortly after, and 5 also were wounded. At 26 General Hospital there were 2 minor casualties amongst the Nursing Staff, and their quarters were partly wrecked. At 46 Stationary Hospital there was one slight casualty, but many of the patients and personnel were killed.'[24] The attack on Doullens was clearly terrifying: No. 3 Canadian Stationary Hospital was bombed and burst into flames. Two surgeons and three sisters were killed instantly, along with several patients and other personnel. Another sister was badly wounded, as was a sister on nearby No. 24 Ambulance Train. McCarthy went on to describe the carnage at the end of the month:

> The raid of the 31st at Etaples was a terrific one. The planes flew low, and used their machine guns. Practically all the hospitals suffered. Those which suffered most heavily were St John's Ambulance Brigade Hospital, where one sister was killed and 5 wounded, besides many patients and personnel. No. 24 General Hospital, where two of the staff were wounded, one severely...No. 46 Stationary Hospital and the two Canadian units which had suffered so severely before, Nos. 1 and 7 Canadian General Hospital. The beautifully equipped St John's Ambulance Brigade Hospital was entirely wrecked.[25]

The courage and endurance of nurses under hostile bombardment was an opportunity for organizations such as the QAIMNS and the TFNS to extol the bravery of their members. The citations of its nurses were recorded in full in a report produced by the Secretary of the TFNS Advisory Council in 1918. The language of the citations is tellingly heroic. On 4 June, for example, Sister Kate Maxey (already a holder of the Royal Red Cross) was awarded the Military Medal for 'gallantry and devotion to duty displayed during a recent hostile bombing raid on a Casualty Clearing Station'. It was said that 'although severely wounded herself, she went to the aid of another Sister, who was fatally wounded and did all she could for her. Later, although suffering severe pain, she showed an example of pluck and endurance which was inspiring to all.'[26]

News of such attacks was greeted with shock at all levels of civilian and military society. Queen Alexandra sent a message of sympathy, expressing the view that 'it is too dreadful to think that our brave Nurses whose lives are devoted to looking after the sick and wounded should have been exposed to such wicked and un-called for trials'.[27] No fewer than forty-four nurses and VADs received the Military Medal for bravery during the air raids of 1918, along with fourteen awards of the French Médaille des Épidémies and two awards of the Belgian Médaille de la Reine Elisabeth.[28]

One of the most exhausting aspects of the bombardments was the need for hospital staff to seek shelter in nearby trenches, tun-nels, or caves. Each time an air-raid warning sounded, day nurses would leave their beds and move to whatever shelter was available, often remaining there for several hours and sometimes having to move several times in the course of one night.[29] Ruth Allan, a sister with the AANS, was with No. 3 AGH in Abbeville in July during several nights of severe bombardment. When air raids began, those patients who could be moved and nurses who were not on duty wore 'tin hats' and sheltered in dugouts. Helpless patients re-mained in their wards, but their beds were lowered to the floors every night at 11 p.m. to place them behind the shelter of sandbags surrounding each tent or hut. At 3 a.m.—the time at which most air raids ceased—the beds were once more raised.[30] Such practices were typical of hospitals in northern France throughout the dan-gerous spring and summer of 1918. Sister M. Hall, based in No. 2 Australian CCS at Blendecques, commented on how,

> every bright night at that time, a working party came round before the hour the planes were due, to put down the beds of all the pa-tients fit to be moved. The legs of the stretchers were knocked under, and the bed gently lowered on to the floor. One could never know if this precaution was of more than mental value, but the idea was that if a splinter bomb fell between the tents, the fragments flying hori-zontally would be turned aside by the sandbags. One had to exercise a great deal of discretion as to who could go down. We found that

the bad leg cases on splints were very uncomfortable there, and they much preferred staying up.[31]

At these times all lights throughout the hospital would be extinguished, creating an eerie atmosphere and making it very difficult for nurses to care adequately for their patients. New Zealand nurse Sybil Surtees found work at Étaples 'really terrifying'; some nights she would shake with fear.[32] Yet the presence of nurses on the wards during air raids appears to have given their helpless patients great reassurance.[33]

Ellen Cuthbert, based at Wimereux, commented that a dugout had been constructed outside the sisters' quarters, but that most sisters preferred to stay in their own rooms throughout the air raids. The work was hard: large convoys of wounded were arriving from the front every night. After the boredom and stagnation of over three years of trench warfare, all the wounded were 'very excited with the retreating and the severity of the fighting'.[34] Elsie May Tranter experienced a narrow escape while getting a pair of boots out of a kit bag in her tent: 'a fairly large piece of shell ripped my tent grazed past my face and passed right between my hands tearing the kit bag and various things that were in it and burying itself in the bag. Of course I was eager to have the piece as a souvenir so felt for it at once—and was rather sorry for my impatience for it was more than comfortably warm to touch.'[35] The nonchalance with which Tranter recounts this story is typical of the ways in which nurses wrote up their diary accounts, and, perhaps, illustrates the way in which they wanted to be viewed by later generations: as brave, calm heroines, unconcerned by the dangers of war.

The 100 nurses who belonged to American Base Hospital No. 41 arrived in Paris on 10 August 1918, just as the tide of war was turning. Casualties from the Marne and Amiens were flooding into the city and influenza was rife. Margaret Cowling and her staff had left Boston on 19 July as part of a large transatlantic convoy, travelling via Liverpool, Southampton, and Le Havre. When they arrived at their destination—the stately eighteenth-century École de la Légion d'Honneur, on the site of a former monastery, attached to the Cathedral at Saint-Denis, near Paris—they were greeted by their medical and 'corpsmen' colleagues, who had established a vast tented hospital in the beautiful parkland surrounding the building.[36] Camilla Louise Wills wrote home to her aunt that she had been posted to 'a very beautiful historical place'.[37] She also commented on the nurses' bathhouse, which she considered 'too funny for anything, about 20 tubs in one room with no screens between them and we all go in and as many as can get in the tubs while the others wait'.[38]

Nurses' quarters were in the old school itself, and Cowling's room was reached 'by a long winding passage' on the wall of which was an inscription, which read: 'Fear not fear.' 'I used to wonder as I read it', Cowling commented, 'whether it was placed there by some one in an ironical mood! At any rate it was most appropriate

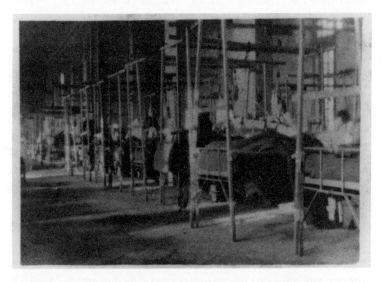

FIGURE 25 Fracture ward at Base Hospital No. 41, Saint-Denis, near Paris (photograph reproduced by kind permission of the Claude Moore Health Sciences Library, the University of Virginia, Charlottesville, VA, USA)

for the weird old building and for the experience that we were
going through and made a good motto for many of us.'[39] Four days
later, the nurses took the words to heart, when Paris was subjected
to a fierce bombardment from the air. At first, the nurses thought
that the explosions and 'sky rockets' were part of local celebrations
of the Feast of the Assumption; then they realized that their neigh-
bourhood was under bombardment. 'I don't mind saying that
I never was so frightened in my life', commented Cowling, adding
however, that, once in the cellars, the hospital staff passed the time
with 'much noise and merriment' to the accompaniment of guitars
and ukeleles.[40] Air raids were not the only trials the nurses had to
endure; Paris was also bombarded by the famous long-distance
cannon 'Big Bertha'. Shells passed directly over the hospital, one
landing nearby. The unit's staff endured several air raids and bombardments during their stay at Saint-Denis. Camilla Louise Wills's
diary entry for 15 September was terse: 'Two air raids tonight. 1st at
2am, 2nd at 4am. Went to cellar both times. Would not let us go
outside. Much bombing.'[41] The disturbance of sleep accompanied
by eleven-hour shifts on the wards was exhausting for staff.

On 12 August, the first convoy of 134 patients had arrived, and
were cared for in the 'receiving room': they were given hot soup,
coffee, and cigarettes, bathed, and had their wounds dressed before
they were moved to a ward. Altogether, the hospital could hold just
under 3,000 patients, some in the main building; the vast majority
in tents. During day shifts, large wards of between 130 and 190 patients were staffed by five to seven nurses, and much of the heavy
work was delegated to corpsmen. At night there was only one
trained nurse on each ward. Corpsman Deming Shear was later to
comment on how he and one trained nurse were the only two
members of staff in a huge fracture ward on night duty, where all
of the patients were in traction and unable to move.[42] Young,
newly-qualified Camilla Louise Wills was in charge of Ward III,
caring for 160 patients, 144 of them receiving Carrel-Dakin treatment. She performed many of the complex dressings herself, with

the help of orderlies such as 'Nate Adams', who, unfortunately, 'fainted' one day 'while doing a bad arm case'. In late September, she had several patients who 'yelled all night'.[43]

As huge numbers of influenza patients began to arrive at the hospital in September and October, nurses found that they had to work under even greater pressure. Eighty of them contracted the disease, and a separate ward had to be used for 'sick nurses'. One became dangerously ill with pneumonia, but was nursed back to health by her colleagues. The most difficult time for the hospital was October 1918. On the 19th, it was obliged to 'take in' patients, even though it already had a complement of 1,765. All the other Paris hospitals had stopped 'receiving' altogether. The hospital admitted 693 sick and wounded men between 4 a.m. on 19 October and 10 a.m. on 22 October. Its staff were 'pretty much exhausted but kept at work persistently'.[44]

## Advance: August–November 1918

The Hundred Days Offensive tested the resolve and ingenuity of nursing staff, perhaps, even more than the spring retreat. One of the most distressing aspects of their work was the care of repatriated prisoners of war, most of whom were in emaciated and neglected states, many suffering from epidemic disease. Their greatest needs were for food, rest, and cleanliness, and nursing work was onerous at a time when large numbers of wounded men were still also pouring into field hospitals. One of the greatest ethical dilemmas at this time was the difficulty of caring for large numbers of German prisoner-patients. The Geneva Convention dictated that 'enemy patients' must be treated with the same consideration as one's own wounded, and nurses recognized that it was their duty to treat German soldiers with humanity. There are no reports of their failing to do so; and yet, some of their personal writings attest to the conflict they experienced when placed in so-called 'German wards'.[45]

At No. 3 British General Hospital, Le Tréport, Edith Appleton was under pressure, caring for casualties of the rapid Allied advance. She commented on how very ill her 'gassed men' were: 'every one of them the colour of a dirty penny, pulses rocky, throats raw—eyes streaming—lids swollen—& off their heads at intervals'. She added that the weather was 'like living in a Green house. It is alright at night, because no one cares if you have nothing on—but the day time! with correct uniform! I ask you!'[46]

In August, Sara McCarron was posted to the Hôtel Dieu, Château Thierry, to a hospital run by Augustinian nuns, which had just been evacuated by the Germans. She and her colleagues 'scrubbed and cleaned all day' in an effort to turn the filthy and dilapidated building into a base hospital. On 14 September, she found herself in charge of six tents, each with twenty-four patients, and 'lots of very sick gas cases'. There was an unexpected rush of patients and she was grateful for the assistance of another nurse, Miss Grant, who 'looked after the eyes so well that nearly all of them opened'. When she went off duty at 9 p.m., she felt 'ready to drop'. The hospital had received and evacuated nearly 300 patients.[47]

The next day, McCarron battled to save the lives of three dangerously-ill patients, one of whom died of gas gangrene. She was sent off duty 'nearly dead'. From this time on, her diary is full of entries relating to the struggle to save the lives of patients with wound infections and severe gas poisoning. On the 23rd she cared for a patient with severe burns over two-thirds of his body, and a 'very sick' chest case; and on 1 October, she was obliged to go into her ward during her morning off to 'special' Private Samuel Meyer, a young boy of 19 with a gunshot wound through the chest. He had contracted pneumonia, and was delirious. She gave him stimulants and oxygen, dressed his wounds, and cared for the tube that was draining fluid from his lung. On 4 October, the date of her last diary entry in France, McCarron was relating how how two ladies from a volunteer unit were visiting Meyer every day, bringing him milk, which was 'about all the nourishment he takes'.[48]

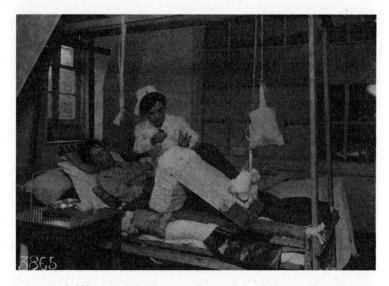

FIGURE 26 US nurse irrigating a patient's wound (photograph reproduced courtesy of the National Library of Medicine, USA)

As medical units advanced eastwards their work was made more onerous by the return of Allied prisoners of war, many in a 'pitiable state of weakness, starvation and filth, some hardly recognisable as men'.[49] The work was always depressing and often shocking. Along with prisoners from both sides of the conflict, British and Dominion army nurses—whose work had always been strictly confined to the care of military personnel—found themselves looking after large numbers of civilian casualties. From the summer onwards, some British and Canadian surgical teams had been loaned to French military hospitals, which had, traditionally, always been more ready to treat civilians. One surgical team from No. 4 Canadian CCS worked at an operating theatre in Arras, caring for large numbers of wounded and gassed civilians. It was found that many elderly patients had been lying in cellars, sheltering from the fighting for several weeks, and were suffering from severe pressure sores.[50]

Air raids and heavy bombardment were not the only hazards to which CCSs were subjected. Overwork and poor conditions also made them vulnerable to serious accidents. On 5 October, a fire was started at No. 36 CCS at Rousbrugge-Haringhe when a lamp overturned in the officers' ward. Five wards and an operating theatre were destroyed. All of the stretcher cases were carried out of the burning buildings by the hospital staff—including the sisters, who, according to Maud McCarthy, 'utterly regardless of their own safety', acted with 'the greatest heroism'. Four were awarded the Albert Medal.[51]

The destruction of No. 36 CCS meant desperately heavy workloads for other CCSs in the area. Head Sister Eleanor Jeffries, based at No. 3 Australian CCS in Haringhe commented that, after the attack on Ypres at the end of that month, the wounded were 'rolling in' and her CCS was barely able to cope. Fortunately, the 'rush' ended soon after the accident at No. 36, and her CCS 'packed up' and moved forward behind the advancing Allied lines. By now, its staff were also nursing large numbers of influenza cases and were barely coping with the work but, on requesting ten additional members of staff, Jeffries was informed that she could only have four, as so many nurses at base were, themselves, ill.[52] Eventually, No. 3 CCS advanced into Germany just behind the Second Army.

Several CCSs moved rapidly eastwards in this way, caring for the wounded of the advancing Allied armies—'leapfrogging' as they went, with each CCS moving forward in turn, while another remained in place to treat and evacuate its wounded.[53] Sister M. Hall, with No. 2 Australian CCS, moved from Blendecques to Hondingen, near Cassel, where the tents were always wet, and the ground was covered in 'deep black mud'. Next, her unit advanced to Saint-Venant, where they were housed in a French asylum. From here, they moved through the devastated areas, amongst 'absolutely destroyed villages', eventually reaching Tournai, in Belgium, where they and other CCSs were housed in a large and beautiful building, which had been used as a German military hospital for four years.[54]

## Nurse-anaesthetists

One of the most important innovations of the war period was the role of the nurse-anaesthetist. Introduced because of the wartime shortage of medical officers, so-called 'lady anaesthetists' created great turbulence and anxiety for the Allied medical services.[55] The role of the nurse-anaesthetist was already recognized in the USA, and many American base hospitals brought their own nurse-anaes-thetists with them to Europe.[56] Jennifer Telford has commented that the rapid increase in the number of patients being cared for at Base Hospital No. 41 and the shortage of surgeons at the hospital meant that nurses were not only giving anaesthetics but also per-forming minor operative procedures, during the autumn of 1918.[57]

For the British military medical services, the position of the 'lady anaesthetist' was a potentially invidious one, as was the position of 'operating team sister'. It was recognized that members of staff who spent much time as part of small and close-knit teams of pro-fessionals, working together on long shifts, might find their loyalties divided. Maud McCarthy reported that 'with regard to discipline, it was found necessary early in the year to issue instructions to all sisters in charge of CCSs to the effect that the team sisters were in no way to be treated differently from the other members of the nursing staff, that they were members of the mess under the con-trol of the sister in charge and when on duty in the operating the-atre, under the control of the sister in charge of the operating theatre'.[58] It was, furthermore, made clear that sisters in charge of operating theatres must on no account leave their own unit for 'team duty'. For McCarthy, the continuity of work within a CCS and the authority of its sister-in-charge were paramount.

On 14 January 1918, the British introduced a strict six-month training in anaesthesia in a base hospital, followed by one month in a casualty clearing station for British and Dominion nurses desig-nated as 'lady anaesthetists'.[59] Seventy-six nurses began training at twenty-five different base hospitals, and sixty-three successfully completed this initial phase of training. They were transferred to CCSs in early March, but many had to be evacuated during the German advance and complete their training at base hospitals. The experience of Australian nurse-anaesthetists was extraordinary, and is illustrated by the career of Australian nurse Elsie Tranter, who did her initial training at American Base Hospital No. 2 (The New York Presbyterian Hospital Unit) in Étretat, and was then sent to No. 29 British Casualty Clearing Station at Grévillers in March. She later moved to Doullens. Following the completion of their training, she and five colleagues found that Sir Neville Howse, Assistant Medical Director of the Australian military medical service, had decided that nurses should not, after all, work as anaesthetists, and they were obliged to return to normal duties.[60] The treatment of the six Australian nurse-anaesthetists was made all the more extraordinary by the fact that significant numbers of American nurses had already been administering anaesthetics in their own units since their arrival in France, the role of the nurse-anaesthetist being well established in the USA.

**Influenza**

The pandemic of influenza which began in the summer of 1918 and ended about a year later, has been described as one of the three most deadly episodes of disease in human history (the other two being the pandemics of bubonic plague in the sixth and fourteenth centuries). It has been estimated that well over 20 million people died.[61] Many of the worst affected were front-line soldiers, whose immune systems had already been compromised by trench life. This, naturally, meant a massive increase in the workloads of nurses who were already under pressure. Maud McCarthy commented in her annual report for 1918 that 'the signing of the Armistice on November 11th did not make any appreciable difference to the work for many weeks. There were no battle casualties, but, though the work changed in character, it was very heavy indeed for some time.'[62] In Tournai, during November 1918, Sister M. Hall, based at No. 2 Australian CCS, was caring for twenty of the worst influenza patients, working 'incessantly' to save the lives of her 'desperately sick' patients. She commented that 'it was work with a great deal of satisfaction, the being able to make them comfortable when they were so utterly helpless, and seeing one and another, as you finished making them so, turn over and have a quiet sleep'.[63]

Influenza affected nurses on all war fronts. New Zealand nurse Winifred Spencer was based at No. 24 British Stationary Hospital, in Palestine. After the signing of the Armistice, patients were still being moved 'down the line' to her hospital: 'the poor boys—the war was ended, peace was declared and they were coming down and dying in hundreds when they were meant to catch their ships to England. It was a really sad ending.'[64] In Salonika, Estelle Armstrong, a staff nurse with the AANS, celebrated the news of the Armistice with a glass of port wine, but was 'so desperately busy that nothing seemed to matter very much'.[65] She was still nursing dangerously ill casualties from the victory at Grande Couronne, and large numbers of patients seriously ill with dysentery were being brought down the line from Serbia and Bulgaria as the Allies advanced through devastated zones in which it was almost impossible to obtain healthy food and water. Prisoners of war in desperate states of malnutrition and emaciation were also beginning to return from Bulgaria. Nurses and orderlies were already exhausted after having nursed large numbers of dysentery patients for several months. Influenza first began to affect patients and staff at the hospital in late September. For patients who were already debilitated by disease, influenza left them with 'practically no chance' of survival.

Influenza affected hospitals on the 'home fronts' too. In Brockenhurst, at the No. 1 New Zealand General Hospital, 68 of the approximately 300 nurses fell ill with influenza and staff shortages led to overwhelming workloads for those still on duty.[66]

## Armistice

A carefully worded note can be found in Maud McCarthy's report for 1918:

> Shortly after the signing of the Armistice on November 11th, innumerable requests were received for permission to be given to the Nursing Staff to dance, in order to celebrate this eventful year in a special way. It was recognised that the rule forbidding dancing had been loyally kept by the vast majority throughout the war, and it was felt that if this pleasure could be granted them, it would be some reward for their remarkable work and behaviour. It was also felt that the task of the matrons in enforcing this rule, so loyally upheld by them, at this particular time would be an almost impossible one, and especially so in those areas where the overseas sisters were stationed, as they, with the exception of the Australians, have always been free to dance in their own messes.[67]

Nurses were duly given permission to dance—and parties were held in both nurses' and medical officers' messes over Christmas. Nurses were also given the opportunity to visit convalescent and rest homes on the French Riviera and in Paris and Deauville, to relax and recuperate after a period of extraordinary endurance and self-sacrifice.[68]

Most military nurses found that their workloads remained very high for several months after the Armistice. Although they no longer encountered new wounds, the sick and debilitated were pouring into their hospitals in their thousands and the work—although different—was as difficult as it had ever been. Indeed, patients now required much more 'core' nursing and less medical treatment, and the burden fell more on nurses than on other hospital staff. The technical work of administering shock treatments, probing and dressing wounds, applying antiseptics, and supervising patients undergoing blood transfusion was giving way to the physically and emotionally draining work of feeding, hydrating, and maintaining comfort and cleanliness in patients who were almost

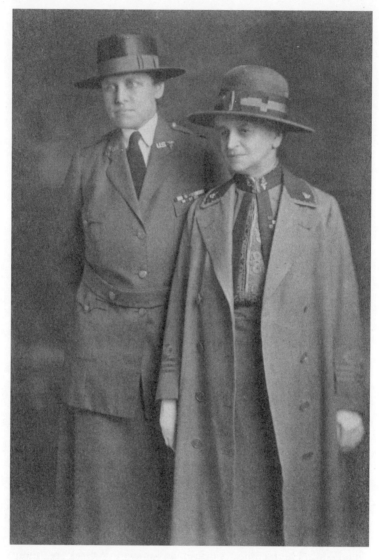

FIGURE 27 Julia Stimson and Maud McCarthy (photograph reproduced by kind permission of the Army Medical Services Museum, Aldershot, UK)

dead with malnutrition, dehydration, and exhaustion. Ellen Cuthbert described her work in Wimereux, with a convoy of over 200 Italian prisoners of war, who had been released from the notorious 'Meschede' camp in Prussia. They were 'in a shocking condition' and it 'made one's heart ache even to look at them'.[69] Some died shortly after arriving at the base hospital.

American Base Hospital No. 41 at Saint-Denis remained busy after the Armistice, and it was not until 28 January 1919 that its last patients were evacuated. The staff then thoroughly cleaned the entire building before leaving for home—part of the contract between the American Red Cross and the French authorities. Its nurses reached New York on 13 March 1919. The personal accounts of some of those who belonged to Base Hospital No. 41 provide an insight into the *esprit de corps* felt by its staff, who continued to hold reunions in Charlottesville well into the second half of the twentieth century. If nurses saw themselves as 'warriors' fighting on a 'second battlefield'—a field where humanitarian effort was pitted against the destruction of conflict and epidemic—then, for many, their war—like that of combatants themselves—was infused with camaraderie and a sense of shared suffering and endurance.

It was not until several months after the Armistice that nurses were demobilized and returned home. Some nurses chose to remain in Europe. Sara McCarron enrolled for a further period of service with the American Red Cross. She was sent to Montenegro (which, following the war, was merged with Serbia); her journey involved a 60-mile ride over the mountains, which she described in her diary as 'very dangerous and thrilling'. In Podgoritza, she worked as a 'district nurse' for eight months and felt that she was able to make a real difference to people's lives. Writing for Lavinia Dock's *History of American Red Cross Nursing*, she described how she and colleagues were able to heal long-standing infected wounds, offer public health advice, improve their patients' housing, and establish a school nursing service.[70]

## Conclusion: 1918, year of endurance and victory

In her report for the year 1918, Maud McCarthy, Matron-in-Chief of the BEF, reflected on the trials suffered by her nursing staff:

> There has been the 'Retreat'. There have been constant and terrifying air raids, and work under shell fire. There has been the 'Great Advance', with its own peculiar horrors, and at the same time the epidemic of influenza and the lack of sufficient Nursing staff to meet the most immediate and pressing demands...There have been some very wonderful examples of endurance and self-sacrifice...The work during the advance was stupendous! Influenza and pneumonia were rampant everywhere, not only among the troops but among women workers and the nursing staff.[71]

McCarthy's rousing relation of the many hardships and dangers faced by her colleagues offers a fascinating insight into the world view of professional nurses during the war. The narrative is a heroic one. There is a sense of heightening tension as the year 1918 advances, with nurses coming more frequently under bombardment and continuing to work as long as possible in CCSs under mortal threat from enemy advance. During the so-called 'Great Advance' they move across dangerous terrain and survive difficult living and working conditions. They risk their lives by nursing patients with influenza. Their matron-in-chief represents British nurses as significant participants in a victorious war-effort. She fails, however, to mention that nurses also extended their skills across normally-accepted professional boundaries, undertaking work normally reserved for surgeons and anaesthetists. Ever the diplomat, McCarthy ensures that, although heroic and highly flattering to the efforts of nurses, her narrative also remains carefully within the bounds of what will prove acceptable to her powerful male medical colleagues.

# Conclusion

Marian Wenzel has commented that 'people willingly go to suffer the horrors of war in the conviction that by so doing they protect those left at home from greater horrors. They often succeed to the extent of obscuring from those protected just what was endured for their sakes.'[1] Wenzel was commenting on the calmness with which the relatives of Mabel Effie Jeffery (1883–1958), who had served with the Scottish Women's Hospitals (in both France and Serbia) and with the French Flag Nursing Corps, viewed her war service. Jeffery had gone to war a young woman of 31 with jet-black hair, but had returned white-haired and exhausted,[2] only to spend much of the rest of her life caring 'single-handed' for her ageing parents in an old rambling Victorian house. Jeffery kept her mementoes of the war—among them, endearing messages of friendship and gratitude from poilus on romantic French postcards. One of the final entries in her notebook states what was, perhaps, an article of faith for this professional nurse who appears to have found the fullest expression of her work in the French field hospitals of the First World War: 'when we come to the end of life the only things that seem worth while our having done, are the sacrifices we have made for others'.[3]

It is only with hindsight that a historian such as Leo van Bergen can describe the essence of warfare as 'the handing over of one's body to the state, giving the government free rein to dispose of it as it sees fit, even if that means it will be grotesquely mutilated by bullets and shells'.[4] The effects on nurses of handling such mutilated bodies—and of placing themselves in difficult, stressful, and often dangerous situations—is only just beginning to be recognized. It is widely accepted that war veterans—both male and female—have difficulty adjusting to peacetime conditions when they return home. Twenty-first-century societies recognize the need for both sensitive support and compensation for those physically or psychologically damaged. Historian Denise Poynter has examined the 'plight of the female veteran in her claim for financial compensation', finding that nurses who suffered damage as a result of their First World War experiences were 'often at the mercy of a new, uncoordinated and complex system'. The 'arbitrary and haphazard' operation of medical boards and the ineffectiveness of the Ministry of Pensions meant that the very real damage suffered by many nurses was neither adequately recognized nor fully redressed.[5] And the sacrifices of many nurses from Allied nations went even further than this. Elizabeth Haldane, writing in 1923, observed that approximately 300 nurses belonging to the British services alone, died or were killed in the course of their duties during the war.[6] Although such sacrifice was acknowledged, the clinical contributions of professional nurses were never fully recognized by the societies they served. Historian Alison Fell has argued that volunteers were more likely than professional women to be remembered as 'the female equivalent to the combatant male' in both Britain and France after the war. She also points out that both types of nurse were viewed as 'self-abnegating, patriotic, and maternal'.[7] On the war memorial in the small Lancashire village of Caton, visitors can still read the name of 'Nurse Clementina Addison'; it appears at the end of a long list of the village's war dead. In large bold letters just below her name is the inscription: 'By Their Sacrifice We Live.'

But the vast majority of professional nurses survived the war, and most do not appear to have remembered their wartime work in terms of self-sacrifice. Some viewed it as an opportunity to prove

their worth—to have their work recognized and their professionalism valued. In some cases this led, understandably, to resentment
towards volunteer nurses who appeared to be claiming the right to
undertake vital life-saving work close to the front lines of war,
without having undergone the training and experience necessary.
In the eyes of many professionals, not only was this dangerous; it
was also an affront to a status that they had gained over three years
of hard labour in the wards of civilian hospitals. Their right to be
'on the front lines' of war had been hard-earned, and its usurpation by volunteers was seen as unjust. In Britain, the myth of the
VAD grew out of this natural mistrust between professional nurses
and VADs, fuelled by writings such as Vera Brittain's *Testament of
Youth*, Irene Rathbone's *We That Were Young*, and Enid Bagnold's
*Diary Without Dates*. VAD Mary Cannan was later to comment on
Vera Brittain's experience: 'I think she was unfortunate.' She added
that the fears of nurses that their profession would be flooded by
the semi-trained after the war were unfounded. Most VADs were
glad to return to their lives away from nursing. This, she added,
was a pity because 'with better relations many might have stayed
on, the "image" of nursing might have been different, and maybe
the present shortage of nurses never happened'.[8] Some professional nurses did try to encourage their VAD assistants to enter
nurse training programmes after the war. Florence Egerton wrote
home to her mother from a Territorial hospital in Leicester during
the war with the news that the sister on her ward was praising her
work and urging her to train as a nurse; but Egerton had already
decided to become an infant teacher, an ambition she was able to
fulfil once the war was over.[9]

The earliest published accounts of war nursing were memoirs
such as Millicent, Duchess of Sutherland's *Six Weeks at the War* and
Sarah Macnaughtan's *A Woman's Diary of the War*; and the earliest
publicity in the national press was for volunteer units such Mabel
St Clair Stobart's Women's Sick and Wounded Convoy Corps.
Hence, the first images to be placed before the eager eyes of a

readership anxious to know that its own 'boys' were safe were those of wealthy volunteers with little experience of nursing work or of highly individualistic freelance ventures. In reality, the efforts of these small units and individual enterprises were rapidly eclipsed by the large-scale clinical interventions of the military nursing services of those countries where nursing was highly developed as a discipline—notably, Britain, Australia, New Zealand, Canada, and South Africa. Yet volunteer nurses remained—and have continued to remain—at the forefront of public perception. The published writings of VADs such as Vera Brittain and Irene Rathbone continue to attract great interest for a number of reasons: these women presented as highly romantic figures in their blue-and-white uniforms; they experienced trials and ordeals which no one who had been properly prepared for the work had to face; and, because of the privilege of education, many were excellent writers.

Wartime mortality and morbidity figures are notoriously difficult to interpret. There are many reasons why some nations experienced disproportionately higher casualty-rates then others. Yet the armies of those nations which had well-organized professional nursing services, do appear to have had better survival rates than those which continued, throughout the war, to rely on large numbers of volunteer nurses. Organized nursing services, staffed by fully trained professionals, appear to have been highly successful in implementing effective wound-management techniques and in preventing epidemics of diseases such as typhus by maintaining control of hospital environments.

Governments and senior medical officers recognized the value of expert nursing and fully trained nurses were at a premium. Those who did not enlist with their own nations' recognized military nursing services but worked instead in a more 'freelance' capacity, either alone or for organizations such as the French Flag Nursing Corps, were in high demand. A classic example was Violetta Thurstan, who chose to go wherever she thought the 'hottest' part of the action would be, and who appears only to have been employed by the official British services in 1917, when as matron of one of the largest hospitals in Belgium she could support victims of one of the war's most destructive battles: Passchendaele.

Some nurses found their work strangely incongruous and troubling. American Ellen LaMotte referred to it as a 'dead end job': patching up the wounded so that they could be sent back to the places of destruction. Yet, for the majority, it appears to have been a highly patriotic endeavour. Belgian nurse Jane De Launoy identified herself with the beguines of former days. For her, returning soldiers to the 'motherland' was an almost divine mission. For many professional nurses the healing of the wounded and sick appears to have had its own rewards. The arrival of a severely damaged man at a field hospital presented a challenge which was both technical and humanitarian: how could the nurse—with the greatest effectiveness and the least risk—save the life and preserve the integrity of this human being? Such work was seen as valuable in its own right, whatever the man's eventual fate; and its successful prosecution was a source of professional pride. The work was infused with clinical and moral dilemmas. Nurses struggled to convert scientific medical prescriptions into effective healing practices in environments that were far from healthy. In 1915, when surgeons were experimenting with a range of different means to combat dangerous anaerobic wound infections such as gas gangrene and tetanus, nurses implemented treatments with precision, while, at the same time, addressing patients' needs for relief and comfort. They also provided essential observational data which would permit treatments to be adjusted and made more effective.

Many of the clinical dilemmas of nurses were understood in terms that mirrored warfare itself: infection-control was a battle against an enemy—the disease germs—that must be wiped out. And many of their dilemmas would never have been encountered in peacetime. In 1917, when bombing raids on bases increased in intensity, it was difficult for nurses to know which was best: to move their heavily splinted patients below the level of the sandbags surrounding their tents, or to leave them 'up' in a position which was healthier for damaged limbs. Whatever they decided for each individual patient, they themselves remained on the wards, offering comfort and support during even the fiercest air raids. And many believed that this ability to display courage and calmness in the face of danger and hardship was one of their most important contributions to the war effort.

Nurses expanded their clinical skills during the war into areas that would probably never have been dreamed of in peacetime. As members of surgical teams, many engaged in minor operative procedures or trained as 'lady anaesthetists'. But even in 'narratives' written for official reasons, they were unlikely to draw attention to their clinical expertise, focusing instead on stories of endurance and courage—of how 'splendidly' everyone had behaved.

Many nurses' writings carry overtones of stoicism and endurance. The 'stiff upper lip', which has become a stereotypical feature of the British soldier, was shared by his female counterpart, the military nurse. And it was a feature which was displayed—albeit in a range of different ways—by nurses of all Allied nations. The diaries and letters of both nurses and VADs contain a conscious cheeriness and determination; they are modelled on heroic tropes. Hence, the 'narrative' of Eveline Vickers-Foote, the Australian nurse, who worked on board the *Assaye* in the Aegean and was then shipwrecked trying to return to Australia, is written with an air of studied nonchalance and embellished with comments such as 'it was exciting all right!'[10] Similarly, the diaries of Jentie Paterson of her work on the Western Front and in the Eastern Mediterranean are infused with a sense of purpose and adventure.

In the winter of 1918–19, nurse-leaders in Allied countries began to look to the future of their profession. Victory and peace had been secured. For a small but significant group of professional nurses in Britain, the battle into which all their energies would now be poured was the battle for nurse registration. Ethel Gordon Fenwick argued vociferously that the country owed its nurses—who

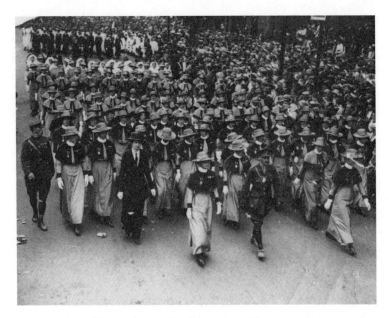

FIGURE 28 Maud McCarthy leads nurses in the 1919 Victory Parade (photograph reproduced by kind permission of Sue Light)

had risked their lives on the front line of war—the political recognition of a closed register. Not only would this protect the public from 'false nurses'; it would also reward 'true nurses' for their unstinting contribution to the war effort. The profession was given the reward it so craved: a register for British nurses passed into legislation on 23 December 1919, as a result of the Nurses Registration Act. In the self-governing Dominions, similar moves were under way. Legislation to provide for the registration of nurses had been passed in all Canadian provinces by 1922, and in all Australian provinces by 1928.[11]

Professional nurses may have won their right to recognition. Yet they continued to exhibit a penchant for self-sacrifice, perhaps believing that their self-effacing demeanour was an asset—one of the elements of their perceived heroism. While working at the South London Hospital for Women in the early 1920s, Kate Luard wrote an article for the *Girl Guides Gazette*, on 'The Importance of Character in Nursing the Sick'. It concludes that 'the watchword in the nursing service is The Patient First, The Hospital Second, Self Last', adding that if her young readers 'act up to this, at whatever cost to yourself, you will be maintaining the great tradition of your profession for those who come after you'.[12] This notion that, by becoming nurses, young women were also becoming a part of something much greater then themselves was one that was to sustain the profession during the difficult interwar years: a time of draconian discipline, poor conditions, and stagnant pay, leading to high attrition and low morale.

For many individual nurses and volunteers, the interwar years were a time of frustration, when their hard-won expertise and prowess was once again buried within a patriarchal society. Although women had acquired the vote, it was to be some time before they would secure the employment rights which would grant them real freedom. Some had been obliged to withdraw from the war effort long before they were due to be discharged from service. The most famous of these was Vera Brittain, who left Étaples in April 1918, in order to care for an ailing mother. Sister Kate Luard was obliged to resign in the late autumn of 1918 to care for her dying father, and Sister Jentie Paterson's diaries end abruptly in 1916 following her father's death. Following her return to 'active service' on 10 January 1917, she was posted to the Cambridge Hospital, Aldershot, but during her time there, she became seriously ill with 'ear and nose problems'. She requested leave to attend an aural surgeon with whom she had worked previously at Guy's Hospital, but Matron-in-Chief Ethel Becher's rather terse response was that 'nurses cannot chose [*sic*] their own specialists while they are in military hospitals'. Having 'no wish to become a chronic case', Paterson tendered her resignation from the QAIMNSR, for the last time, on 11 July 1917.[13] Personal illness, or the need to return home to take up the role of family carer, caused considerable disruption for many women both during and after the war.

In the British Dominions, nurse-leaders were following a very similar path to that taken by campaigning British nurses such as Ethel Gordon Fenwick. In an era long before the concept of cultural sensitivity, the International Council of Nurses (ICN) encouraged the idea that there could be a global understanding of professionalism in nursing and that practice in all countries should be based on a Western notion of good educational standards and legally sanctioned systems of regulation. Jane Child, who had travelled to Europe in 1915 at the head of the first contingent of South African nurses to serve with the Allied medical services, became South Africa's representative on the ICN in 1921. In 1931, she expressed, in a foreword to the 'jubilee edition' of the *South African Nursing Journal,* her sense of the need for nurses to remain vigilant about the educational standards and ethical purity of their profession. She did so in heroic terms, which were strangely redolent of much of the language used by nurses during the war: 'I would send you a watchword for the future—let it be "Courage"; let courage defend what has been won, let it be the staff with which you go to meet the future in all your professional concerns...keep your Register pure and your professional and ethical standards high.'[14]

In Belgium the move to develop effective schools of nursing—which war had so abruptly halted—resumed. But one of the country's most effective nurse-educators—Edith Cavell—had been lost, and the struggle to reorganize nurse training was just one part of a long and slow national recovery. Queen Elisabeth of the Belgians, one of the most potent symbols of wartime nursing, continued to support the work of developing a nascent nursing profession, but the process was a difficult one. Decades after the war, Belgium was still one of the 'devastated lands'—a place to which tourists came to view extant trenches and shell holes, and in which the children of farmers could still be horribly mutilated by unexploded shells.

In France, the campaign for the professionalization of nursing had, from the start, been more fragmented and less successful than in Britain and its Dominions. Individual, highly-successful secular

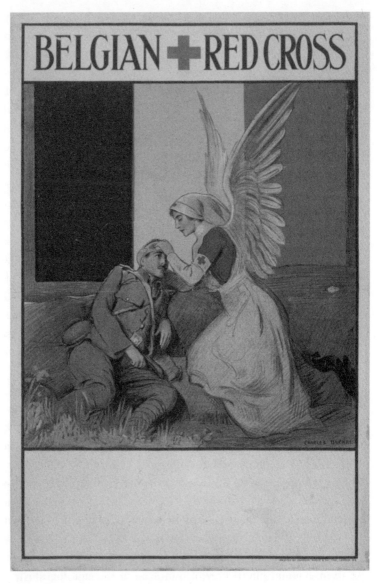

FIGURE 29 Image from a Belgian Red Cross poster (©Archives Belgian Red Cross, Brussels)

training schools, such as those established by Désiré Bourneville in Paris and Anna Hamilton in Bordeaux, had not acted as models for a national reform of nurse training. Nor had small pockets of professional activity or frequent calls for employment rights led to any large-scale movement for professionalization. The flooding of military hospitals with 'Red Cross ladies' had proved an even greater problem for the French than for the British, dissolving the boundaries between professional and amateur, and fuelling the patriarchal belief that nursing was a low-status, innately feminine activity rather than an expert professional pursuit, requiring train-ing and regulation. The profile of the nurse had, indeed, been raised by the activities of both trained and 'amateur' care-givers during the war years; but the wartime image of the nurse—of womanly duty and patriotic self-sacrifice—was one that could not be sustained in peacetime. What was needed now was a cadre of thoroughly knowledgeable and committed professionals.[15]

In the four years following the Armistice a small handful of cam-paigners fought to rebuild the nascent professional boundaries which the war 'had so effectively erased'.[16] Léonie Chaptal, direc-trice of a small nursing school in Paris, and Anna Hamilton, vet-eran campaigner for nurse education, took advantage of the serious shortage of nurses created by the desertion of those tens of thou-sands of 'amateurs' whose motives had been purely patriotic. At the same time, the involvement of trained nurses in public health projects, such as the campaign against tuberculosis, demonstrated to both the government and the medical elites that a fully profes-sional nursing service was a requirement for any modern state. On 27 June 1922 a state decree established the official title of 'Licensed Nurse of the French State'. Licensure was dependent upon train-ing in a recognized nursing school for two years and the passing of an examination. The decree also created a 'Council for the Im-provement of Nursing Schools'.[17] But the passing of legislation which effectively closed the boundaries of professional nursing did not place control of that profession into the hands of nurses themselves. Membership of the council was composed almost entirely of hospital administrators and doctors; not one of its members was a practising nurse. Furthermore, the law did not state that only holders of a nursing diploma could practise as nurses. Anyone who chose to could still call themselves a 'nurse' and secure work caring for patients.

Fully trained US nurses seem to have fared somewhat better than their European counterparts. Margaret Cowling returned to the USA with the nurses of Base Hospital No. 41 in March 1919. By 1920 she was back in her powerful and highly respected role as Superintendent of Nurses of the University of Virginia Hospital.[18] Sara McCarron—a woman of clearly adventurous tastes—signed up for further Red Cross service following the Armistice, travelling directly from France to the war-blighted and impoverished town of Podgoritza.[19] Her taste for travel and adventure was not incompatible with her desire—and her ability—to offer public health support to devastated populations. Following her return to the USA, she worked as a public health nurse in New York City, but thirteen years after her retirement she was taken seriously ill and hospitalized. The affection and respect her family held for her is revealed by their fight to prevent the authorities from moving her to Baltimore, several hundred miles from her home. Her niece Lillian Behringer wrote to, among others, President Kennedy, appealing on her aunt's behalf, stating that a proposed move away from her family would 'break her heart', and adding that 'my Aunt, who has given so much to the cause of humanity, deserves humane treatment for herself at this time when her need is great'. Behringer was successful in having McCarron transferred to a VA Hospital on 23rd Street, New York City and her aunt died three years later, in 1964, in the heart of the city whose population she had nursed and close to the relatives who had held her in such high esteem.

Nurses in the USA seemed to overleap some of the obstacles that had been proving so intransigent in Britain. In an article published long before the war, American nurse-leader Lavinia Dock had commented that registration was 'not only a nurses' affair. It is an educational question. It is a woman's question. It is a part of the vast human advance.'[20] The first university course for nurses had been established in 1892 at Columbia University, New York, and Adelaide Nutting, the USA's first professor of nursing, was appointed in 1910. The US Army Nurse Corps had been founded in 1901, and although military nurses were not to be afforded officer status until the 1940s, they were recognized as an important element of the military medical services. In November 1914, Mary Messer had declared, in an article published in the *American Journal of Nursing*, that 'the graduate nurse today must be educated in all lines. She must be broad-minded and of a high character so that she may successfully cope with the problems of the day.'[21] The formation of the Army School of Nursing during the war enabled US nurse-leaders to avoid the disruption that was caused in Britain by the abrupt cessation of the wave of enthusiasm for nursing among untrained women which had characterized the war. American nurse-leaders had had time to plan. The Atlantic Ocean stood between them and the armies of the Central Powers. Their nursing services had not been hastily assembled in the face of a sudden national emergency. A smaller proportion of the population was directly affected by death and mutilation, and no lands were devastated. The development of a nursing service was able to continue without the distortions that traumatic upheaval had occasioned in Europe.

In Russia and Eastern Europe, the development of an autonomous nursing profession was curtailed by the emergence of peculiarly patriarchal and chauvinistic forms of communist government. In Russia, the 'All-Union Congress of Russian Sisters of Mercy', an organization which had formed under pressure of wartime need, was dissolved by the Bolshevik government in 1919 and so-called 'red sisters' with only two months' training were appointed to care for soldiers on the Civil War front.[22] Professional recovery was a long and painfully slow progress, which did not really begin to take hold until the later twentieth century.

Maria Bucur has argued that, in Romania—a nation that suffered tremendous casualties and was rapidly overrun by the Central Powers—a myth of the wartime nurse as war heroine was deliberately fostered by women-writers in an attempt to counterbalance a narrative of the war as an exclusively male enterprise. Bucur has commented on the emphasis on 'women's dignified and selfless participation in the war effort' as a common motif in their writings.[23] One of the best-known such autobiographies was Queen Marie's *Ordeal: The Story of My Life*, which bore witness to the suffering of civilians.[24] Such writings deliberately questioned the assumption that heroism could only be associated with combat, by emphasizing the bravery inherent in performing the grinding and exhausting work of caring for the wounded and enduring with fortitude the privations of daily life as a nurse. But, in doing so, they rendered the stories of wartime nurses into heroic romances rather than catalogues of achievement. While the actions of doctors—along with their beneficial effects—were detailed in 'official histories' of the wartime medical services, those of nurses were obscured by romantic and often fanciful interpretations. Queen Marie's own memoir, while a testament to her dedication to her nation and devotion to her people, is also a skilful piece of self-promoting propaganda. She writes of the winter of 1916/17 as 'a period of almost superhuman stress, when the exultation of sacrifice multiplied my usual strength, so that I never at any time completely broke down'.[25] Her memoir is punctuated with Hollywood-style images of herself in her Red Cross uniform (see Figure 30). The epitome of the 'warrior-queen', Marie stands as one of the most powerful images of the wartime nurse. She, perhaps, provides the glamorized counterfoil of practising professional nurses such as Kate Luard, who became head sister of the Advanced Abdominal Centre at Brandhoek during the Battle of Passchendaele, and Matron Grace Wilson, who somehow ran an effective Australian General Hospital on the Island of Lemnos, in spite of drought, flies, dystentery, and male medical chauvinism.

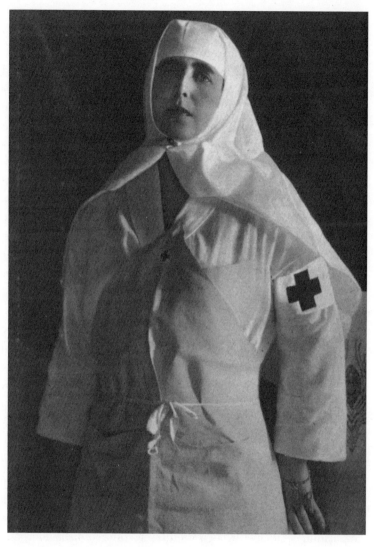

FIGURE 30 Queen Marie of Romania (image from her book: *Ordeal: The Story of My Life* (New York: Charles Scribner's Sons, 1935)). Caption reads: 'My white Red Cross dress had become a symbol'.

Yet such images also distort our understanding of women's achieve-ments, overlaying the reality of the professional nurse with an image of the fantasy-nurse.

The white-veiled woman sitting at the bedside of the wounded soldier is a potent image—one that was exploited during and after the war by propagandists, novelists, and film-makers anxious to evoke an emotional rather than a rational response. For some, the nurse was a nurse simply because she was female and *there*. Her mere presence at the bedside of the wounded and sick could evoke healing. There was an assumption that, as a woman, she would know what to do, and this knowledge would be all the more pro-found if she had the 'breeding' of an upper-class lady. For many professional nurses, this image was a distorting, even insulting, one. They knew that it was not their mere presence at the bedside of the wounded that mattered, but their knowledgeable, skilled, and intel-ligent presence. Such qualities, welded to compassion, ensured that their patients were both safe and comfortable.

Yet, for many members of the military, the presence of any woman—trained or untrained—at the bedside of the wounded soldier was dangerous: the female military nurse put not only her-self but her patient and, indeed, the whole army in danger, be-cause she disturbed the masculine balance of warfare—confusing the thinking of the male combatant and softening his approach to his mission.

The right for nurses simply to be where they were most needed was hard-won. Overcoming the image of the camp-follower, who was little better than a prostitute, had not been straightforward, and had not yet been fully achieved. It required the careful ma-nipulation of image through the use of costume, behaviour, and discipline. But this image was all too easy to subvert. Authors, film-makers, and politicians alike would choose to see innate qual-ities of pure femininity rather than a hard-won professionalism. Or, at least, if they portrayed the latter, it would be personified by the hard, embittered spinster-nurse, who acted as a foil to the heroine-volunteer. Thus, the image of the nurse as a mere cipher, a luminous and rather unreal presence in a world where men were the main actors was perpetuated. Powerful fictional men such as Frederic Henry in Hemingway's *A Farewell to Arms* and Yuri Zhivago in Pasternak's *Doctor Zhivago* wooed fragile, ethereal heroines such as Catherine Barkley and Larissa Antipova. And the power of nursing itself was, largely, overlooked by all but a handful of articulate former VADs whose experiences of the turbulence within the nursing profession had left them with at best ambivalent and at worst highly negative perspectives. Still, even for them, nursing was more than a mere passive transmission of healing from nurse to patient. It was, rather, an awakening of awareness and consciousness—a transformative encounter with suffering.

In the twenty-first century, there are indications that a few popular fiction writers are beginning to explore the potentialities of the fully trained professional nurse of the First World War as a gritty and characterful—though still romantic—figure. Thomas Keneally's powerful story of the 'Durance sisters'—two fictional professional nurses who travelled to the Eastern Mediterranean and the Western Front with the Australian Army Nursing Service—contains searching, and yet dramatic, episodes relating a range of technical and ethical dilemmas faced by trained nurses. Yet Naomi and Sally Durance—for all their aloofness and professional demeanour—are also romantic heroines, whose experiences are moving and whose fates are poignant.[26]

And First World War nurses are, once again, the subjects of drama. In 2013, as I write this book, directors and producers sit in a BBC cutting room producing the final edits for a new BBC drama, *The Crimson Field*, to be released in 2014.[27] Although, on the face of it, the central characters in the series are the beautiful and youthful VADs in their gorgeous (but not entirely authentic) blue-and-white costumes, one of the goals of the project is to capture the characters of professional nurses with sympathy and artistry. At least some of the programme's plot lines give precedence to the experiences of trained nurses. At a base hospital somewhere on the north coast of France, Matron Grace Carter struggles to hold together a disparate and challenging nursing workforce, consisting of trained nurses, VADs, and orderlies. Her impressive colleague, Joan Livesey, offers an impeccably professional nursing service to patients, while facing her own troubling personal struggle. The dilemmas faced by *The Crimson Field*'s characters are a blend of the clinical and the personal, and some of its emphases are on the drama of nursing itself.

Professional nurses provide authors and scriptwriters with perfect 'heroines': many travelled far from home and endured danger and deprivation; they presented themselves as idealistic, compassionate, and unselfish; and they undertook work that brought them into intimate contact with the war and its wounded. Yet only recently have writers begun to pay attention to what it meant to be a professional nurse. Perhaps only now, in the twenty-first century, can writers and directors allow themselves to view independent, self-contained—and often very powerful—professional women as worthy material for popular fiction.

Yet, even though it is separated from them by a gulf of one hundred years, the modern perspective is not so different from those of the nurses themselves. In the second decade of the twentieth century, nurses of all Allied nations appear to have been inspired by the ideal of 'heroism' and it seems that many modelled their behaviour in accordance with the notion that if soldiers could be heroes, then so too could nurses. The propagandist writings of journalists served to keep this image in the minds of populations and of nurses themselves—yet they also subtly undermined it. Stories of women trekking over the Albanian Alps in 1915 and poignant tales of the courage of *Marquette* victims in professional nursing journals promoted the image of the nurse-heroine, an image that was further propagated—and yet also subverted—by mainstream national newspapers. When a *Manchester Guardian* journalist wrote of 'ragged, dishevelled women and girls' in 'gay west end shops', he managed to put the nurses of the Serbian units back into their places as females in a male-dominated society, by subtly colouring their heroic exploits with shades of victimhood and shopping.

The nursing services of the First World War were a heterogeneous group: composed, as they were, of many nationalities and drawn from every social class, their common mission was distorted by their lack of common identity. They were nursing on many geographical fronts; and their emotional, moral, and professional struggles took many forms. For the duration of the war, their greatest effort was poured into the struggle to keep alive millions of casualties on the 'second battlefield' of the world's military hospitals. But they also fought a more hidden and subversive battle: for their own identity as professional women in a male-dominated and class-driven world. And, even as they joined forces to defeat their common enemies—injury, disease, and despair—they also turned inwards against each other. The lack of any formal political or social recognition for their work meant that fully trained professional nurses resented the presence of volunteer nurses on their wards, even as they valued some of their contributions. Volunteers themselves—many of whom were of high social status—often failed to recognize the artistry and expertise inherent in nursing work, or the importance of a three-year training in making such work possible. Nurses were fighting a multi-layered battle: for lives, for recognition, and for equality. Their struggles would continue well beyond the Armistice of 11 November 1918.

# Notes

## Introduction

1. Vera Brittain, *Testament of Youth: An Autobiographical Study of the Years 1900–1925* (1933; London: Virago, 2004), 75.

2. Vera Brittain, *Chronicle of Youth* (1981; London: Phoenix Press, 2000), 230.

3. One of the most significant analyses of mythology was offered by one of the First World War's most famous survivors: Robert Graves. See Robert Graves, *The Greek Myths* (1955; London: Penguin, 1992). On the power of mythology, see also Joseph Campbell, *The Hero with a Thousand Faces* (1949; London: Fontana, 1993). On collective memory of the First World War, see Paul Fussell, *The Great War and Modern Memory* (1975; Oxford: Oxford University Press, 2000); Robert Wohl, *The Generation of 1914* (London: Weidenfeld and Nicolson, 1980); Jay Winter, *Sites of Memory, Sites of Mourning: The Great War in European Cultural History* (Cambridge: Cambridge University Press, 1995).

4. Brittain, *Testament of Youth*; Enid Bagnold, *A Diary Without Dates* (1918; London: Virago, 1978); Irene Rathbone, *We That Were Young: A Novel* (1932; New York: The Feminist Press, 1989). For a fuller discussion of the impact of these three writings, see Christine E. Hallett, '"Emotional Nursing": Involvement, Engagement, and Detachment in the Writings of First World War Nurses and VADs', in Alison S. Fell and Hallett (eds.), *First World War Nursing: New Perspectives* (New York: Routledge, 2013), 87–102.

5. On the idea that the young men who fought in the First World War were 'Lions led by Donkeys' see Alan Clark, *The Donkeys* (1961; London: Pimlico, 1991). For an analysis of this myth, see Dan Todman, *The Great War: Myth and Memory* (London: Hambledon Continuum, 2005), 73–120.

6. On the relationships between trained nurses and VADs, see Sharon Ouditt, *Fighting Forces, Writing Women: Identity and Ideology in the First World War* (London: Routledge, 1994); Janet S. K. Watson, 'Wars in the Wards: The Social Construction of Medical Work in First World War Britain', *Journal of British Studies*, 41 (2002), 484–510; Janet S. K. Watson, *Fighting Different Wars: Experience, Memory and the First World War in Britain* (Cambridge: Cambridge University Press, 2004), 59–104; Christine E. Hallett, *Containing Trauma: Nursing Work in the First World War* (Manchester: Manchester University Press, 2009), 201; Hallett, ' "Emotional Nursing" ', 87–102.

7. On the character of nurse-training in the late nineteenth and early twentieth centuries, see Ann Bradshaw, *The Nurse Apprentice, 1860–1977* (Aldershot: Ashgate, 2001); Christine Hallett, 'Nursing, 1840–1920: Forging a Profession', in Anne Borsay and Billie Hunter (eds.), *Nursing and Midwifery in Britain Since 1700* (London: Palgrave Macmillan, 2012), 46–73; Christine Hallett and Hannah Cooke, *Historical Investigations into the Professional Self-Regulation of Nursing and Midwifery*, i. *Nursing* (London: Nursing and Midwifery Council, 2011), available at the Archives of the Nursing and Midwifery Council, 23 Portland Place, London.

8. Ernest Hemingway, *A Farewell to Arms* (New York: Charles Scribner's Sons, 1929).

9. Henry Serrano Villard and James Nagel, *Hemingway in Love and War: The Lost Diary of Agnes von Kurowsky, Her Letters and Correspondence of Ernest Hemingway* (Boston: Northeastern University Press, 1989).

10. Hallett, *Containing Trauma*, 155–93.

11. *A Farewell to Arms* (1932), directed by Frank Borzage; *A Farewell to Arms* (1957), directed by John Huston and Charles Vidor.

12. *In Love and War* (1996), directed by Richard Attenborough.

13. Boris Pasternak, *Doctor Zhivago*, trans. Max Hayward and Manya Harari (1958; London: Vintage Books, 2002), 32.

14. Pasternak, *Doctor Zhivago*, quotes on pp. 104, 106.

15. On the outbreak of the First World War, and the readiness of populations to fight, see Paul Fussell, *The Great War and Modern Memory*, 18–29; Hew Strachan, *The First World War* (2003; London: Pocket Books, 2006), 60–3; Adrian Gregory, *The Last Great War: British Society and the First World War* (Cambridge: Cambridge University Press, 2008), 9–39.

16. On the perspectives of women, see Gail Braybon, *Women Workers in the First World War: The British Experience* (London: Croom Helm, 1981); Claire Tylee, *The Great War and Women's Consciousness: Images of Militarism and Womanhood in Women's Writings, 1914–1964* (Houndmills: Macmillan 1990), 20; Ouditt, *Fighting Forces, Writing Women*; Margaret Higonnet, *Lines of Fire: Women Writers of World War I* (Harmondsworth: Penguin, 1999); Susan Grayzel, *Women's Identities at War: Gender, Motherhood, and Politics in Britain and France during the First World War* (Chapel Hill, NC: University of North Carolina Press, 1999).

17. On the fight for women's suffrage, see Ray Strachey, *The Cause: A Short History of the Women's Movement in Great Britain* (Bath: Cedric Chivers, 1928); A. Fell and I. Sharp (eds.), *The Women's Movement in Wartime: International Perspectives 1914–1918* (Basingstoke: Palgrave, 2007).

18. In the USA, the term 'woman suffrage' was used: see Ellen Carol Dubois, *Woman Suffrage and Women's Rights* (New York: New York University Press, 1998). On the march for woman suffrage, see Kimberly Jensen, *Mobilizing Minerva: American Women in the First World War* (Urbana and Chicago: University of Illinois Press, 2008), 1–10.

19. On the perspectives of nurses, see Anne Marie Rafferty and Diana Solano, 'The Rise and Demise of the Colonial Nursing Service: British Nurses in the Colonies, 1896–1966', *Nursing History Review*, 15 (2007), 147–54.

20. On 'Daughters of the Empire' see Katie Pickles, *Female Imperialism and National Identity: Imperial Order Daughters of the Empire* (Manchester: Manchester University Press, 2002).

21. On the Russian women's battalions, see Laurie Stoff, *They Fought for the Motherland: Russia's Women Soldiers in World War I and Revolution* (Lawrence, Kan.: University of Kansas Press, 2006).

22. Angela Smith, *Women's Writing of the First World War* (Manchester: Manchester University Press, 2000), 179.

23. Numerous letters of complaint were published in the three main nursing journals during the early months of the war: *British Journal of Nursing* (available online at the Royal College of Nursing Archives); *Nursing Times*; *Nursing Mirror and Midwives Journal*. For examples, see Hallett, ' "Emotional Nursing" ', 87–102.

24. Millicent, Duchess of Sutherland, *Six Weeks at the War* (London: *The Times*, 1914); Mary Borden, *The Forbidden Zone* (London: William Heinemann Ltd, 1929).

25. Borden, *The Forbidden Zone*, 147.

26. Mary was very serious about her ambition to become a nurse. On her 21st birthday, 25 April 1918, she applied to Great Ormond Street Hospital in London, to train as a children's nurse: Mary Mackie, *Sky Wards: A History of the Princess Mary's Royal Air Force Nursing Service* (London: Robert Hale, 2001), 47.

27. Luc de Munck and Luc Vandeweyer, *Het Hospitaal van de Koningin: Rode Kruis, L'Océan en De Panne* (De Panne: Gemeetebestuur De Panne en de auteurs, 2012), 112. I am indebted to Luc de Munck and Lionel Roosemont for translations of material from this book.

28. Marie told her own story in Marie, Queen of Roumania, *Ordeal: The Story of My Life* (New York: Charles Scribner's Sons, 1935).

29. On Edith Cavell's life and work, see A. A. Hoehling, *Edith Cavell* (London: Cassel and Company, 1958); Jonathan Evans, *Edith Cavell* (London: The London Hospital Museum, 2008); Diana Souhami, *Edith Cavell* (London: Quercus, 2010): on Cavell's work at the Training School for Nurses, Rue de la Culture, Brussels, see pp. 93–109.

30. *Nurse Edith Cavell*, directed by Herbert Wilcox and starring Anna Neagle (USA, 1939).

31. Baroness de T'Serclaes, *Flanders and Other Fields* (London: George G. Harrap and Co. Ltd, 1964); G. E. Mitton (ed.), *The Cellar-House of Pervyse: A Tale of Uncommon Things from the Journals and Letters of the Baroness De T'Serclaes and Mairi Chisholm* (London: A and E Black, 1916); Diane Atkinson, *Elsie and Mairi Go To War: Two Extraordinary Women on the Western Front* (London: Preface Publishing, 2009). On heroism in nursing, see also Tammy M. Proctor, ' "Patriotism is not enough": Women, Citizenship and the First World War', *Journal of Women's History*, 17/2 (2005), 169–76.

32. Brian Abel-Smith, *A History of the Nursing Profession* (London: Heinemann, 1960); Susan McGann, *The Battle of the Nurses: A Study of Eight Women Who Influenced the Development of Professional Nursing, 1880–1930* (London: Scutari Press, 1992); Anne Marie Rafferty, *The Politics of Nursing Knowledge* (London: Routledge, 1996).

33. In Cape Colony, South Africa, a register had been attained as part of a Medical and Pharmacy Act in 1891. In New Zealand a Nurses' Registration Act was passed in 1901 (in NZ, women, by this time, also had the vote): Lavinia Dock, 'The Progress of Registration', *American Journal of Nursing*, 6/5 (Feb. 1906), 297–305.

34. On the life and work of Ethel Bedford Fenwick, see Winifred Hector, *The Work of Mrs Bedford Fenwick and the Rise of Professional Nursing* (London: Royal College of Nursing, 1973). On the *British Journal of Nursing* as an organ of professionalization, see Christine E. Hallett, '"Intelligent interest in their own affairs": The First World War, the *British Journal of Nursing* and the Pursuit of Nursing Knowledge', in P. D'Antonio, J. Fairman, and J. Whelan (eds.), *Routledge Handbook on the Global History of Nursing* (London and New York: Routledge, 2013), 95–113.

35. On the International Council of Nurses, see Barbara Brush et al., *Nurses of All Nations: A History of the International Council of Nurses, 1899–1999* (Philadelphia: Lippincott, Williams and Wilkins, 1999).

36. Mark Bostridge, *Florence Nightingale: The Woman and Her Legend* (London: Viking, 2008), 502–6. See also McGann, *The Battle of the Nurses*; Rafferty, *The Politics of Nursing Knowledge*.

37. Hallett and Cooke, *Historical Investigations into the Professional Self-Regulation of Nursing and Midwifery*.

38. Strachey, *The Cause*, 337.

39. Fenwick included a column on the women's movement, entitled 'Outside the Gates', in every issue of the *British Journal of Nursing*. All three nursing journals are available at the Royal College of Nursing Archives, Edinburgh. The *British Journal of Nursing* is, additionally, available online at <http://rcnarchive.rcn.org.uk/>.

40. On the Australian Army Nursing Services see Jan Bassett, *Guns and Brooches: Australian Army Nursing from the Boer War to the Gulf War* (Melbourne: Oxford University Press, 1992), 1–31; Ruth Rae, *Scarlet Poppies: The Army Experience of Australian Nurses during World War One* (Burwood, NSW: College of Nursing, 2004); Ruth Rae, *Veiled Lives: Threading Australian Nursing History into the Fabric of the First World War* (Burwood, NSW: College of Nursing, 2009); Kirsty Harris, *More than Bombs and Bandages: Australian Army Nurses at Work in World War I* (Newport, NSW: Big Sky Publishing, 2011). On the New Zealand Army Nursing Service,

see Sherayl Kendall and David Corbett, *New Zealand Military Nursing: A History of the Royal New Zealand Nursing Corps, Boer War to Present Day* (Auckland: Sherayl Kendall and David Corbett, 1990); Jan Rodgers, 'Potential for Professional Profit: The Making of the New Zealand Army Nursing Service, 1914–1915', *Nursing Praxis in New Zealand*, 11/2 (July 1996), 4–12; Jill Clendon, 'New Zealand Military Nurses' Fight for Recognition: World War I–World War II', *Nursing Praxis in New Zealand*, 12/1 (Mar. 1997), 24–8; Anna Rogers, *While You're Away: New Zealand Nurses At War, 1899–1948* (Auckland: Auckland University Press, 2003). On the Canadian nursing services, see Shawna M. Quinn, *Agnes Warner and the Nursing Sisters of the Great War* (Fredericton, New Brunswick: Goose Lane Editions, 2010).

41. Mary T. Sarnecky, *A History of the U.S. Army Nurse Corps* (Philadelphia: University of Pennsylvania Press, 1999), 51.
42. It should be noted that the Canadian military nursing service did incorporate small numbers of 'VADs' into its ranks. See Linda Quiney, 'Assistant Angels: Canadian Voluntary Aid Detachment Nurses in the Great War', *Canadian Bulletin of Medical History*, 15/1 (1998), 189–206.
43. On the formation of the VAD movement, see Thelka Bowser, *The Story of British VAD Work in the Great War* (1917; London: Imperial War Museum, 2003); Anne Summers, *Angels and Citizens: British Women as Military Nurses, 1854–1914* (London: Routledge and Kegan Paul, 1988), 237–70.
44. On the founding of the QAIMNS see Summers, *Angels and Citizens*, 220–36. The Indian Nursing Service, which was renamed the Queen Alexandra's Military Nursing Service in India, remained independent: Elizabeth S. Haldane, *The British Nurse in Peace and War* (London: John Murray, 1923), 168. On the QARNNS, see Kathleen Harland, *A History of Queen Alexandra's Royal Naval Nursing Service* (Portsmouth: *Journal of the Royal Naval Medical Service*, n.d.), 24–8.
45. Sue Light, 'British Military Nurses and the Great War: A Guide to the Services', *Western Front Association Forum* (7 Feb. 2010), 4; sourced at <http://www.westernfrontassociation.com> [accessed 30 Oct. 2012].
46. Anon. (ed.), *Reminiscent Sketches, 1914 to 1919 by Members of Her Majesty Queen Alexandra's Imperial Military Nursing Service* (London: John Bale, Sons and Danielsson, Ltd, 1922), preface, p. iii. On the foundation of

the QAIMNSR in 1908, see Haldane, *The British Nurse in Peace and War*, 167.

47. Light, 'British Military Nurses and the Great War'. The actual number has been placed at 10,404: Anon. (ed.), *Reminiscent Sketches*, p. iv; Haldane, *The British Nurse in Peace and War*, 187. On the British military nursing services at the outset of the war, see also Christine E. Hallett and Alison S. Fell, 'Introduction: New Perspectives on First World War Nursing', in Fell and Hallett (eds.), *First World War Nursing: New Perspectives* (New York: Routledge, 2013), 1–2.

48. Anon (ed.), *Reminiscent Sketches*, p. iv.

49. Emma Maud McCarthy left Britain for France on 14 August 1914. In 1915, she was installed at Abbeville as matron-in-chief of the British Expeditionary Force in France and Flanders. Her wartime reports can be found at Dame Maud McCarthy, Matron-in-Chief, British Expeditionary Force in France, Reports on Nursing Services, 1918, Box 10, 43/1985, Army Medical Services Museum Archives, Aldershot, UK. See also H. S. Gillespie, 'McCarthy, Dame (Emma) Maud (1858–1949)', in *Oxford Dictionary of National Biography* (Oxford: Oxford University Press, 2004–13); Perdita McCarthy, 'McCarthy, Dame Emma Maud (1859–1949)', in *Australian Dictionary of National Biography*, available online at <http://adb.anu.edu.au/biography/mccarthy-dame-emma-maud-7306> [accessed 24 Aug. 2013]. The Official War Diary of Maud McCarthy is available in The National Archives, Kew, UK: WO95/3988, WO95/3989, WO95/3990, WO95/3991. A full transcript of the diaries can be viewed online at <http://www.scarletfinders.co.uk/25.html> [last accessed 24 Aug. 2013].

50. Harland, *A History of Queen Alexandra's Royal Naval Nursing Service*, 29.

51. Sidney Browne had also helped found the QAIMNS, and had been its first matron-in-chief, before transferring her services to the Territorial Force Nursing Service on its formation in 1908. For documentary evidence relating to her career and a list of Territorial Force matrons and their hospitals, see Dame Sidney Jane Browne, Papers, Box 1, Army Medical Services Museum Archives, Aldershot, UK. For criticism of the matron of the First London General Hospital, see Brittain, *Testament of Youth*; Rathbone, *We That Were Young*. For a commentary on these issues, see Hallett, '"Emotional Nursing"', 87–102.

52. Circular Memorandum No. 83, War Office, 7 Aug. 1908. See also Report on the TFNS (1918). Both available in Dame Sidney Jane Browne, Papers, Box 1, Army Medical Services Museum Archives, Aldershot, UK.

53. The archives and published record contain slightly inconsistent figures: a 1918 report on the TFNS refers to a total number of 7,145, whilst the Secretary's Report to a meeting of the Advisory Council in the same year gives the figure as 7,269: Dame Sidney Jane Browne, Papers, Box 1, Army Medical Services Museum Archives, Aldershot, UK. Elizabeth Haldane claimed that 'by the end of the war the number enrolled was 8,140, of whom 2,280 served abroad': Haldane, *The British Nurse in Peace and War*, 179, 187.

54. Henriette Donner, 'Under the Cross—Why VADs Performed the Filthiest Tasks in the Dirtiest War: Red Cross Women Volunteers, 1914–1918', *Journal of Social History*, 30/3 (1997), 687–704; Watson, 'Wars in the Wards', 484–510; Hallett, *Containing Trauma*, 201.

55. Hallett, *Containing Trauma*, 201.

56. On the inadequacies of the nursing services during the Anglo-Boer War, see Summers, *Angels and Citizens*, 205–20.

57. Mark Harrison, *The Medical War: British Military Medicine in the First World War* (Oxford: Oxford University Press, 2010), 5.

58. The formation of a military nursing service for Belgium is discussed in Chapter 1 of this book. On the development of professional nursing in France, see Katrin Schultheiss, *Bodies and Souls: Politics and the Professionalization of Nursing in France, 1880–1922* (Cambridge, Mass.: Harvard University Press, 2001); Margaret Darrow, 'French Volunteer Nursing and the Myth of War Experience in World War I', *American Historical Review*, 101/1 (1996), 80–106.

59. Schultheiss, *Bodies and Souls*, 4–5, 30–4, 52, 85–115.

60. Schultheiss, *Bodies and Souls*, 4.

61. The three organizations which collectively made up the French Red Cross were the Société de Secours aux Blessés Militaires, the Association des Dames Françaises, and the Union des Femmes de France: Schultheiss, *Bodies and Souls*, 153; Hallett and Fell, 'Introduction: New Perspectives on First World War Nursing', 1–14.

62. R. Thamin, *Revue des deux mondes* (Nov.–Dec. 1919), quoted in Schultheiss, *Bodies and Souls*, 145.

63. Margaret H. Darrow, 'The Making of Sister Julie: The Origin of First World War French Nursing Heroines in Franco-Prussian War Stories', in Fell and Hallett (eds.), *First World War Nursing: New Perspectives*, 17–34.

64. Christine E. Hallett, 'Russian Romances: Emotionalism and Spirituality in the Writings of "Eastern Front" Nurses, 1914–1918', *Nursing History Review*, 17 (2009), 101–28; Susan Grant, 'Nursing in Russia and the Soviet Union, 1914–1941: An Overview of the Development of a Soviet Nursing System', *Bulletin of the UK Association for the History of Nursing*, 2 (2012), 21–33; Laurie Stoff, 'The "Myth of the War Experience" and Russian Wartime Nursing in World War I', *Aspasia: The International Yearbook of Central Eastern, and Southeastern European Women's and Gender History*, 6 (2012), 96–116.

65. Harrison, *The Medical War*, 11. On the medical services in the First World War see Sir William Grant Macpherson, *History of the Great War Based on Official Documents by Direction of the Historical Section of the Committee of Imperial Defence; Medical Services: General History*, i, ii, and iii (London: Macmillan, 1921, 1923, 1924).

66. Janet Butler, ' "Very busy in Bosches Alley": One Day of the Somme in Sister Kit McNaughton's Diary', *Health and History: Journal of the Australian Society of the History of Medicine*, 6/2 (2004), 18–32.

67. Christine E. Hallett, 'The Personal Writings of First World War Nurses: A Study of the Interplay of Authorial Intention and Scholarly Interpretation', *Nursing Inquiry*, 14/4 (2007), 320–9. On nurses' wartime writings, see also Christine E. Hallett, 'Portrayals of Suffering: Perceptions of Trauma in the Writings of First World War Nurses and Volunteers', *Canadian Bulletin of the History of Medicine*, 27/1 (2011), 65–84.

68. The published narratives are in Anon., *Reminiscent Sketches*; the unpublished larger collection is held at Army Medical Services Museum Archives, Aldershot, UK (QARANC Collection).

69. Nurses' Narratives, Butler Collection (including interviews conducted by Matron Kellett, 1919–20), AWM41, Australian War Memorial, Canberra, Australia; Arthur G. Butler, *Official History of the Australian Army Medical Services, 1914–1918*, i. *Gallipoli, Palestine and New Guinea* (2nd edn., Melbourne: Australian War Memorial, 1938); Arthur G. Butler, *Official History of the Australian Army Medical Services, 1914–1918*, ii. *The Western Front* (Canberra: Australian War Memorial, 1940); Arthur G.

Butler, *Official History of the Australian Army Medical Services, 1914–1918*, iii. *Special Problems and Services* (Melbourne: Australian War Memorial, 1943).

70. Borden, *The Forbidden Zone*, 147. 'The Second Battlefield' was taken as the title of an influential book on nurses' writings: Angela Smith, *The Second Battlefield: Women, Modernism and the First World War* (Manchester: Manchester University Press, 2000).

## Chapter 1

1. Adrian Gregory has indicated that over 100,000 had enlisted by 22 August 1914: Adrian Gregory, *The Last Great War: British Society and the First World War* (Cambridge: Cambridge University Press, 2008), 31. See also Allan Mallinson, *Fight The Good Fight: Britain, The Army and The Coming of the First World War* (London: Bantam Press, 2013).

2. I am indebted to Alison Fell for this information. On French nurses see Alison S. Fell, ' "Fallen Angels?" The Red Cross Nurse in First World War Discourse', in Maggie Allison and Yvette Rocheron (eds.), *The Resilient Female Body: Health and Malaise in Twentieth-Century France* (Bern: Peter Lang, 2007). On preparations for war in France, see also Susan Grayzel, *Women's Identities at War: Gender, Motherhood and Politics in Britain and France during the First World War* (Chapel Hill, NC: University of North Carolina Press, 1999); Susan R. Grayzel, ' "The Souls of Soldiers": Civilians Under Fire in First World War France', *Journal of Modern History*, 78/3 (2006), 588–622.

3. Katrin Schultheiss has observed that 300 FFNC nurses had been hired within the first few months of the war. Many were placed in supervisory positions, and a brand new 700-bed military hospital in Talence, near Bordeaux, was staffed entirely by FFNC nurses, until it was taken over by an American unit in 1917: Katrin Schultheiss, *Bodies and Souls: Politics and the Professionalization of Nursing in France, 1880–1922* (Cambridge, Mass.: Harvard University Press, 2001), 170.

4. Anon., 'The Work of the St John Ambulance Association', *British Journal of Nursing* (5 Sept. 1914), 189.

5. Millicent, Duchess of Sutherland, *Six Weeks at the War* (London: *The Times*, 1914); Diane Atkinson, *Elsie and Mairi Go To War: Two Extraordinary Women on the Western Front* (London: Preface Publishing, 2009);

Andrew Hallam and Nicola Hallam, *Lady Under Fire on the Western Front: The Great War Letters of Lady Dorothie Fielding* (Barnsley: Pen and Sword Books, 2010).

6. On Rachel Williams, see Monica Baly, *Florence Nightingale and the Nursing Legacy* (1986; London, Whurr Publishers, 1997), 164–5; Lynn McDonald (ed.), *Florence Nightingale: Extending Nursing* (Waterloo: Wilfrid Laurier University Press, 2009), 103–43.

7. Violetta Thurstan, *Field Hospital and Flying Column: Being the Journal of an English Nursing Sister in Belgium and Russia* (London: G. P. Putnam's Sons, 1915), 5.

8. Sarah Macnaughtan, *A Woman's Diary of the War* (London: Thomas Nelson, 1915), 22–4.

9. M. N. Oxford, *Nursing in Wartime: Lessons for the Inexperienced* (London: Methuen and Co., 1914), 14. On complaints in professional nursing journals, see Christine E. Hallett, ' "Emotional Nursing": Involvement, Engagement, and Detachment in the Writings of First World War Nurses and VADs', in Alison S. Fell and Hallett (eds.), *First World War Nursing: New Perspectives* (New York: Routledge, 2013), 87–102.

10. Margaret Darrow, 'French Volunteer Nursing and the Myth of War Experience in World War I', *American Historical Review*, 101 (1996), 81–4. See also Margaret H. Darrow, 'The Making of Sister Julie: The Origin of First World War French Nursing Heroines in Franco-Prussian War Stories', in Fell and Hallett (eds.), *First World War Nursing: New Perspectives*, 17–34.

11. Luc de Munck and Luc Vandeweyer, *Het Hospital van de Koningin: Rode Kruis, L'Océan en De Panne* (De Panne: Gemeetebestuur De Panne en de auteurs, 2012).

12. Dorothy Seymour, Private Papers: Diary and Letters, documents.3210, 95/28/1, Imperial War Museum, London, UK. Seymour was granddaughter of Admiral of the Fleet, Sir George Francis Seymour and a 'Woman of the Bedchamber' to Princess Christian. On Mary Borden, see Jane Conway, *Mary Borden: A Woman of Two Wars* (Chippenham: Munday Books, 2010). On Millicent, Duchess of Sutherland, see Denis Stuart, *Dear Duchess: Millicent Duchess of Sutherland (1867–1955)* (Newton Abbot: David and Charles, 1982).

13. Alan Kramer, *Dynamic of Destruction: Culture and Mass Killing in the First World War* (Oxford: Oxford University Press, 2007), 6–30.

14. Millicent, Duchess of Sutherland, *Six Weeks at the War*: published extracts from diary for 23 Aug. 1914.

15. Macnaughtan, *A Woman's Diary of the War*, 41–2.

16. Lawrence Sondhaus, *World War I: The Global Revolution* (Cambridge: Cambridge University Press, 2011). Sondhaus has observed that the First Battle of Ypres 'accounted for over two-thirds of Britain's casualties for 1914 and destroyed most of what was left of the original BEF, Britain's fully-trained prewar professional army': quote on p. 79.

17. For Violetta Thurstan's two differing accounts of her experience in Belgium, see Thurstan, *Field Hospital and Flying Column*, 10–91; Thurstan, *The Hounds of War Unleashed* (St Ives: United Writers, 1978), 13–28 (for the episode relating to caring for German soldiers' feet, see pp. 16–17).

18. Miss M. D. Vernon Allen, Private Papers: Diary and extracts from letters, documents. 4575, 81/13/1, Imperial War Museum, London, UK.

19. The hospital was to treat approximately 26,000 patients before its closure at the end of 1919: Leah Leneman, 'Medical Women at War, 1914–1918', *Medical History*, 38 (1994), 160–77; Jennian Geddes, 'Deeds and Words in the Suffrage Military Hospital in Endell Street', *Medical History*, 51/1 (2007), 79–98.

20. Claire Tylee, *The Great War and Women's Consciousness: Images of Militarism and Womanhood in Women's Writings, 1914–1964* (Houndmills: Macmillan 1990), 7. Elsie Inglis's units were formed with the support of the Scottish Federation of Women's Suffrage Societies, part of the non-militant National Union of Women's Suffrage Societies. By the end of the war, the SWH would have established units in France, Serbia, Salonika, Corsica, Macedonia, Russia, and Romania: Leneman, 'Medical Women at War', 166–8.

21. Eileen Crofton, *The Women of Royaumont: A Scottish Women's Hospital on the Western Front* (East Linton: Tuckwell Press, 1997); Leah Leneman, *In the Service of Life: The Story of Elsie Inglis and the Scottish Women's Hospitals* (Edinburgh: Mercat Press, 1998).

22. On the Abbaye de Royaumont, see Marian Wenzel and John Cornish, *Auntie Mabel's War: An Account of Her Part in the Hostilities of 1914–1918* (London: Allen Lane, 1980), 24–6.

23. Professional nurses and VADs also each had their own separate table. See Wenzel and Cornish, *Auntie Mabel's War*, 39. Note: a few men did work at Royaumont.

24. On Stobart's 'narrow escape' see Mabel St Clair Stobart, *The Flaming Sword in Serbia and Elsewhere* (London: Hodder and Stoughton, 1916), 6–9. On the later work of volunteer units, see Leneman, 'Medical Women at War', 165. See also Harriet Blodgett, 'Stobart, Mabel Annie St Clair', in *Oxford Dictionary of National Biography* (Oxford: Oxford University Press, 2004–13).

25. Later in the war—in 1917—the hospital was shelled and had to be evacuated.

26. John Van Schaick Jr., *The Little Corner Never Conquered: The Story of the American Red Cross War Work for Belgium* (New York: Macmillan Company, 1922), 63.

27. On the history of L'Hôpital de l'Océan, see de Munck and Vandeweyer, *Het Hospital van de Koningin*; Pierre Boonefaes and Willy Vilain, *Eenwig in eben vloed* (De Panne: Municipality of De Panne, 2011). I am indebted to Luc de Munck and Lionel Roosemont for translating sections of these books into English for me.

28. On the role of Queen Elisabeth, see de Munck and Vandeweyer, *Het Hospital van de Koningin*, 112.

29. Boonefaes and Vilain, *Eenwig in eben vloed*, 130, trans. Lionel Roosemont.

30. Jane De Launoy, *Infirmières de guerre en service commande (Front de 14 à 18)* (Brussels: L'Édition universelle, 1937), 62.

31. De Launoy, *Infirmières de guerre*, 62–8, 10–11.

32. Mark Harrison, *The Medical War: British Military Medicine in the First World War* (Oxford: Oxford University Press, 2010), 16–24.

33. Anon. [Kate Luard], *Diary of a Nursing Sister on the Western Front* (Edinburgh: William Blackwood and Sons, 1915), 1–80.

34. Many of Kate Luard's letters, and replies received from members of her family, are available at Luard Family Papers, Files 55/13/1-4, D/Dlu 58, Essex Record Office, Colchester, UK. See also Kate Luard, Service Record, WO 399/5023, The National Archives, Kew, UK.

35. Sister E. Dodd, 'At an Officers Hospital in France', Nurses' Accounts, Army Medical Services Museum Archives, Aldershot, UK.

36. Anon., *A Matron's Experiences of Work at a Base Hospital, France, 1914–1915*, Nurses' Accounts, Army Medical Services Museum Archives, Aldershot, UK. This anonymous account referred to the 'sugar sheds' being located in Wimereux—in fact, these were in Boulogne, although the hospital did relocate to Wimereux later in the war. I am indebted to Sue Light for drawing this fact to my attention.

37. Christine Hallett, *Containing Trauma: Nursing Work in the First World War* (Manchester: Manchester University Press, 2009), 49–59; Harrison, *The Medical War*, 27–9.

38. Harrison, *The Medical War*, 25–6, 33.

39. Dame Maud McCarthy, Matron-in-Chief, BEF, File of Correspondence relating to CCS, 1914, Box 10, Army Medical Services Museum Archives, Aldershot, UK.

40. Harrison, *The Medical War*, 33.

41. Dame Maud McCarthy, Matron-in-Chief, BEF, File of Correspondence relating to CCS, 1914–15, Box 10, Army Medical Services Museum Archives, Aldershot, UK.

42. Paterson's War Office Record indicates that she joined the Reserves on 17 August 1914: Jentie Paterson, Service Record, WO 399/6503, The National Archives, Kew, UK.

43. Sister Jentie Paterson, Private Papers: Diaries, documents.378, 90/10/1, Imperial War Museum, London, UK.

44. Paterson, Diaries.

45. Paterson, Diaries [emphasis in the original].

46. Paterson, Diaries.

47. Sister Jentie Paterson, Private Papers: Letter to 'Martha', documents.378, 90/10/1 Imperial War Museum, London, UK.

48. Paterson, Letter to 'Martha'.

49. Paterson, Letter to 'Martha'.

50. Sister Jentie Paterson, Private Papers: Newspaper clipping, documents.378, 90/10/1, Imperial War Museum, London, UK.

51. Tylee, *The Great War and Women's Consciousness*; Trudi Tate, *Modernism, History and the First World War* (Manchester: Manchester University Press, 1998), 41–62.

52. Anon. [Luard], *Diary of a Nursing Sister*, 46–7.

53. Harrison, *The Medical War*, 38–41.

54. Anon. [Luard], *Diary of a Nursing Sister*, 52–3. On Kate Luard, see also Yvonne McEwen, 'Behind and Between the Lines: The War Diary of Evelyn Kate Luard, Nursing Sister on the Western Front and Unofficial Correspondent', in McEwen and Fiona Fisken (eds.), *War, Journalism and History: War Correspondents in the Two World Wars* (Bern: Peter Lang, 2012), 73–93.

55. Miss Bickmore, Private Papers: 'Life on an Ambulance Train in France, 1914–1917', documents.3814, 85/51/1, Imperial War Museum, London, UK.

56. Bickmore, 'Life on an Ambulance Train in France, 1914–1917'.

57. Bickmore, 'Life on an Ambulance Train in France, 1914–1917'.

58. Bickmore, 'Life on an Ambulance Train in France, 1914–1917'.

59. Bickmore, 'Life on an Ambulance Train in France, 1914–1917'; Sister Elsie Dobson, Nurses' Narratives, Butler Collection, AWM41/964, Australian War Memorial, Canberra, Australia.

60. Sister H. Chadwick, Narrative account of No. 26 Ambulance Train, Nurses' Narratives, Butler Collection, AWM41/953, Australian War Memorial, Canberra, Australia. On work on hospital trains, see also J. A. Connal, Sister TFNS, Account; J. Orchardson, TFNS, *Work on an Ambulance Train*; Sister K. Flower, QAIMNSR, Account: all in Nurses' Accounts, Army Medical Services Museum Archives, Aldershot, UK.

61. Harrison, *The Medical War*, 49.

62. Mrs Louie Johnson, oral history interview, conducted on 5 Mar. 1974, IWM330, Imperial War Museum, London, UK.

63. Mrs Louie Johnson, oral history interview, conducted on 5 Mar. 1974.

64. The hospital remained open for the first six months of the war. See Album of mementoes of the London/28 detachment (Kensington) of the VAD, 1914–1925, Red Cross Archives, London, UK, 2423/1.

65. Harrison, *The Medical War*, 50. On the work of the Joint War Committee, see also E. F. Schneider, 'The British Red Cross Wounded and Missing Enquiry Bureau: A Case of Truth-Telling in the Great War', *War in History*, 4/3 (July 1997), 296–315.

66. May W. Cannan, *Recollections of a British Red Cross Voluntary Aid Detachment No 12, Oxford University, March 26th 1911–April 24th 1919*, Red Cross Archives, London, UK.

67. Cannan, *Recollections of a British Red Cross Voluntary Aid Detachment No 12*.

68. Van Straubenzee obtained a posting at Clandon Park hospital in October 1916: Margaret Van Straubenzee, Account, X/142, LIB 88/595, T2(STR), Red Cross Archives, London, UK.

69. Mrs Fussell, Early account of the Australian Army Nursing Service, unnumbered file, Imperial War Museum, London, UK.

70. Anna Rogers, *While You're Away: New Zealand Nurses At War, 1899–1948* (Auckland: Auckland University Press, 2003), 55; Sherayl Kendall and David Corbett, *New Zealand Military Nursing: A History of the Royal New Zealand Nursing Corps, Boer War to the Present Day* (Auckland: S. Kendall and D. Corbett, 1990).

71. Anon., 'Miss J. C. Child's Career', *South African Nursing Journal* (Sept. 1939), 594.

72. The papers of Dorothy Cotton are available online from Library and Archives Canada, Ottawa: <www.collectionscanada.gc.ca/nursing-sisters/025013-2200-e.html>.

73. Linda Quiney, 'Assistant Angels: Canadian Voluntary Aid Detachment Nurses in the Great War', *Canadian Bulletin of Medical History*, 15/1 (1998), 189–206; Cynthia Toman, ' "Help us, serve England": First World War Military Nursing and National Identities', *Canadian Bulletin of Medical History*, 30/1 (2013), 156–7.

74. Letter written by McCarron's niece-by-marriage: Sara McCarron Collection, Barbara Bates Center for the Study of the History of Nursing, University of Pennsylvania, Philadelphia, USA.

75. The American Red Cross sent ten units in total, each composed of twelve nurses and three surgeons. The SS *Red Cross* left New York on 2 September 1914: Papers of Base Hospital 41, 1905–2009, Accession Number MS-17, Historical Collections, Claude Moore Health Sciences Library (Historical Collections), the University of Virginia, Charlottesville, USA.

76. Diary, Sarah McCarron Collection, Barbara Bates Center.

77. Diary, Sarah McCarron Collection, Barbara Bates Center.

78. Lavinia L. Dock et al., *History of American Red Cross Nursing* (New York: Macmillan Company, 1922).

79. Margaret Cowling, 'A Red Cross Nurse', incorporated into Deming J. Shear, 'Historical Sketch of Base Hospital #41', File 2, Box 1, Papers of Base Hospital 41, 1905–2009, Accession Number MS-17, Claude

Moore Health Sciences Library (Historical Collections), University of Virginia, Charlottesville, USA.

80. Harrison, *The Medical War*, 33.

81. Elizabeth Haldane noted that, by the end of 1914, there were General Hospitals at Le Havre, Étretat, Rouen, Boulogne, Wimereux, Versailles, Le Tréport, Dieppe, and Abbeville: Elizabeth S. Haldane, *The British Nurse in Peace and War* (London: John Murray, 1923), 191.

## Chapter 2

1. Glen E. Torrey, 'L'Affaire de Soissons, January 1915', *War in History*, 4/4 (1997), 398–410; Lawrence Sondhaus, *World War I: The Global Revolution* (Cambridge: Cambridge University Press, 2011), 130.

2. Estelle and Thérèse Bieswal, *Journal: Années 1914 à 1918*, 34, 46, Royal Museum of the Armed Forces and of Military History, Brussels. I am indebted to Luc de Munck for translating this manuscript source for me.

3. Jane De Launoy, *Infirmières de guerre en service commande (Front de 14 à 18)* (Brussels: L'Édition universelle, 1937), 82, 94.

4. Luc de Munck and Luc Vandeweyer, *Het Hospital van de Koningin: Rode Kruis, L'Océan en De Panne* (De Panne: Gemeetebestuur De Panne en de auteurs, 2012), 69; on Jane De Launoy, see also p. 71.

5. Pierre Boonefaes and Willy Vilain, *Eenwig in eben vloed* (De Panne: Municipality of De Panne, 2011), 128. I am indebted to Lionel Roosemont for his translation of this passage.

6. Grace Ellison, 'Nursing at the French Front', in Gilbert Stone (ed.), *Women War Workers: Accounts Contributed by Representative Workers of the Work Done by Women in the More Important Branches of War Employment* (London: George G. Harrap and Co., 1917), 155–80.

7. Ellen N. La Motte, *The Backwash of War: The Human Wreckage of the Battlefield as Witnessed by an American Hospital Nurse* (New York: G. P. Putnam's Sons, The Knickerbocker Press, 1916).

8. See e.g. Anon. [Kate Luard], *Diary of a Nursing Sister on the Western Front 1914–1915* (Edinburgh: William Blackwood and Sons, 1915), 111–42. On the reactions of nurses to caring for 'colonial' troops, see Alison S. Fell, 'Nursing the Other: The Representations of Colonial Troops in French and British First World War Nursing Memoirs', in Santanu Das (ed.),

*Race, Empire and First World War Writing* (Cambridge: Cambridge University Press, 2011), 158–74. The term *poilu* was used to refer to the regular French private soldier in much the same way that 'Tommy' was used to refer to a British soldier.

9. This letter was actually sent in 1917: Evelyn Proctor, Private Papers: Manuscript letters, documents.1039, 88/16/1, Imperial War Museum, London, UK.

10. Marjorie Starr, Private Papers: Documents.4572, 81/12/1, Imperial War Museum, London, UK.

11. Marian Wenzel and John Cornish, *Auntie Mabel's War: An Account of Her Part in the Hostilities of 1914–1918* (London: Allen Lane, 1980), 17. The documentary source materials used in Wenzel and Cornish's book are held at the Imperial War Museum, London, UK: Miss Mabel Jeffery, Private Papers: Draft of the book, 'Auntie Mabel's War', containing original documents relating to Miss Jeffery's service as a qualified nurse, documents.6461, 81/38/2&2A.

12. Wenzel and Cornish, *Auntie Mabel's War*, 38.

13. Wenzel and Cornish, *Auntie Mabel's War*, quote on p. 47; on Jeffery's time at Royaumont, see pp. 24–55.

14. Wenzel and Cornish, *Auntie Mabel's War*, 48.

15. Wenzel and Cornish, *Auntie Mabel's War*, 24–55.

16. Christine E. Hallett, *Containing Trauma: Nursing Work in the First World War* (Manchester: Manchester University Press, 2009), 28; Mark Harrison, *The Medical War: British Military Medicine in the First World War* (Oxford: Oxford University Press, 2010), 35–6.

17. On the treatment of shock, see Hallett, *Containing Trauma*, 28–35; Harrison, *The Medical War*, 105; E. Ann Robertson, 'Anaesthesia, Shock and Resuscitation', in Thomas Scotland and Steven Heys (eds.), *War Surgery 1914–1918* (Solihull: Helion and Co. Ltd, 2012), 85–115. On blood transfusion, see Kim Pelis, 'Taking Credit: The Canadian Army Medical Corps and the British Conversion to Blood Transfusion in World War I', *Journal of the History of Medicine and Allied Health Sciences*, 56 (2001), 238–77.

18. Harrison, *The Medical War*, 42.

19. Sister M. Peterkin, QAIMNSR, *Work on a Hospital Barge in France*, Nurses' Accounts, Army Medical Services Museum Archives, Aldershot, UK.

20. Peterkin, QAIMNSR, *Work on a Hospital Barge in France*.
21. This quotation is taken from Luard's published diary, which she produced by putting together (with minor edits) a series of 'journals' which she had written and sent home to her family. Anon. [Luard], *Diary of a Nursing Sister*, 283.
22. Anon. [Luard] *Diary of a Nursing Sister*, 284.
23. Many of Kate Luard's letters, including this one, and replies received from members of her family, are available at Luard Family Papers, Files 55/13/1–4, D/Dlu 58, Essex Record Office, Colchester, UK. I am indebted to Tim Luard for forwarding me transcripts of excerpts from these letters.
24. Luard Family Papers, Files 55/13/1–4, D/Dlu 58.
25. Luard Family Papers, Files 55/13/1–4, D/Dlu 58.
26. Luard Family Papers, Files 55/13/1–4, D/Dlu 58.
27. Kate E. Luard, *Unknown Warriors* (London: Chatto and Windus, 1930), 77.
28. On the deployment of chemical weapons see Steve Sturdy, 'War as Experiment: Physiology, Innovation and Administration in Britain, 1914–1918: The Case of Chemical Warfare', in Roger Cooter, Mark Harrison, and Sturdy (eds.), *War, Medicine and Modernity* (Stroud: Sutton Publishing, 1998), 65–84; Martin Goodman, *Suffer and Survive* (London: Simon and Schuster, 2007); Gerard Fitzgerald, 'Chemical Warfare and the Medical Response during World War I', *American Journal of Public Health*, 98/4 (Apr. 2008), 611–25.
29. J. Elliot Black, Elliot T. Glenny, and J. W. McNee, 'Observations on 685 Cases of Poisoning by Noxious Gases Used by the Enemy', *British Medical Journal* (31 July 1915), 165–7.
30. Violetta Thurstan, *A Text Book of War Nursing* (London: G. P. Putnam's Sons, 1917), 167–9.
31. Dame Maud McCarthy, Matron-in-Chief, BEF, File of Correspondence relating to CCSs, 1914–15, Box 10, Army Medical Services Museum Archives, Aldershot, UK.
32. Harrison, *The Medical War*, 34.
33. On base hospitals see Harrison, *The Medical War*, 43–58; figures quoted are given on p. 44.
34. There was also, from 1915, a unit from Chicago: Elizabeth S. Haldane, *The British Nurse in Peace and War* (London: John Murray, 1923), 196.

35. British Medical Association, *British Medicine in the War, 1914–1917: Being Essays on the Problems of Medicine, Surgery and Pathology Arising Among the British Armed Forces Engaged in This War and the Manner of Their Solution* (London: British Medical Association, 1917); Medical Research Committee, *Report on the Anaerobic Bacteria and Infections: Report on the Anaerobic Infections of Wounds and the Bacteriological and Serological Problems Arising Therefrom* (London: HMSO, 1919).

36. Thurstan, *A Text Book of War Nursing*, 129–32.

37. Sister Jentie Paterson, Private Papers: Diaries, documents.378, 90/10/1, Imperial War Museum, London, UK.

38. Paterson, Diaries.

39. Jentie Paterson, Service Record, WO 399/6503, The National Archives, Kew, UK.

40. R. Manning, Private Papers: Account, documents.4763, 80/21/1, Imperial War Museum, London, UK.

41. Dorothy Seymour, Private Papers: Diary and Letters, documents.3210, 95/28/1, Imperial War Museum, London, UK.

42. Dorothy Seymour, Diary and Letters.

43. E. C. Barton, *Hints to VAD Members in Hospitals* (London: *Nursing Times* Publishing, 1915). The quotation is taken from a review of the book: Anon., 'For VAD Probationers', *Nursing Times*, 12/557 (1916), 48.

44. Edith Appleton, *Diaries*, Private Collection of Dick Robinson, entry for 29 Nov. 1915. An abridged version of Appleton's diaries is available as Ruth Cowen (ed.), *War Diaries—A Nurse at the Front: The Great War Diaries of Sister Edith Appleton* (London: Simon and Schuster, 2012), quotation on pp. 81–2.

45. Thomas R. Scotland, 'Evacuation Pathway for the Wounded', in Scotland and Steven Heys (eds.), *War Surgery 1914–1918* (Solihull: Helion and Co. Ltd, 2012), 51–84.

46. Hallett, *Containing Trauma*, 41.

47. Harrison, *The Medical War*, 29.

48. On treatment controversy, see Christine E. Hallett, '"Intelligent interest in their own affairs": The First World War, the *British Journal of Nursing* and the Pursuit of Nursing Knowledge', in P. D'Antonio, J. Fairman, and J. Whelan (eds.), *Routledge Handbook on the Global History of Nursing* (London and New York: Routledge, 2013), 95–113. On the work of Almroth Wright, see Harrison, *The Medical War*, 95–9.

49. Hallett, '"Intelligent interest in their own affairs"'. On Henry Gray, see Thomas R. Scotland, 'Developments in Orthopaedic Surgery', in Scotland and Steven Heys (eds.), *War Surgery 1914–1918* (Solihull: Helion and Co. Ltd, 2012), 148–77, at 151–2.

50. Thurstan, *A Text Book of War Nursing*, 114–15. See also the citation of this text in Hallett, '"Intelligent interest in their own affairs"', 107–8.

51. Hallett, *Containing Trauma*, 49–59.

52. One of the most evocative descriptions of a dressing technique can be found in Irene Rathbone, *We That Were Young* (1932; New York: The Feminist Press, 1989), 196–9.

53. Hallett, *Containing Trauma*, 56–8; Harrison, *The Medical War*, 31.

54. Anon., 'Nursing at La Panne', *British Journal of Nursing* (10 Mar. 1917), 169. On L'Hôpital de l'Océan, see also Anon., 'Care of the Wounded', *British Journal of Nursing* (14 Apr. 1917), 253; Anon., Column, *British Journal of Nursing* (16 June 1917).

55. Nurses were also responsible for mixing Dakin's solution to produce the antiseptic. A description of how to 'make up' a supply of Dakin's solution and deliver it through the Carrel apparatus can be found in Thurstan, *A Text Book of War Nursing*, 118–19.

56. Hallett, *Containing Trauma*, 101–6.

57. Mark Harrison, *The Medical War*; on specialization see pp. 99–109; on abdominal surgery pp. 102–3; on orthopaedics pp. 100–1. On orthopaedics and the introduction of the Thomas Splint, see Scotland, 'Developments in Orthopaedic Surgery', 148–77.

58. Mary Clarke, Diary, 84/46/1, Imperial War Museum, London, UK.

59. On trench conditions, see Richard van Emden, *The Trench: Experiencing Life on the Front Line, 1916* (London: Corgi, 2002), *passim*; E. P. F. Lynch, *Somme Mud: The Experiences of an Infantryman in France, 1916–1919* (London: Bantam Books, 2006), *passim*.

60. On trench foot and measures to prevent it, see Harrison, *The Medical War*, 129. On the squalor of trench conditions, see Richard Holmes, *Tommy: The British Soldier on the Western Front, 1914–1918* (London: HarperCollins, 2004), 285–8; van Emden, *The Trench*, 163–78.

61. Hallett, *Containing Trauma*, 85–92.

62. On the nursing of patients with infectious diseases on all fronts, see Hallett, *Containing Trauma*, 140–8. On the treatment and prevention of infection on the Western Front, see Harrison, *The Medical War*, 131–70.

63. Thomas Lewis, *The Soldier's Heart and the Effort Syndrome* (London: Shaw and Sons, 1918).

64. Joel D. Howell, ' "Soldier's Heart": The Redefinition of Heart Disease and Speciality Formation in Early Twentieth-Century Great Britain', in Roger Cooter, Mark Harrison, and Steve Sturdy (eds.), *War, Medicine and Modernity* (Stroud: Sutton Publishing, 1998), 85–105; Harrison, *The Medical War*, 106.

65. For modern analyses on the nature and causes of shell shock, see Martin Stone, 'Shellshock and the Psychologists', in W. F. Bynum, R. Porter, and M. Shepherd (eds.), *The Anatomy of Madness: Essays on the History of Psychiatry*, ii (New York and London: Tavistock, 1985), 242–71; Eric J. Leed, *No Man's Land: Combat and Identity in World War I* (Cambridge: Cambridge University Press, 1979); Elaine Showalter, *The Female Malady: Woman, Madness and English Culture, 1830–1980* (London: Virago, 1993); Ben Shephard, *A War of Nerves: Soldiers and Psychiatrists, 1914–1994* (2000; London: Pimlico, 2002); P. J. Leese, *Shell Shock: Traumatic Neurosis and the British Soldiers of the First World War* (London: Palgrave Macmillan, 2002).

66. Shephard, *A War of Nerves*, 22.

67. Shephard, *A War of Nerves*, 29. On 'malingering', see Roger Cooter, 'Malingering in Modernity: Psychological Scripts and Adversarial Encounters during the First World War', in Cooter, Mark Harrison, and Steve Sturdy (eds.), *War, Medicine and Modernity* (Stroud: Sutton Publishing, 1998), 125–48; Joanna Bourke, *Dismembering the Male: Men's Bodies, Britain and the Great War* (London: Reaktion Books, 1996), 89–107.

68. Edmund Blunden, *Undertones of War* (1928; London: Penguin, 2000); Robert Graves, *Goodbye to All That* (1929; London: Penguin, 2000); Erich Maria Remarque, *All Quiet on the Western Front* (1929; London: Vintage, 1996).

69. Douglas Bell, *A Soldier's Diary of the Great War* (London: Faber and Gwyer, 1929), 121–3. On the emotional trauma of war, see Santanu Das, *Touch and Intimacy in First World War Literature* (Cambridge: Cambridge University Press, 2005), *passim*; Michael Roper, *The Secret Battle: Emotional Survival in the Great War* (Manchester: Manchester University Press, 2009), *passim*.

70. Bell, *A Soldier's Diary*, 120–5.

71. Bell, *A Soldier's Diary*, 142.

72. Shephard, *A War of Nerves*, 31–2.

73. This approach was used later in the war—from about 1917 onwards: Harrison, *The Medical War*, 113.

74. Thurstan, *A Text Book of War Nursing*, 138–9.

75. Elizabeth Haldane pointed out that there were also private convalescent homes for nurses at Paris Plage, Wimereux, Étaples, Boulogne, and Camiers. There were also thirteen Princess Victoria's Rest Clubs for Nurses: Haldane, *The British Nurse in Peace and War*, 197.

76. A. Essington-Nelson, Private Papers: Documents.2784, 86/48/1, Imperial War Museum, London, UK. Nurses' rest homes and convalescent homes appear to have been the result of philanthropic donation of houses by wealthy patrons. Other examples included 'Lady Desborough's house at Taplow, and Mr Moseley's at Hadley Wood': Anon., 'The Care of War Nurses: Rest and Holiday Homes', *The Times* (28 Mar. 1916), cited in Denise J. Poynter, ' "The Report on her Transfer was Shell-Shock": A Study of the Psychological Disorders of Nurses and Female Voluntary Aid Detachments Who Served Alongside the British and Allied Expeditionary Forces during the First World War, 1914–1918' (unpublished PhD thesis, University of Northampton, 2008), 144.

77. Essington-Nelson, Private Papers: Documents.2784, 86/48/1.

78. Elizabeth Haldane, Letter, *The Times* (27 Mar. 1915), cited in Poynter, ' "The Report on her Transfer was Shell-Shock" ', 173. British nurses did eventually receive disability pensions. Similarly, in France, the Military Pensions Act of 31 January 1919 made possible the award of disability pensions to French nurses. I am indebted to Alison Fell for drawing my attention to this fact.

79. From a contemporary Press Report quoted in *Reveille: Lancaster Military Heritage Group*; available at <http://lancasterwarmemorials.org.uk/essays/e27.htm>. I am indebted to Tim Padfied of BBC Radio Lancashire for drawing my attention to this source.

80. Anon., Column, *British Journal of Nursing* (22 July 1916), 68.

81. Poynter, ' "The Report on her Transfer was Shell-Shock" '. On the trauma experienced by nurses, see Ariela Freedman, 'Mary Borden's *Forbidden Zone*: Women's Writing from No-Man's Land', *Modernism/modernity*,

9/1 (2002), 109–24; Margaret Higonnet, 'Authenticity and Art in Trauma Narratives of World War I', *Modernism/modernity*, 9/1 (2002), 91–107.

82. On the trauma-writings of First World War nurses, see Christine E. Hallett, 'Portrayals of Suffering: Perceptions of Trauma in the Writings of First World War Nurses and Volunteers', *Canadian Bulletin of the History of Medicine*, 27/1 (2010), 65–84.

## Chapter 3

1. For an account of the war on the 'Eastern Front' see Peter Gatrell, *Russia's First World War: A Social and Economic History* (New York: Pearson Longman, 2005). See also Bertram D. Wolfe, 'Titans Locked in Combat, Part II', *Russian Review*, 24/1 (Jan. 1965); Michael Hughes, ' "Revolution Was in the Air": British Officials in Russia during the First World War', *Journal of Contemporary History*, 31/1 (1996), 75–97; John Keegan, *The First World War* (1998; London: Hutchinson, 1999), 151–87.

2. Graydon A. Tunstall, *Blood on the Snow: The Carpathian Winter War of 1915* (Lawrence, Kan.: University of Kansas Press, 2010), 1.

3. Tunstall, *Blood on the Snow*, 1, 212.

4. Lawrence Sondhaus, *World War I: The Global Revolution* (Cambridge: Cambridge University Press, 2011), 154; Keegan, *The First World War*, 246–8; A. J. P. Taylor, *The First World War: An Illustrated History* (1963; London, Penguin, 1966), 89–90.

5. Susan Grant, 'Nursing in Russia and the Soviet Union 1914–1941: An Overview of the Development of a Soviet Nursing System', *Bulletin of the UK Association for the History of Nursing*, 2 (2012), 21–33, at 22.

6. Very little has been written in English on this subject, but there appear to have been no references in contemporary sources to Russian nursing associations or journals. See Grant, 'Nursing in Russia and the Soviet Union', 21–33, at 21–4.

7. On Russia's First World War nurses, see Laurie Stoff, 'The "Myth of the War Experience" and Russian Wartime Nursing in World War I', *Aspasia: The International Yearbook of Central Eastern, and Southeastern European Women's and Gender History*, 6 (2012), 96–116.

8. On Russian women's wartime work, see Alfred Meyer, 'The Impact of World War I on Russian Women's Lives', in Barbara Clements, Barbara

Engel, and Christine Worobec (eds.), *Russia's Women: Accommodation, Resistance, Transformation* (Berkeley and Los Angeles: University of California Press, 1991); Barbara Engel, *Women in Russia, 1700–2000* (Cambridge: Cambridge University Press, 2004); Peter Gatrell, 'The Epic and the Domestic: Women and War in Russia, 1914–1917', in Gail Braybon (ed.), *Evidence, History and the Great War: Historians and the Impact of 1914–1918* (New York: Berghahn Books, 2003); Rochelle Ruthchild, *Equality and Revolution: Women's Rights in the Russian Empire, 1905–1917* (Pittsburgh: University of Pittsburgh Press, 2010).

9. Florence Farmborough, *Nurse at the Russian Front: A Diary 1914–1918* (London: Book Club Associates, 1974). This book was republished in a new edition: Florence Farmborough, *With the Armies of the Tsar: A Nurse at the Russian Front in War and Revolution, 1914–1918* (New York: Cooper Square Press, 2000). Farmborough's original diaries are held at the Imperial War Museum, London, UK: Florence Farmborough, Private Papers: Diaries, documents.1381. Two interviews with Florence Farmborough are available: Florence Farmborough, interview conducted by Margaret Brooks, 1975, IMW312, Imperial War Museum, London, UK; Florence Farmborough, interview conducted by Peter Liddle, July 1975 (tape 302), RUS 11, Liddle Collection, Brotherton Library, University of Leeds, UK. See also Violetta Thurstan, *Field Hospital and Flying Column: Being the Journal of an English Nursing Sister in Belgium and Russia* (London: G. P. Putnam's Sons, 1915).

10. Farmborough, *Nurse at the Russian Front*, 28–9.

11. Mary Britnieva, *One Woman's Story* (London: Arthur Baker, 1934); Thurstan, *Field Hospital and Flying Column*.

12. Michael Harmer, *The Forgotten Hospital: An Essay* (London: Springwood Books, 1982).

13. Harmer, *The Forgotten Hospital*, 5.

14. Anon., 'The Anglo-Russian Hospital', *Nursing Times*, 12/557 (1916), 181.

15. Dorothy Seymour, Private Papers: Diary and Letters, documents.3210, 95/28/1, Imperial War Museum, London, UK.

16. Hodges also stayed at the hospital on her return from the front: Miss K. Hodges, Private Papers: Documents.1974, 92/22/1, pp. 65, 100, Imperial War Museum, London, UK.

17. Margaret H. Barber, *A British Nurse in Bolshevik Russia: The Narrative of Margaret H. Barber, April 1916–December 1919* (London: A. C. Fifield, 1920).

18. On Margaret Macdonald, see Susan Mann, *Margaret Macdonald: Imperial Daughter* (Montreal: McGill Queen's University Press, 2010).

19. Anon., Column, *British Journal of Nursing* (9 Oct. 1915), 294. Cotton left the hospital itself on 10 June, to form part of a field hospital travelling to the 'front'.

20. Dorothy Cotton, Diary, available online from Library and Archives Canada, Ottawa: <www.collectionscanada.gc.ca/nursing-sisters/025013-2200-e.html> [last accessed 17 May 2013].

21. Anon., Column, *British Journal of Nursing* (9 Oct. 1915) 294.

22. Thurstan, *Field Hospital and Flying Column*, 115–116; Cotton, Diary, 25; Miss K. Hodges, Private Papers: Diary, 83.

23. Irene Rathbone, *We That Were Young* (1932; New York: The Feminist Press, 1989), 196–9.

24. Cotton, Diary, 45.

25. Cotton, Diary, 27.

26. Cotton, Diary, 28.

27. Cotton, Diary, 45. See also Violetta Thurstan, *The People Who Run, Being the Tragedy of the Refugees in Russia* (London: G. P. Putnam's Sons, 1916).

28. Harmer, *The Forgotten Hospital*.

29. Cotton explains in her diary that a 'verst' is roughly equivalent to two-thirds of a mile. Hence the field hospital was about the same distance from the Russian Front as a CCS might be from the British or French sectors of the Western Front. Cotton, Diary, 36.

30. Cotton, Diary, 39–40; quote on p. 39.

31. Christine E. Hallett, 'Russian Romances: Emotionalism and Spirituality in the Writings of "Eastern Front" Nurses, 1914–1918', *Nursing History Review*, 17 (2009), 101–28.

32. Thurstan, *Field Hospital and Flying Column*.

33. Miss Elizabeth Agnes Greg, Private Papers: Letters, documents.8337, 01/17/1, Imperial War Museum, London, UK.

34. Thurstan, *Field Hospital and Flying Column*, 113–78.

35. Farmborough, *Nurse at the Russian Front*, 44.

36. Peter Liddle, *Captured Memories 1900–1918: Across the Threshold of War* (Barnsley: Pen and Sword Military, 2010), 237.

37. Britnieva, *One Woman's Story*, 10.

38. Britnieva, *One Woman's Story*, 10.

39. F. E. Latham, 'With the First British Field Hospital in Serbia', *Nursing Times*, 12/557 (1916), 93–4.

40. Mabel St Clair Stobart, *The Flaming Sword in Serbia and Elsewhere* (London: Hodder and Stoughton, 1916), 13–122.

41. On the fate of these units, see Angela K. Smith, '"Beacons of British-ness": British Nurses and Female Doctors as Prisoners of War', in Alison S. Fell and Christine E. Hallett (eds.), *First World War Nursing: New Perspectives* (New York: Routledge, 2013), 35–50. On Lady Paget's unit, see also Anon., 'British Nurses in Serbia', *Nursing Times*, 12 (1916), 63; Lady Paget, *With Our Serbian Allies, Second Report*, printed for private circulation, available in Miss F. Scott, Private Papers: Documents.6977, 77/15/1, Imperial War Museum, London, UK.

42. Miss M. Barclay, Private Papers: Letter, documents.4320, 82/1/1, Imperial War Museum, London, UK.

43. Anon., 'Back from Serbia: An Interview with Miss Caldwell', *Nursing Times*, 12 (1916), 291.

44. Anon., 'Return of Two Scottish Units from Serbia: Adventure and Imprisonment', *Nursing Times*, 12 (1916), 210–13.

45. Latham, 'With the First British Field Hospital in Serbia', 93–4.

46. Anon., 'Arrival of Nurses from Serbia', *Nursing Times*, 12 (1916), 11.

47. Cited in Anon., 'Arrival of Nurses from Serbia', 11.

48. Stobart, *The Flaming Sword in Serbia and Elsewhere*, frontispiece; on the journey taken by Stobart's unit through Albania and Montenegro, see pp. 186–288.

49. Anon., 'Another Story of the Flight', *Nursing Times*, 12 (1916), 61.

50. Anon., 'Arrival of Nurses from Serbia', 11.

51. Anon., 'Arrival of Nurses from Serbia', 11.

52. Cited in Anon., 'Arrival of Nurses from Serbia', 12.

53. Cited in Anon., 'Arrival of Nurses from Serbia', 15.

54. Miss K. Hodges, Private Papers: Diary, 68. These incidents were also reported in Anon., 'Arrival of Nurses from Serbia', *Nursing Times*, 12 (1916), 15; Anon., 'News from the Front: Thrilling Experiences in Serbia', *Nursing Times*, 12 (1916), 269.

## Chapter 4

1. On the Gallipoli campaign, see John Masefield, *Gallipoli* (London: W. Heinemann, 1916); Peter Hart, *Gallipoli* (London: Profile, 2011); Edward J. Erickson, *Gallipoli and the Middle East, 1914–1918: From the Dardanelles to Mesopotamia* (London: Amber, 2008); Edward J. Erickson, *Gallipoli: The Ottoman Campaign* (Barnsley: Pen and Sword Military, 2010); Lawrence Sondhaus, *World War I: The Global Revolution* (Cambridge: Cambridge University Press, 2011), 133.

2. More correctly referred to as the 'Mediterranean Expeditionary Force'. S. E. Oram, Late Matron-in-Chief, Egyptian Expeditionary Force, 'Nursing in Egypt and Palestine 1915–1919', Army Medical Services Museum Archives, Aldershot, UK. Sue Light advises that her official title was 'Acting Matron-in-Chief'.

3. Mark Harrison, *The Medical War: British Military Medicine in the First World War* (Oxford: Oxford University Press, 2010), 171. See also the official medical histories of the campaign: W. G. Macpherson and W. J. Mitchell (eds.), *History of the Great War based on Official Documents; Medical Services, General History*, iv. *Medical Services on the Gallipoli Peninsula; in Macedonia; in Mesopotamia and North-West Persia; in East Africa; in the Aden Protectorate, and in North Russia; Ambulance Transport during the War* (London: Macmillan, 1924); Arthur G. Butler, *Official History of the Australian Army Medical Services, 1914–1918*, i. *Gallipoli, Palestine and New Guinea* (2nd edn., Melbourne: Australian War Memorial, 1938).

4. Harrison, *The Medical War*, 171–4; on the findings of the Dardanelles Commission, see pp. 198–203.

5. Oram, 'Nursing in Egypt and Palestine 1915–1919'.

6. Harrison, *The Medical War*, 191.

7. Sondhaus, *World War I*, 138.

8. Lavinia Dock, 'The Progress of Registration', *American Journal of Nursing*, 6/5 (Feb. 1906), 297–305, at 300–2.

9. On the formation of the Australian Army Nursing Service, see Jan Bassett, *Guns and Brooches: Australian Army Nursing from the Boer War to the Gulf War* (Melbourne: Oxford University Press, 1992), 1–31; Ruth Rae, *Scarlet Poppies: The Army Experience of Australian Nurses during World War One* (Burwood, NSW: College of Nursing, 2004); Ruth Rae, *Veiled Lives:*

*Threading Australian Nursing History into the Fabric of the First World War* (Burwood, NSW: College of Nursing, 2009); Kirsty Harris, *More than Bombs and Bandages: Australian Army Nurses at Work in World War I* (Newport, NSW: Big Sky Publishing, 2011). On the poor treatment of Australian nurses by the army, see Katie Holmes, 'Between the Lines: The Letters and Diaries of First World War Australian Nurses' (unpublished honours thesis, Department of History, University of Melbourne). On the formation of the New Zealand Army Nursing Service, see Sherayl Kendall and David Corbett, *New Zealand Military Nursing: A History of the Royal New Zealand Nursing Corps, Boer War to Present Day* (Auckland: Sherayl Kendall and David Corbett, 1990); Jan Rodgers, 'Potential for Professional Profit: The Making of the New Zealand Army Nursing Service, 1914–1915', *Nursing Praxis in New Zealand*, 11/2 (July 1996), 4–12; Jill Clendon, 'New Zealand Military Nurses' Fight for Recognition: World War I–World War II', *Nursing Praxis in New Zealand*, 12/1 (Mar. 1997), 24–8; Anna Rogers, *While You're Away: New Zealand Nurses At War, 1899–1948* (Auckland: Auckland University Press, 2003).

10. Matron Ellen Gould, Nurses' Narratives, Butler Collection, AWM41/975, Australian War Memorial, Canberra, Australia. On the work of the earliest Australian units, see Bassett, *Guns and Brooches*.

11. See, for example, the narrative of Ellen Cuthbert, in which she refers to her 'pioneering work': Sister Ellen Cuthbert, Nurses' Narratives, Butler Collection, AWM41/958, Australian War Memorial, Canberra, Australia. On the work of Australian army nurses, see Kirsty Harris, '"All for the Boys": The Nurse–Patient Relationship of Australian Army Nurses in the First World War', in Alison S. Fell and Christine E. Hallett (eds.), *First World War Nursing: New Perspectives* (New York: Routledge, 2013), 71–86.

12. For a description of Luna Park, see Bassett, *Guns and Brooches*, 36.

13. Gertrude M. Doherty, Nurses' Narratives, Butler Collection, AWM41/966, Australian War Memorial, Canberra, Australia. Sister E. McClelland commented that the wicker beds were replaced with iron bedsteads after a few months: Sister E. McClelland, Nurses' Narratives, Butler Collection, AWM41/1000, Australian War Memorial, Canberra, Australia.

14. Bassett, *Guns and Brooches*, 41–4.

15. Head Sister N. Morrice, Nurses' Narratives, Butler Collection, AWM41/1013, Australian War Memorial, Canberra, Australia.

16. Gould, Nurses' Narratives, AWM41/975.

17. Sister E. Vickers-Foote, Nurses' Narratives, Butler Collection, AWM41/1054, Australian War Memorial, Canberra, Australia. There are various versions of Vickers-Foote's name in the records, including Vickers Foot and Vicars Foote.

18. Papers relating to the efforts to form a New Zealand Army Nursing Service from 1908 onwards can be found at Archives New Zealand, Wellington, NZ: New Zealand Army Nursing Service, General File June 1910–August 1925, AD64 1. Jan Rodgers describes these attempts. For six years, the service consisted only of a 'matron-in-chief' and its development was blocked by Colonel J. Purdy, the army's director of medical services. His successor, W. Will, was more supportive of the service, and vigorous campaigning by the Trained Nurses' Association following the outbreak of war prompted its development: Rodgers, 'Potential for Professional Profit', 4–12.

19. Although it should be noted that six nurses had accompanied the Advanced Expeditionary Force to Samoa in August 1914, and twelve had accompanied the Australian Army Nursing Service, leaving New Zealand on 1 April 1915: Rodgers, 'Potential for Professional Profit', 4–12; Kendall and Corbett, *New Zealand Military Nursing*, 19–26; Rogers, *While You're Away*, 43–59. Hester Maclean's own account of these events was published in 1932: Maclean, *Nursing in New Zealand—History and Reminiscences* (Wellington, NZ: Tolan Printing Co., 1932).

20. New Zealand Army Nursing Service, General File, June 1910–August 1925, AD64 1, Archives New Zealand, Wellington, NZ; Clendon, 'New Zealand Military Nurses' Fight for Recognition', 24–8, at 25–6.

21. Rogers, *While You're Away*, 60–72.

22. Daphne Rona Commons, Letters, MS-Papers-1582-09, Alexander Turnbull Library, Wellington, NZ.

23. Commons, Letters, MS-Papers-1582-09.

24. Fanny Speedy, Diary, MS-Papers-1703, Alexander Turnbull Library, Wellington, NZ. A copy of Speedy's diary is also available in the Liddle Collection at the Brotherton Library, University of Leeds: Five diary transcripts (1915–1919), ANZAC (NZ). On the large numbers of

patients in Alexandria hospitals, see also May Chalmer, McDuff Notes on Sister May Chalmer, MS-Papers-8058, Alexander Turnbull Library, Wellington, NZ.

25. Louisa Higginson, Diary, MS-Papers-2477, Folders 1 and 2, Alexander Turnbull Library, Wellington, NZ.

26. Oram, 'Nursing in Egypt and Palestine'. On the work of No. 3 AGH on Lemnos, see Margaret Aitken, Nurses' Narratives, Butler Collection, AWM41/937, Australian War Memorial, Canberra, Australia.

27. Harris, *More Than Bombs and Bandages*, 95.

28. Sister M. E. Webster, *Notes on the Gallipoli Campaign* (written in 1920), Nurses' Accounts, Army Medical Services Museum Archives, Aldershot, UK.

29. Sister I. G. Lovell, Nurses' Narratives, Butler Collection, AWM41/998, Australian War Memorial, Canberra, Australia.

30. Bassett, *Guns and Brooches*, 44–8.

31. Matron Grace Wilson, Nurses' Narratives, Butler Collection, AWM41/1059, Australian War Memorial, Canberra, Australia.

32. Sister E. W. B. Lea, Private Papers: Letters (letter dated 6 Jan. 1916), documents.510 Con Shelf, Imperial War Museum, London, UK.

33. Harrison, *The Medical War*, 175.

34. Harrison, *The Medical War*, 175–84.

35. Webster compiled her diary entries, possibly with some editing, into an account for the Queen Alexandra's Imperial Nursing Service: Webster, *Notes on the Gallipoli Campaign*.

36. M. A. Brown, Private Papers: Three MS diaries covering her service in Egypt, Palestine, and on hospital ships, *Devanha* and *Delta*, documents.1001, 88/7/1, Diary 1, Imperial War Museum, London, UK.

37. Rogers, *While You're Away*, 73–93.

38. Charlotte Le Gallais, recording of her letters, rec. Sept. 1983, New Zealand Nursing Education and Research Foundation Oral History Project, OHC-157, listening copy no. LC-4645, Alexander Turnbull Library, Wellington, NZ. On work on board the *Maheno*, see also Amy Copeland, interviewed by H. Campbell, rec. 17 Mar. 1983, New Zealand Nursing Education and Research Foundation Oral History Project, OHInt-0014/040, original no. OHC-81a, listening copy no. LC-8113, Alexander Turnbull Library, Wellington, NZ.

39. Le Gallais, recording of her letters, rec. Sept. 1983.

40. Vickers-Foote, Nurses' Narratives, AWM41/1054.

41. Vickers-Foote, Nurses' Narratives, AWM41/1054.

42. Lovell, Nurses' Narratives, AWM41/998.

43. Lea, Letters.

44. Jentie Paterson, Service Record, WO 399/6503, The National Archives, Kew, UK. Paterson had 'signed on' once more for active service, on 9 November 1915.

45. Sister Jentie Paterson, Private Papers: Diaries, documents.378, 90/10/1, Imperial War Museum, London, UK.

46. Paterson, Diaries [emphasis in the original].

47. Paterson, Diaries.

48. Paterson, Diaries [emphasis in the original].

49. Cutting from the *Daily Sketch* (25 Nov. 1916). Contained in Paterson, Private Papers: Documents.378, 90/10/1, Imperial War Museum, London, UK.

50. M. A. Brown, Three MS diaries, Diary 1; Service Record for Mary Ann Brown, WO 399/1023, The National Archives, Kew, UK.

51. Sister Ruth Taylor, Nurses' Narratives, Butler Collection, AWM41/1051, Australian War Memorial, Canberra, Australia.

52. Head Sister Jeffries, Nurses' Narratives, Butler Collection, AWM41, Australian War Memorial, Canberra, Australia.

53. Barbara Mildred Tilly, Letters, MS-Papers-1451, Alexander Turnbull Library, Wellington, NZ.

54. Rodgers, 'Potential for Professional Profit', 4–12; Kendall and Corbett, *New Zealand Military Nursing*, 37–42; Rogers, *While You're Away*, ch. 6; Oram, 'Nursing in Egypt and Palestine 1915–1919'.

55. Major Wylie's statement was published in the New Zealand journal *Kai Tiaki*, and reproduced in the *British Journal of Nursing*: Anon., Column, *British Journal of Nursing* (15 Apr. 1916), 336.

56. Emily Hodges, interviewed by H. Campbell, rec. 25 June and 5 Sept. 1982, New Zealand Nursing Education and Research Foundation Oral History Project, OHInt-0014/074, listening copy no. LC-8112, Alexander Turnbull Library, Wellington, NZ.

57. Anon., Column, *British Journal of Nursing* (15 Apr. 1916), 336.

58. Anon., 'Sinking of the Marquette', *Marlborough Express*, 49/278 (24 Nov. 1915), 5.

59. Rogers, *While You're Away*, 108.

60. The report of the cheering nurses on deck can be found in Anon., 'Sinking of the Marquette', 5.

61. Anon., Column, *Auckland Weekly News* (11 Nov. 1915), cited at <http://freepages.genealogy.rootsweb.ancestry.com/~sooty/awnppnov1915.html>.

62. Rogers, *While You're Away*, 111–12.

63. See, for example, Aitken, Nurses' Narratives, AWM41/937.

64. In fact, Mark Harrison states that of all campaigns conducted outside Western Europe 'the Palestine campaign of 1917–18 was by far the most impressive from a medical point of view': Harrison, *The Medical War*, 254. See also a similar comment on p. 78. For an overview of the medical services in the Palestine Campaign see pp. 254–9.

65. Oram, 'Nursing in Egypt and Palestine'.

66. Winifred Ellen Spencer, interviewed by Yvonne Shadbolt, rec. 16 Apr. 1983, New Zealand Nursing Education and Research Foundation Oral History Project, OHInt-0014/156, Alexander Turnbull Library, Wellington, NZ.

67. Oram, 'Nursing in Egypt and Palestine 1915–1919'.

68. Oram, 'Nursing in Egypt and Palestine'.

69. Harrison, *The Medical War*, 239–54.

70. On the inadequacy of the evacuation lines in Mesopotamia, see Harrison, *The Medical War*, 206–20.

71. Sister A. J. Low, Nurses' Narratives, Butler Collection, AWM41/999, Australian War Memorial, Canberra, Australia.

72. On the measures taken to reform the lines of evacuation in Mesopotamia, see Harrison, *The Medical War*, 262–90.

73. Winifred Lemere-Goff, Oral History Interview, 1986, IWM9523, Imperial War Museum, London, UK.

74. This incident did not find its way into any of the official accounts of the wartime nursing services. Ruth Rae, 'Reading between Unwritten Lines: Australian Army Nurses in India, 1916–19', *Journal of the Australian War Memorial Canberra*, 36 (4 May 2002).

75. On conditions in and around Salonika, and Allied medical services' efforts to eradicate malaria, see Harrison, *The Medical War*, 228–39.

76. Winifred Seymour, Private Papers: Documents.7165, 97/34/1, Imperial War Museum, London, UK.

77. Mrs E. B. Moor, Private Papers: Diary and Letters, documents.7779, 98/9/1, Imperial War Museum, London, UK.
78. Moor, Diary and Letters.
79. Sister K. E. Maloney, Nurses' Narratives, Butler Collection, AWM41/ 1005, Australian War Memorial, Canberra, Australia.
80. Mary Millicent Rumney, Oral History Interview 1984, IWM739, Imperial War Museum, London, UK.
81. Osborne was actually referring to conditions following her units move into Macedonia: R. Osborne, 'Nursing with the British Salonika Force and Army of the Black Sea, August 1917 to July 1920', in Anon. (ed.), *Reminiscent Sketches, 1914–1919* (London: John Bale, Sons and Danielsson, Ltd, 1922), 17.
82. Sister Wray, Nurses' Narratives, Butler Collection, AWM41/1062, Australian War Memorial, Canberra, Australia.
83. Staff Nurse C. E. Strom, Letters, Nurses' Narratives, Butler Collection, AWM41/1068, Australian War Memorial, Canberra, Australia.
84. Strom, Letters, Nurses' Narratives, AWM41/1068.
85. Strom, Letters, Nurses' Narratives, AWM41/1068.
86. Strom, Letters, Nurses' Narratives, AWM41/1068. On conditions in Salonika, see also Sister Linda Watson, AANS, PR01246, Australian War Memorial, Canberra, Australia. However, see also the narrative of Sister Maloney who 'loved' the camp life and work at Salonika: Sister K. E Maloney, Nurses' Narratives, AWM 41/1005.
87. Strom, Letters, Nurses' Narratives, AWM41/1068.

**Chapter 5**
1. T. Travers, *The Killing Ground: The British Army, the Western Front and the Emergence of Modern Warfare, 1900–1918* (London: Allen & Unwin, 1987); Alan Kramer, *Dynamic of Destruction: Culture and Mass Killing in the First World War* (Oxford: Oxford University Press, 2007).
2. On Verdun, see Alistair Horne, *The Price of Glory: Verdun 1916* (1962; London: Penguin, 1993); Kramer, *Dynamic of Destruction*, 216–21; Marc Ferro, *The Great War 1914–1918*, trans. Nicole Stone (1973; London: Routledge, 2002), 83–93; Lawrence Sondhaus, *World War I: The Global Revolution* (Cambridge: Cambridge University Press, 2011), 207–8.
3. Gary Sheffield, *The Somme* (2003; London, Cassell, 2004), 13–19.

4. On the 'Battle of the Somme', see Lynn Macdonald, *Somme* (1983; London: Penguin, 1993), *passim*; Norman Stone, *World War One: A Short History* (2007; London: Penguin, 2008), 100–6.

5. Kramer, *Dynamic of Destruction*, 214–15.

6. Sondhaus, *World War I*, 213.

7. Kramer, *Dynamic of Destruction*, 211.

8. Charles H. Horton, *Stretcher Bearer! Fighting for Life in the Trenches*, ed. Dale Le Vack (Oxford: Lion Hudson, 2013), 55–68.

9. Sondhaus, *World War I*, 216.

10. Geoff Dyer, *The Missing of the Somme* (London: Penguin, 1994).

11. Dan Todman, *The Great War: Myth and Memory* (London: Hambledon Continuum, 2005), 80, 111–13.

12. Sheffield, *The Somme, passim*; Gary Sheffield, *Forgotten Victory: The First World War: Myths and Realities* (2001; London: Headline Book Publishing, 2002), 159–89.

13. Anon., Column, *British Journal of Nursing* (22 Apr. 1916), 358; Anon., 'French Flag Nursing Corps: Meeting at the Indian Empire Club', *British Journal of Nursing* (20 May 1916), 437–8.

14. Anon., 'French Flag Nursing Corps: Meeting at the Indian Empire Club', 437. Some British-trained and volunteer nurses also worked in an independent capacity for the French Red Cross.

15. Anon., 'French Flag Nursing Corps: Meeting at the Indian Empire Club', 437.

16. Anon., 'Echoes of the Great War: The Chivalrous Poilu', *British Journal of Nursing*, 88 (Mar. 1940), 39.

17. Anon., Letter, *British Journal of Nursing* (18 Mar. 1916), 244.

18. Dorothy Cator, *In a French Military Hospital* (London: Longman, Green and Co., 1915).

19. Anon., 'A French Military Hospital', *Nursing Times* (15 Jan. 1916), 60.

20. Anon., 'French Flag Nursing Corps: Meeting at the Indian Empire Club', 437.

21. Anon., 'French Flag Nursing Corps', *British Journal of Nursing* (1 Apr. 1916), 290.

22. Anon., 'Echoes of the Great War: The Chivalrous Poilu', 39.

23. Anon., 'Nursing and the War', *British Journal of Nursing* (15 Apr. 1916), 335.

24. Anon., 'Echoes of the Great War: The Chivalrous Poilu', 39.

25. Anon., 'French Flag Nursing Corps', 290.

26. Anon., 'Nursing and the War', 335–6.

27. Marian Wenzel and John Cornish, *Auntie Mabel's War: An Account of Her Part in the Hostilities of 1914–1918* (London: Allen Lane, 1980), 72.

28. Wenzel and Cornish, *Auntie Mabel's War*, 72–3.

29. Wenzel and Cornish, *Auntie Mabel's War*, 78.

30. Sister Jentie Paterson, Private Papers: Diaries, documents.378, 90/10/1, Imperial War Museum, London, UK.

31. Letter to Matron-in-Chief, dated 30 Apr. 1916: Jentie Paterson, Service Record, WO 399/6503, The National Archives, Kew, UK.

32. Elizabeth S. Haldane, *The British Nurse in Peace and War* (London: John Murray, 1923), 197.

33. Edith Appleton, *Diaries*, Private Collection of Dick Robinson, entry for 13 Mar. 1916. An abridged version of Appleton's diaries is available as Ruth Cowen (ed.), *War Diaries—A Nurse at the Front; The Great War Diaries of Sister Edith Appleton* (London: Simon and Schuster, 2012): this episode appears on pp. 110–11.

34. Sister Ellen Cuthbert, Nurses' Narratives, Butler Collection, AWM41/958, Australian War Memorial, Canberra, Australia.

35. Gertrude M. Doherty, Nurses' Narratives, Butler Collection, AWM41/966, Australian War Memorial, Canberra, Australia.

36. Cuthbert, Nurses' Narratives, AWM41/958.

37. Mark Harrison, *The Medical War* (Oxford: Oxford University Press, 2010), 66–9.

38. On the system of evacuation on the Western Front, see Christine Hallett, *Containing Trauma: Nursing Work in the First World War* (Manchester: Manchester University Press, 2009), 15–17; Harrison, *The Medical War*, 66–91.

39. Sister M. A. C. Blair, QA, *Reminiscences of a Nursing Sister in the Great War*, Nurses' Accounts, Army Medical Services Museum Archives, Aldershot, UK.

40. Sister Elsie Dobson, Nurses' Narratives, Butler Collection, AWM41/964, Australian War Memorial, Canberra, Australia.

41. Dobson, Nurses' Narratives, AWM41/964.

42. Sister Leila Smith, *Life on an Ambulance Train*, Nurses' Narratives, Butler Collection, AWM41/1043, Australian War Memorial, Canberra, Australia. Smith refers to 'Germaincourt' in her narrative. There is no

record of such a CCS, and she may be referring to Gezaincourt. I am indebted to Sue Light for this information.

43. Matron Ellen Gould, Nurses' Narratives, Butler Collection, AWM41/975, Australian War Memorial, Canberra, Australia.

44. Appleton, *Diaries*, 3 July 1916; in Cowen (ed.), *War Diaries*, quotation on p. 160.

45. Appleton, *Diaries*, 4 July 1916; in Cowen (ed.), *War Diaries*, 161.

46. Appleton, *Diaries*, entries for various dates in July 1916; in Cowen (ed.), *War Diaries*, 161.

47. Appleton, *Diaries*, entries from 13 July to 8 Aug. 1916; in Cowen (ed.), *War Diaries*, 166–83.

48. Appleton, *Diaries*, 23 Aug. 1916; in Cowen (ed.), *War Diaries*, 183.

49. Appleton, *Diaries*, 28 Aug. and 9 Sept. 1916; in Cowen (ed.), *War Diaries*, 183.

50. Lyn Macdonald, *The Roses of No Man's Land* (1980; London: Penguin, 1993), 172.

51. On patient-feeding see Hallett, *Containing Trauma*, 106–11.

52. Jan Bassett, *Guns and Brooches: Australian Army Nursing from the Boer War to the Gulf War* (Melbourne: Oxford University Press, 1992), 56–7.

53. Bassett, *Guns and Brooches*, 58–9.

54. Anon., *The Edith Cavell Nurse from Massachusetts: A Record of One Year's Personal Service with the British Expeditionary Force in France; Boulogne–The Somme, 1916–1917; With an Account of the Imprisonment, Trial and Death of Edith Cavell* (Boston: W. A. Butterfield, 1917); Anon., 'An Edith Cavell Memorial Nurse', *British Journal of Nursing* (4 Mar. 1916), 214.

55. Alice Howell Friedman, 'Fitzgerald, Alice Louise, Florence', in Martin Kaufman (ed.), *Dictionary of American Nursing Biography* (New York: Greenwood Press, 1988), 121–3.

56. Alice Fitzgerald, Unpublished Memoirs incorporating War Diary, Alice Fitzgerald Papers, MdHR M2633 and MdHR M 2634 (unpaginated), Maryland Historical Society, Baltimore, USA.

57. Alice Fitzgerald, Unpublished Memoirs incorporating War Diary.

58. Alice Fitzgerald, Unpublished Memoirs incorporating War Diary.

59. Harrison, *The Medical War*, 37–8.

60. Alice Fitzgerald, Unpublished Memoirs incorporating War Diary.

61. Alice Fitzgerald, Unpublished Memoirs incorporating War Diary.

62. Mary Borden, *The Forbidden Zone* (London: William Heinemann Ltd, 1929), 143.

63. Janet Butler, ' "Very busy in Bosches Alley": One Day of the Somme in Sister Kit McNaughton's Diary', *Health and History: Journal of the Australian Society of the History of Medicine*, 6/2 (2004), 18–32, at 26–7. See also Janet Butler, *Kitty's War: The Remarkable Wartime Experiences of Kit McNaughton* (St Lucia, Queensland: University of Queensland Press, 2013).

64. Gerard Fitzgerald, 'Chemical Warfare and the Medical Response during World War I', *American Journal of Public Health*, 98/4 (Apr. 2008), 611–25; Harrison, *The Medical War*, 107. Prior to this, poison gas had been released as 'cloud gas' rather than via shells.

65. See, for example, Julia Stimson, *Finding Themselves: The Letters of an American Army Chief Nurse at a British Hospital in France* (New York: Macmillan Company, 1927), 79–80.

66. On deaths from gas poisoning, see T. J. Mitchell and G. M. Smith, *History of the Great War Based on Official Documents: Medical Services* (Uckfield, West Sussex: The Naval and Military Press, Ltd with the Imperial War Museum; facsimile of book first published in 1931), 111. On the long-term effects of gas poisoning: Adolphe Abrahams, 'The Later Effects of Gas Poisoning', *The Lancet*, 200/5174 (28 Oct. 1922), 933–4; Harold Vallow, 'The Later Effects of Gas Poisoning', *The Lancet*, 200/5175 (4 Nov. 1922), 985.

67. Wenzel and Cornish, *Auntie Mabel's War*, 76.

68. Janet Irene Miller, *Recollections of a Military Hospital, Manchester*, AACC 0459, 92/19, T2 (MIL), Red Cross Archives, London, UK.

69. No. 2 NZ General Hospital was located at Oatlands Park, Walton-on-Thames, and No. 3 NZ General Hospital at Codford St Mary in Wiltshire: Anon., *New Zealanders in Brockenhurst: The No 1 New Zealand General Hospital 1916–1919*, 2nd edn., with foreword by David Brewster (Brockenhurst: Frost Printers, 2006), 3.

70. Anon., *New Zealanders in Brockenhurst*, 4. On Lady Haringe's original hospital and the establishment of the No. 1 NZ General Hospital, see also John Cockram (ed.), *Brockenhurst and the Two World Wars* (Brockenhurst: Cockram, n.d.), 48.

71. Anon., *New Zealanders in Brockenhurst*, 10.

72. Anon., *New Zealanders in Brockenhurst*, 10. On Brockenhurst, see also Florence Le Lievre, interviewed by Mary Grant, rec. 8 Nov. 1983, New Zealand Nursing Education and Research Foundation Oral History Project, OHC-184, listening copy no. LC-6172, Alexander Turnbull Library, Wellington, NZ; Charlotte Leslie McIntyre, interviewed by Yvonne Shadbolt, rec. 29 June 1983, New Zealand Nursing Education and Research Foundation Oral History Project, OHInt-0014/103, Alexander Turnbull Library, Wellington, NZ.

73. May Chalmer, Letter, *Kai Tiaki* (Jan. 1917). See also May Chalmer, 'NZ Hospital at Walton: A New Extension', *Kai Tiaki* (Apr. 1917); May Chalmer, Letter, *Kai Tiaki* (Apr. 1917).

## Chapter 6

1. Norman Stone, *World War One* (2007; London: Penguin, 2008), 118; Michael Howard, *The First World War* (Oxford: Oxford University Press, 2002), 81–4.

2. Marie, Queen of Roumania, *Ordeal: The Story of My Life* (New York: Charles Scribner's Sons, 1935).

3. On the Russian Revolution and its impact on the First World War, see Ronald Hingley, *Russian Revolution* (London: Bodley Head, 1970); Richard Pipes, *The Russian Revolution, 1899–1919* (London: Collins Harvill, 1990); Rex A. Wade, *The Russian Revolution, 1917* (Cambridge: Cambridge University Press, 2000); Sheila Fitzpatrick, *The Russian Revolution* (3rd edn., Oxford: Oxford University Press, 2008); Douglas Smith, *Former People: The Last Days of the Russian Aristocracy* (London: Macmillan, 2012).

4. Robert H. Ferrell, *America's Deadliest Battle: Meuse-Argonne, 1918* (Lawrence, Kan.: University Press of Kansas, 2007), 1.

5. Edward Hungerford, *With the Doughboy in France* (New York: Macmillan Company, 1920); John Van Schaick Jr., *The Little Corner Never Conquered: The Story of the American Red Cross War Work for Belgium* (New York: Macmillan Company, 1922).

6. On the 'Zimmermann Telegram' see Stone, *World War One*, 124–5. On the USA's entry into the war, see Lawrence Sondhaus, *World War I: The Global Revolution* (Cambridge: Cambridge University Press, 2011), 321.

7. On the 'Nivelle Offensive' see A. J. P. Taylor, *The First World War* (1963; London: Penguin, 1966), 165–9; Hew Strachan, *The First World*

*War* (2003; London: Pocket Books, 2006), 238–44; Sondhaus, *World War I*, 255.

8. Sondhaus, *World War I*, 256.

9. On the Third Battle of Ypres, see Lyn Macdonald, *They Called it Passchendaele* (London: Penguin, 1978); A. J. P. Taylor, *The First World War*, 191–5; David Stephenson, *1914–1918: The History of the First World War* (London: Allen Lane, 2004), 334–6.

10. Mark Harrison, *The Medical War: British Military Medicine in the First World War* (Oxford: Oxford University Press, 2010), 66–77.

11. Harrison, *The Medical War*, 77.

12. The medal was actually awarded on 26 November: Secretary's Report at a meeting of the Advisory Council of the TFNS (1918); available in Dame Sidney Jane Browne, Papers, Box 1, Army Medical Services Museum Archives, Aldershot, UK. Herbert was working at No. 35 General Hospital, Calais, at the time of this incident, which took place on the night of 3/4 September 1917.

13. Harrison, *The Medical War*, 82.

14. Gertrude M. Doherty, Nurses' Narratives, Butler Collection, AWM41/ 966, Australian War Memorial, Canberra, Australia.

15. Doherty, Nurses' Narratives, AW41/966.

16. Sister A. N. Smith, Nurses' Narratives, Butler Collection, AWM41/1041, Australian War Memorial, Canberra, Australia.

17. Sister A. N. Smith, Nurses' Narratives, AWM41/1041. See also Sister V. M. Payne, Nurses' Narratives, Butler Collection, AWM41/1021, Australian War Memorial, Canberra, Australia.

18. Sister A. N. Smith, Nurses' Narratives, AWM41/1041. On CCS work in 1917, see also L. Ida G. Willis, *A Nurse Remembers* (Lower Hutt, NZ: AK Wilson, 1968).

19. Sister A. N. Smith, Nurses' Narratives, AWM41/1041.

20. Although Sassoon directly experienced the Third Battle of Ypres, Owen was just returning, after being hospitalized for shell shock, to another sector of the front, during the battle.

21. Leo van Bergen, *Before My Helpless Sight: Suffering, Dying and Military Medicine on the Western Front, 1914–1918*, trans. Liz Waters (Farnham: Ashgate, 2009), 455.

22. On abdominal surgery during the war, see Steven D. Heys, 'Abdominal Wounds: Evolution of Management and Establishment of Surgical

Treatments', in Thomas Scotland and Heys (eds.), *War Surgery 1914–1918* (Solihull: Helion and Co. Ltd, 2012), 178–211; Harrison, *The Medical War*, 102–4.

23. Harvey Cushing, *From a Surgeon's Journal, 1915–1918* (Boston: Little, Brown and Company, 1936), 170.

24. Direct quotation taken from Ann Clayton, *Chavasse Double VC* (1992; Barnsley: Pen and Sword Books, 2008), 207–8.

25. Four other CCSs (British 10 and 17 and Candian 2 and 3) were actually located at 'Remy Siding' itself: Thomas R. Scotland, 'Evacuation Pathway for the Wounded', in Scotland and Steven Heys (eds.), *War Surgery 1914–1918* (Solihull: Helion and Co. Ltd, 2012), 51–84, at 66.

26. Kate Luard, *Unknown Warriors* (London: Chatto and Windus, 1930), 230–1.

27. Jan and Katrien Louagie-Nolf, *Talbot House Poperinge: De Eerste Halte na de Hel* (Lannoo: Tielt, 1998), 240. I am indebted to Geertjan Remerie for this and other translations from the Louagie-Nolfs' book, and to Lionel Roosemont for important insights into Remy Siding and Lijssenthoek.

28. Cushing, *From a Surgeon's Journal*, 194.

29. Doherty, Nurses' Narratives, AWM41/966.

30. Christine Hallett, *Containing Trauma: Nursing Work in the First World War* (Manchester: Manchester University Press, 2009), 60.

31. On the use of mustard gas, see Gerard Fitzgerald, 'Chemical Warfare and Medical Response During World War I', *American Journal of Public Health*, 98/4 (Apr. 2008), 611–25; Harrison, *The Medical War*, 81.

32. Leah Leneman, 'Medical Women at War, 1914–1918', *Medical History*, 38 (1994), 167.

33. Elizabeth S. Haldane, *The British Nurse in Peace and War* (London: John Murray, 1923), 212.

34. Elsie May Tranter, Diary, Nurses' Narratives, Butler Collection, 3 DRL 4081/A, AWM419/22/21, Australian War Memorial, Canberra, Australia.

35. Sister Elsie Dobson, Nurses' Narratives, Butler Collection, AWM41/964, Australian War Memorial, Canberra, Australia.

36. Vera Brittain, *Testament of Youth: An Autobiographical Study of the Years 1900–1925* (1933; London: Virago, 2004), 340–3.

37. Sister E. L. Steadman, Nurses' Narratives, Butler Collection, AWM41/1046, Australian War Memorial, Canberra, Australia.

38. Steadman, Nurses' Narratives, AWM41/1046. For examples of Allied nurses describing their experiences of caring for German or Austrian patients, see also Anon., *Twenty Months a VAD* (Sheffield: J. Northen, n.d.), 29–30, available at the Red Cross Archive, London; Henrietta Tayler, *A Scottish Nurse at War: Being a Record of Four and a Half Years of War* (London: John Lane, 1920), 75; Shirley Millard, *I Saw Them Die: Diary and Recollections of Shirley Millard*, ed. Adele Comandini (London: George G. Harrap and Co., 1936), 37–8.

39. Sister Ellen Cuthbert, Nurses' Narratives, Butler Collection, AWM41/958, Australian War Memorial, Canberra, Australia.

40. Minnie Goodnow, *War Nursing: A Text-Book for the Auxiliary Nurse* (Philadelphia and London: W. B. Saunders Company, 1917), 11.

41. Violetta Thurstan, *A Text Book of War Nursing* (London: G. P. Putnam's Sons, 1917), 57.

42. Florence Egerton, Papers, 812/1-11, Red Cross Archives, London, UK.

43. Sir Wilmot P. Herringham, 'Gas Poisoning', *The Lancet*, 195/5034 (21 Feb. 1920), 423–4; Gerard Fitzgerald, 'Chemical Warfare and Medical Response', 611–25.

44. Head Sister N. Morrice, Nurses' Narratives, Butler Collection, AWM41/1013, Australian War Memorial, Canberra, Australia.

45. Matron Ellen Gould, Nurses' Narratives, Butler Collection, AWM41/975, Australian War Memorial, Canberra, Australia.

46. Marie, Queen of Roumania, *Ordeal*. Contemporary sources refer to 'Roumania'; hence, this spelling has been retained for direct quotations.

47. Marie, Queen of Roumania, *Ordeal*, 55–6.

48. Marie, Queen of Roumania, *Ordeal*, 58.

49. Marie, Queen of Roumania, *Ordeal*, 81.

50. Marie, Queen of Roumania, *Ordeal*, 177.

51. Marie, Queen of Roumania, *Ordeal*, 148.

52. Miss K. Hodges, Private Papers: Diary, documents.1974, 92/22/1, p. 67, Imperial War Museum, London, UK.

53. Miss K. Hodges, Private Papers: Diary, 70.

54. Miss K. Hodges, Private Papers: Diary, 85; Dorothy Cotton, Diary. 28, available online from Library and Archives Canada, Ottawa:

&lt;www.collectionscanada.gc.ca/nursing-sisters/025013-2200-e.html&gt; [last accessed 17 May 2013]; Thurstan, *A Text Book of War Nursing*, 114. See also Hallett, *Containing Trauma*, 139.

55. Miss K. Hodges, Private Papers: Diary, 85–6.
56. Dorothy Cotton, Letter to 'Elsie', available online from Library and Archives Canada, Ottawa: www.collectionscanada.gc.ca/nursing-sisters/025013-2200-e.html [last accessed 17 May 2013].
57. Miss K. Hodges, Private Papers: Diary, 87.
58. Miss K. Hodges, Private Papers: Diary, 83–4, 87.
59. Miss K. Hodges, Private Papers: Diary, 85.
60. Farmborough's book was written several decades after the events it describes and, although it is guided by her original contemporaneously-written diary, it is probably influenced by later hindsight. For this quotation and more information on the propaganda being circulated among Russian soldiers in the spring of 1917, see Florence Farmborough, *Nurse at the Russian Front: A Diary, 1914–1918* (London: Book Club Associates, 1974), 264.
61. Farmborough, *Nurse at the Russian Front*, 271; Peter Liddle, *Captured Memories 1900–1918: Across the Threshold of War* (Barnsley: Pen and Sword Military, 2010), 240.
62. Farmborough, *Nurse at the Russian Front*, 277–8.
63. Sanitars were hospital orderlies, responsible for the cleanliness and order of the hospital and for providing personal care to patients under the supervision of nurses.
64. Miss K. Hodges, Private Papers: Diary, 97–9.
65. Miss K. Hodges, Private Papers: Diary, 103.
66. Dorothy Seymour, Private Papers: Diary and Letters, documents.3210, 95/28/1, Imperial War Museum, London, UK.
67. Farmborough, *Nurse at the Russian Front*, 373–409.
68. Margaret H. Barber, *A British Nurse in Bolshevik Russia: The Narrative of Margaret H. Barber, April 1916–December 1919* (London: A. C. Fifield, 1920), 11.
69. Barber, *A British Nurse in Bolshevik Russia*, 11.
70. Barber, *A British Nurse in Bolshevik Russia*, 25.
71. Barber, *A British Nurse in Bolshevik Russia*, 59–60.
72. Mary Britnieva, *One Woman's Story* (London: Arthur Baker, 1934), 265–87.

73. On the work of American volunteer nurses, see Jane Potter, ' "I feel as a Normal Being Should, in Spite of the Blood and Anguish in Which I Move": American Women's First World War Nursing Memoirs', in Alison S. Fell and Christine E. Hallett (eds.), *First World War Nursing: New Perspectives* (New York: Routledge, 2013), 51–68.

74. Mary Sarnecky, *A History of the U.S. Army Nurse Corps* (Philadelphia: University of Pennsylvania Press, 1999); George W. Crile, *George Crile: An Autobiography* (Philadelphia: J. B. Lippincott, 1947); Anon., *Medical Department of the United States Army in the World War* (Washington, DC; US Surgeon General's Office, 1921–9).

75. On the formation of the base hospitals and the role of trained nurses in them, see Kimberly Jensen, 'A Base Hospital is not a Coney Island Dance Hall: American Women Nurses, Hostile Work Environment, and Military Rank in the First World War', *Frontiers*, 26/2 (2005), 206–35, at 211; Sarnecky, *A History of the Army Nurse Corps*, 80–1. On the formation of Base Hospital No. 10, see Anon., *History of the Pennsylvania Hospital Unit (Base Hospital No. 10, USA) In the Great War* (New York: Paul B. Hoeber, 1921).

76. Jennifer Casavant Telford, 'American Red Cross Nursing during World War I: Opportunities and Obstacles' (unpublished PhD thesis, University of Virginia, 2007), 149–55; Susan Zeiger, *In Uncle Sam's Service: Women Workers with the American Expeditionary Force, 1917–1919* (Philadelphia: University of Pennsylvania Press, 1999), 27.

77. Sarnecky, *A History of the Army Nurse Corps*, 92–3.

78. Memorandum from the Surgeon General of the Army to the Secretary of War: Establishment of an Army School of Nursing, in Annie Warburton Goodrich Papers, MC 4, Box 1, Barbara Bates Center for the Study of the History of Nursing, University of Pennsylvania, Philadelphia, USA.

79. Annie Warburton Goodrich Papers, MC 4, Box 1. Mary Sarnecky has argued that two of the most influential senior army nurses, Jane Delano (Chair of the American Red Cross Nursing Service) and Dora Thompson (Superintendent of the Army Nurse Corps), had been in favour of the use of 'nurses aides' in base hospitals overseas, but had lost a vote at a Convention of the National Nursing Organizations in Cleveland Ohio on this issue in May 1918: Sarnecky, *A History of the U.S. Army Nurse Corps*, 85.

80. Paper on the formation of the ASN, in Annie Warburton Goodrich Papers, MC 4, Box 1.

81. Paper on the formation of the ASN, in Annie Warburton Goodrich Papers, MC 4, Box 1. On the formation of the Army School of Nursing, see Sarnecky, *A History of the U.S. Army Nurse Corps*, 86–9; on 'Vassar Training Camp', the other significant training school for nurses established to serve the needs of war, see pp. 89–91.

82. Margaret Cowling, 'A Red Cross Nurse', incorporated into Deming J. Shear, 'Historical Sketch of Base Hospital #41', File 2, Box 1, Papers of Base Hospital 41, 1905–2009, Accession Number MS-17, Claude Moore Health Sciences Library (Historical Collections), University of Virginia, Charlottesville, USA.

83. Letter written by Julian M. Cabell to Dr Stephen Watts, 10 Jan. 1919, File 2, Box 3, Papers of Base Hospital 41, 1905–2009, Accession Number MS-17, Claude Moore Health Sciences Library (Historical Collection), University of Virginia, Charlottesville, USA.

84. Camilla Louise Wills, Letter to 'Aunt Mamie', date unknown, Box 1, Folder 9, Camilla Louise Wills Collection, Eleanor Crowder Bjoring Center for Nursing Historical Inquiry, University of Virginia, Charlottesville, USA. Also cited by Telford, 'American Red Cross Nursing during World War I', 129. The American Red Cross Nursing Service certificate of 'Katie Louise Wills' is dated 16 March 1918: Camilla Louise Wills Collection.

85. Camilla Louise Wills, Letter to 'Aunt Mamie', 17 Apr. 1918, Box 1, Folder 5, Camilla Louise Wills Collection. Also cited by Telford, 'American Red Cross Nursing during World War I', 124.

86. Telford, 'American Red Cross Nursing during World War I', 126.

87. Camilla Louise Wills, Letter to 'Aunt Mamie', 12 July 1918, Box 1, Folder 9, Camilla Louise Wills Collection.

88. Julia Stimson, *Finding Themselves: The Letters of an American Army Chief Nurse at a British Hospital in France* (New York: Macmillan Company, 1927), 3–4.

89. Alice Howell Friedman, 'Stimson, Julia Catherine', in Martin Kaufman (ed.), *Dictionary of American Nursing Biography* (New York: Greenwood Press, 1988), 350–1.

90. Jensen, 'A Base Hospital is not a Coney Island Dance Hall', 206–35; Kimberly Jensen, *Mobilizing Minerva: American Women in the First World War* (Urbana and Chicago: University of Illinois Press, 2008).

91. Camilla Louise Wills, Letter to 'Aunt Mamie', 9 Oct. 1918, Box 1, Folder 9, Camilla Louise Wills Collection. Also cited by Telford, 'American Red Cross Nursing during World War I', 135–6.

92. Vera Woodroffe, Private Papers: Letters, documents.3262, 95/31/1, Imperial War Museum, London, UK.

93. Woodroffe, Letters. On the use of X-rays, see Alexander MacDonald, 'X-Rays during the Great War', in Thomas Scotland and Steven Heys (eds.), *War Surgery 1914–1918* (Solihull: Helion and Co. Ltd, 2012), 134–47.

94. S. Reeves, Private Papers: Account, documents.133, 89/10/1, Imperial War Museum, London, UK.

95. Woodroffe, Letters; on the campaigns in Italy, see also Anon., *With the Italian Expeditionary Force*, Nurses' Accounts, Army Medical Services Museum Archives, Aldershot, UK.

96. Reeves, Account.

97. Sister E. Vickers-Foote, Nurses' Narratives, Butler Collection, AWM41/1054, Australian War Memorial, Canberra, Australia.

98. Vickers-Foote, Nurses' Narratives, AWM41/1054.

## Chapter 7

1. Malcolm Brown, *1918 Year of Victory* (London: Pan Books with Imperial War Museum, 1998), 45–141; Lawrence Sondhaus, *World War I: The Global Revolution* (Cambridge: Cambridge University Press, 2011), 406–12.

2. Robert H. Ferrell, *America's Deadliest Battle: Meuse-Argonne, 1918* (Lawrence, Kan.: University Press of Kansas, 2007), p. xi.

3. Sondhaus, *World War I*, 430.

4. Carol R. Byerly, *Fever of War: The Influenza Epidemic in the U.S. Army During World War I* (New York: Viking, 1991). The origin of the influenza pandemic is not well understood, and its emergence in Kansas is only one of a number of theories. See also Niall Johnson, *Britain and the 1918–1919 Influenza Pandemic* (London: Routledge, 2006); Howard Phillips and David Killingray, *The Spanish Influenza Pandemic of 1918–1919:*

*New Perspectives* (London: Routledge, 2003). On the importance of nursing care for influenza victims, see A. Keeling, ' "Alert to the Necessities of the Emergency": U.S. Nursing during the 1918 Influenza Pandemic', *Public Health Reports: Special Supplement on Pandemic Influenza* (2010), 125, 105–12.

5. On the influenza pandemic, see Margaret Van Straubenzee, Extract from Memoirs, *c.*1916–1919, X/142, LIB 88/595, T2 (STR), Red Cross Archives, London, UK; Joyce Sapwell, 'The Reminiscences of a VAD in Two World Wars', T2 SAP, Red Cross Archives, London, UK; Henrietta Tayler, *A Scottish Nurse at Work: Being a Record of Four and a Half Years of War* (London: John Lane, 1920), 86–7.

6. Dame Sidney Jane Browne, Papers, Box 1, Army Medical Services Museum Archives, Aldershot, UK.

7. Mark Harrison, *The Medical War: British Military Medicine in the First World War* (Oxford: Oxford University Press, 2010), 84.

8. Sister Ella Redman, Nurses' Narratives, Butler Collection, AWM 41/1027, Australian War Memorial, Canberra, Australia. There is also a shortened version of Redman's account in Anon., *Australian Nursing Services During the First World War*, Misc 47, Item 790, Imperial War Museum, London, UK.

9. Redman, Nurses' Narratives, AWM 41/1027.

10. Redman, Nurses' Narratives, AWM 41/1027.

11. Dame Maud McCarthy, Matron-in-Chief, British Expeditionary Force in France, Reports on Nursing Services, 1918, Box 10, 43/1985, Army Medical Services Museum Archives, Aldershot, UK, 27. Morbidity was said to have been caused largely by infectious diseases, made worse by overwork and exhaustion. The influenza pandemic was beginning to account for many of the morbidities.

12. Dame Maud McCarthy, Reports on Nursing Services, 1918, 4.

13. On the creation of specialist roles and the pressures this placed on the nursing workforce, see Dame Maud McCarthy, Reports on Nursing Services, 1918, 12.

14. Dame Maud McCarthy, Reports on Nursing Services, 1918, 21.

15. Christine E. Hallett, *Containing Trauma: Nursing Work in the First World War* (Manchester: Manchester University Press, 2009), 114–16.

16. Mary Mackie, *Sky Wards: A History of the Princess Mary's Royal Air Force Nursing Service* (London: Robert Hale, 2001), 22–54.

17. Dame Maud McCarthy, Reports on Nursing Services, 1918, 22–3.

18. Patient 111: Pte Johnstone; Catherine Eva Bennett, *Record of the Patients of Stamford Hospital, April 24th 1917–Jan 24th 1919, written for the Earl of Stamford*, Archives of Dunham Massey Hall, Cheshire, John Rylands Library, University of Manchester, UK. Reproduced by kind permission of the National Trust. I am indebted to Laura Wilson and Charlotte Smithson for providing me with a copy of this source.

19. By this time McCarron was a member of the US Army Nurse Corps and had served for six months at Fort Bliss, near the US–Mexican border: Sara McCarron Collection, Barbara Bates Center for the Study of the History of Nursing, University of Pennsylvania, Philadelphia, USA.

20. Sara McCarron Collection, Barbara Bates Center.

21. Jane De Launoy, *Infirmières de guerre en service commandé (Front de 14 à 18)* (Brussels, L'Édition universelle, 1937), 226.

22. Dame Maud McCarthy, Reports on Nursing Services, 1918, 20–1. Julia Stimson's own account of her work with Base Hospital No. 21 can be found in a collection of her letters; Julia Stimson, *Finding Themselves: The Letters of an American Army Chief Nurse in a British Hospital in France* (New York: Macmillan Company, 1927).

23. Marian Wenzel and John Cornish, *Auntie Mabel's War: An Account of Her Part in the Hostilities of 1914–1918* (London: Allen Lane, 1980), 93–5.

24. Dame Maud McCarthy, Reports on Nursing Services, 1918, 27.

25. Dame Maud McCarthy, Reports on Nursing Services, 1918, 28.

26. The Secretary's Report at a meeting of the Advisory Council of the TFNS, 1918, available in Dame Sidney Jane Browne, Papers, Box 1, Army Medical Services Museum Archives, Aldershot, UK.

27. Dame Maud McCarthy, Reports on Nursing Services, 1918, 28.

28. Dame Maud McCarthy, Reports on Nursing Services, 1918, 41.

29. See, for example, the account of VAD Dorothy Seymour: Private Papers: Diary and Letters, documents.3210, 95/28/1, Imperial War Museum, London, UK.

30. Ruth Allan, Nurses' Narratives, Butler Collection, AWM41/938, Australian War Memorial, Canberra, Australia.

31. Sister M. E. Hall, Nurses' Narratives, Butler Collection, AWM41/979, Australian War Memorial, Canberra, Australia.

32. Sybil Surtees, interviewed by Hugo Manson, NZOHA Sunlight Centenarians Oral History Project, OHColl-0004, Alexander Turnbull Library, Wellington, NZ.

33. Sister E. McClelland, Nurses' Narratives, Butler Collection, AWM41/1000, Australian War Memorial, Canberra, Australia.

34. Sister Ellen Cuthbert, Nurses' Narratives, Butler Collection, AWM41/958, Australian War Memorial, Canberra, Australia.

35. Elsie May Tranter, Diary, Nurses' Narratives, Butler Collection, 3DRL 4081/A, AWM 419/22/21, Australian War Memorial, Canberra, Australia.

36. Deming J. Shear, 'Historical Sketch of Base Hospital #41', File 2, Box 1, Papers of Base Hospital 41, 1905–2009, Accession Number MS-17, Claude Moore Health Sciences Library (Historical Collections), University of Virginia, Charlottesville, USA. See also Base Hospital 41's own newsletter: *Between Convoys*, 1 (Dec. 1918), Papers of Base Hospital 41, 1905–2009, Accession Number MS-17, Claude Moore Health Sciences Library (Historical Collections), University of Virginia, Charlottesville, USA.

37. Camilla Louise Wills, Letter to 'Aunt Mamie', 19 Aug. 1918, Box 1, Folder 9, Camilla Louise Wills Collection, Eleanor Crowder Bjoring Center for Nursing Historical Inquiry, University of Virginia, Charlottesville, USA. Also cited by Jennifer Casavant Telford, 'American Red Cross Nursing during World War I: Opportunities and Obstacles' (unpublished PhD thesis, University of Virginia, 2007), 120.

38. Camilla Louise Wills, Letter to 'Aunt Mamie', 19 Aug. 1918. Also cited by Telford, 'American Red Cross Nursing during World War I', 131.

39. Margaret Cowling, 'A Red Cross Nurse', incorporated into Deming J. Shear, 'Historical Sketch of Base Hospital #41', File 2, Box 1, Papers of Base Hospital 41, 1905–2009, Accession Number MS-17, Claude Moore Health Sciences Library (Historical Collections), University of Virginia, Charlottesville, USA.

40. Cowling, 'A Red Cross Nurse'.

41. Camilla Louise Wills, Diary, 15 Sept. 1918, Box 1, Folder 1, Camilla Louise Wills Collection. Also cited by Telford, 'American Red Cross Nursing during World War I', 133.

42. Deming J. Shear, 'Historical Sketch of Base Hospital #41'.

43. Camilla Louise Wills, Diary entries for 20–30 Sept. 1918, Box 1, Folder 9, Camilla Louise Wills Collection. Also cited by Telford, 'American Red Cross Nursing during World War I', 138–9.

44. Deming J. Shear, 'Historical Sketch of Base Hospital #41', 17.

45. See Chapter 5.

46. Edith Appleton, *Diaries*, Private Collection of Dick Robinson, entry for 22 Aug. 1918. An abridged version of Appleton's diaries is available as Ruth Cowen (ed.), *War Diaries—A Nurse at the Front: The Great War Diaries of Sister Edith Appleton* (London: Simon and Schuster, 2012): the reference to 'gassed men' is on p. 245; the reference to the heat has been omitted from the published version.

47. Diary, Sara McCarron Collection, Barbara Bates Center.

48. Diary, Sara McCarron Collection, Barbara Bates Center.

49. Dame Maud McCarthy, Reports on Nursing Services, 1918, 47.

50. Dame Maud McCarthy, Reports on Nursing Services, 1918, 16–17.

51. Dame Maud McCarthy, Reports on Nursing Services, 1918, 39–40.

52. Head Sister Jeffries, Nurses' Narratives, Butler Collection, AWM41, Australian War Memorial, Canberra, Australia.

53. Harrison, *The Medical War*, 88.

54. Hall, Nurses' Narratives, AWM41/979; Staff Nurse Leila Brown, Nurses' Narratives, Butler Collection, AWM41/946, Australian War Memorial, Canberra, Australia.

55. The term 'lady anaesthetist' was used by Maud McCarthy in her report on the year 1918: Dame Maud McCarthy, Reports on Nursing Services, 1918, 7.

56. Arlene W. Keeling, *Nursing and the Privilege of Prescription, 1893–2000* (Columbus: Ohio State University Press, 2007): see ch. 2: 'Practicing Medicine without a Licence? Nurse Anesthetists, 1900–1938', 28–48.

57. Telford, 'American Red Cross Nursing during World War I', 134–5.

58. Dame Maud McCarthy, Reports on Nursing Services, 1918, 7.

59. Dame Maud McCarthy, Reports on Nursing Services, 1918, 7–8.

60. Tranter's war experience was reported in her diary: Elsie May Tranter, Diary, 3 DRL 4081/A, AWM419/22/21, Australian War Memorial, Canberra, Australia. The episode involving the nurse-anaesthetists was reported by Jan Bassett, *Guns and Brooches: Australian Army Nursing from the Boer War to the Gulf War* (Melbourne: Oxford

University Press, 1992), 61–2. See also Margaret Aitken, Nurses' Narratives, Butler Collection, AWM41/937, Australian War Memorial, Canberra, Australia.

61. Leo van Bergen, *Before My Helpless Sight: Suffering, Dying and Military Medicine on the Western Front, 1914–1918*, trans. Liz Waters (Farnham: Ashgate, 2009), 160.

62. Dame Maud McCarthy, Reports on Nursing Services, 1918.

63. Hall, Nurses' Narratives, AWM41/979.

64. Winifred Ellen Spencer, interviewed by Yvonne Shadbolt, rec. 16 Apr. 1983, New Zealand Nursing Education and Research Foundation Oral History Project, OHInt-0014/156, Alexander Turnbull Library, Wellington, NZ.

65. Staff Nurse Estelle M. Armstrong, Nurses' Narratives, Butler Collection, AWM41/940, Australian War Memorial, Canberra, Australia.

66. Anon., *New Zealanders in Brockenhurst: The No 1 New Zealand General Hospital 1916–1919*, 2nd edn., with foreword by David Brewster (Brockenhurst: Frost Printers, 2006), 10.

67. Dame Maud McCarthy, Reports on Nursing Services, 1918, 30.

68. Dame Maud McCarthy, Reports on Nursing Services, 1918, 30–5.

69. Cuthbert, Nurses' Narratives, AWM41/958.

70. Lavinia L. Dock et al., *History of American Red Cross Nursing* (New York: Macmillan Company, 1922), 1104.

71. Dame Maud McCarthy, Reports on Nursing Services, 1918, 41–6.

## Conclusion Notes

1. Introduction to Marian Wenzel and John Cornish, *Auntie Mabel's War: An Account of Her Part in the Hostilities of 1914–1918* (London: Allen Lane, 1980), 6.

2. Wenzel and Cornish, *Auntie Mabel's War*, 8.

3. Wenzel and Cornish, *Auntie Mabel's War*, 120.

4. Leo van Bergen, *Before My Helpless Sight: Suffering, Dying and Military Medicine on the Western Front, 1914–1918*, trans. Liz Waters (Farnham: Ashgate, 2009), 168.

5. Denise J. Poynter, '"The Report on her Transfer was Shell-Shock": A Study of the Psychological Disorders of Nurses and Female Voluntary Aid Detachments Who Served alongside the British and Allied

Expeditionary Forces during the First World War, 1914–1918' (unpublished PhD thesis, University of Northampton, 2008), quotations on pp. 37–8 and 196.

6. Elizabeth S. Haldane, *The British Nurse in Peace and War* (London: John Murray, 1923), 173.

7. Alison S. Fell, 'Afterword: Remembering the First World War Nurse in Britain and France', in Fell and Christine E. Hallett (eds.), *First World War Nursing: New Perspectives* (New York: Routledge, 2013), 173–92.

8. Cannan's *Recollections* appear to have been written in the interwar period, when the nursing profession was experiencing a recruitment crisis: May W. Cannan, *Recollections of a British Red Cross Voluntary Aid Detachment No 12, Oxford University, March 26th 1911–April 24th 1919*, Red Cross Archives, London, UK.

9. Florence Egerton, Papers, 812/1–11, Red Cross Archives, London, UK.

10. Sister E. Vickers-Foote, Nurses' Narratives, Butler Collection, AWM41/1054, Australian War Memorial, Canberra, Australia.

11. On Canadian nurse-registration see Diane Mansell and Dianne Dodd, 'Professionalism and Canadian Nursing', in Christina Bates, Dianne Dodd, and Nicole Rousseau (eds.), *On All Frontiers: Four Centuries of Canadian Nursing* (Ottawa: University of Ottawa Press, 2005), 197–211 at 200; on Australia, see Lavinia Dock and Isabel Stewart, *A Short History of Nursing* (4th edn., New York: G. P. Putnam's Sons, 1938), 259.

12. Luard Family Papers, Files 55/13/1–4, D/DLu 58/1, Essex Record Office, Colchester, UK. Material taken from transcripts provided by Tim Luard.

13. Correspondence in Jentie Paterson, Service Record, WO 399/6503, The National Archives, Kew, UK.

14. Anon., 'Miss J. C. Child's Career', *South African Nursing Journal* (Sept. 1939), 594.

15. Katrin Schultheiss, *Bodies and Souls: Politics and the Professionalization of Nursing in France, 1880–1922* (Cambridge, Mass.: Harvard University Press, 2001), *passim*.

16. Schultheiss, *Bodies and Souls*, 175.

17. Schultheiss, *Bodies and Souls*, 188–9.

18. Exhibition information on Margaret Brand Cowling, File 5, Box 3, Papers of Base Hospital 41, 1905–2009, Accession Number MS-17,

Claude Moore Health Sciences Library (Historical Collections), University of Virginia, Charlottesville, USA.

19. Lavinia L. Dock et al., *History of American Red Cross Nursing* (New York: Macmillan Company, 1922), 1104.

20. Lavinia Dock, 'The Progress of Registration', *American Journal of Nursing*, 6/5 (Feb. 1906), 297–305, at 305.

21. Mary Messer, 'Is Nursing a Profession?', *American Journal of Nursing*, 15/2 (Nov. 1914), 122–5.

22. Susan Grant, 'Nursing in Russia and the Soviet Union: 1914–1941: An Overview of the Development of a Soviet Nursing System', *Bulletin of the UK Association for the History of Nursing*, 2 (2012) 21–33, at 21–4.

23. Maria Bucur, 'Women's Stories as Sites of Memory: Gender and Remembering Romania's World Wars', in N. M. Wingfield and Bucur, *Gender and War in Twentieth-Century Eastern Europe* (Bloomington: Indiana University Press, 2006), 171–92.

24. Marie, Queen of Roumania, *Ordeal: The Story of My Life* (New York: C. Scribner's Sons, 1935). See also Hannah Pakula, *Queen of Roumania: The Life of Princess Marie, Grand-daughter of Queen Victoria* (London: Eland Publishing, 1989); Hannah Pakula, *The Last Romantic: A Biography of Queen Marie of Roumania* (London: Weidenfeld and Nicolson, 1996).

25. Marie, Queen of Roumania, *Ordeal*, 149.

26. Thomas Keneally, *The Daughters of Mars* (London: Hodder and Stoughton, 2012).

27. British Broadcasting Corporation, *The Crimson Field*; writer: Sarah Phelps; script editor: Victoria Brown; directors: David Evans, Richard Clark, Thaddeus O'Sullivan; Matron Grace Carter: Hermione Norris; Sister Joan Livesey: Suranne Jones; VAD Kitty Trevelyan: Oona Chaplin.

# Bibliography

**Manuscript Sources**

*Alexander Turnbull Library, Wellington, NZ*

Chalmer, Sister May, MS-Papers-8058.

Commons, Daphne Rona, Letters, MS-Papers-1582-09.

Higginson, Louisa, Diary, MS-Papers-2477, Folders 1 and 2.

Speedy, Fanny, Diary, MS-Papers-1703.

Tilly, Barbara Mildred, Letters, MS-Papers-1451.

Oral History Recordings

*New Zealand Nursing Education and Research Foundation Oral History Project:*

Copeland, Amy, interviewed by H. Campbell, rec. 17 Mar. 1983, OHInt-0014/040, original no. OHC-81a, listening copy no. LC-8113.

Hodges, Emily, interviewed by H. Campbell, rec. 25 June 1982 and 5 Sept. 1982, OHInt-0014/074, listening copy no. LC-8112.

Le Gallais, Charlotte, recording of her letters, rec. Sept. 1983, OHC-157, listening copy no. LC-4645.

Le Lievre, Florence, interviewed by Mary Grant, rec. 8 Nov. 1983, OHC-184, listening copy no. LC-6172.

McIntyre, Charlotte Leslie, interviewed by Yvonne Shadbolt, rec. 29 June 1983, OHInt-0014/103.

Spencer, Winifred Ellen, interviewed by Yvonne Shadbolt, rec. 16 Apr. 1983, OHInt-0014/156.

*NZOHA Sunlight Centenarians Oral History Project:*

Surtees, Sybil, interviewed by Hugo Manson, OHColl-0004.

*Archives New Zealand, Wellington, NZ*

New Zealand Army Nursing Service, General File June 1910–Aug. 1925, AD64 1.

*Army Medical Services Museum Archives, Aldershot, UK*

Browne, Dame Sidney Jane, Papers, Box 1, Army Medical Services Museum.
McCarthy, Dame Maud, Matron-in-Chief, British Expeditionary Force in France, Reports on Nursing Services, 1918, Box 10, 43/1985.
McCarthy, Dame Maud, Matron-in-Chief, British Expeditionary Force, File of Correspondence relating to CCS, 1914–15, Box 10.

Nurses' Accounts

Anon., *A Matron's Experiences of Work at a Base Hospital, France, 1914–1915.*
Anon., *With the Italian Expeditionary Force.*
Blair, Sister M. A. C., QA, *Reminiscences of a Nursing Sister in the Great War.*
Connal, J. A., Sister TFNS, *Account.*
Dodd, Sister E., *At an Officers Hospital in France.*
Flower, Sister K., QAIMNSR, *Account.*
Oram, S. E., Late Matron-in-Chief, Egyptian Expeditionary Force, *Nursing in Egypt and Palestine 1915–1919.*
Orchardson, J., TFNS, *Work on an Ambulance Train.*
Peterkin, Sister M., QAIMNSR, *Work on a Hospital Barge in France.*
Webster, Sister M. E., *Notes on the Gallipoli Campaign.*

*Australian War Memorial, Canberra, Australia*

Nurses' Narratives, Butler Collection, AWM41
Aitken, Margaret, AWM41/937.
Allan, Ruth, AWM41/938.
Armstrong, Staff Nurse Estelle M., AWM41/940.
Brown, Staff Nurse Leila, AWM41/946.
Chadwick, Sister H., Narrative account of No. 26 Ambulance Train, AWM41/953.
Cuthbert, Sister Ellen, AWM41/958.
Dobson, Sister Elsie, AWM41/964.
Doherty, Gertrude M., AWM41/966.
Gould, Matron Ellen, AWM41/975.
Hall, Sister M. E., AWM41/979.
Jeffries, Head Sister, AWM41.
Lovell, Sister I. G., AWM41/998.
Low, Sister A. J., AWM41/999.
McClelland, Sister E., AWM41/1000.

Maloney, Sister K. E., AWM41/1005.
Morrice, Head Sister N., AWM41/1013.
Payne, Sister V. M., AWM41/1021.
Redman, Sister Ella, AWM 41/1027.
Smith, Sister A. N., AWM41/1041.
Smith, Sister Leila, *Life on an Ambulance Train*, AWM41/1043.
Steadman, Sister E. L., AWM41/1046.
Strom, Staff Nurse C. E., Letters, AWM41/1068.
Taylor, Sister Ruth, AWM41/1051.
Tranter, Elsie May, Diary, 3 DRL 4081/A, AWM419/22/21.
Vickers-Foote, Sister E., AWM41/1054.
Wilson, Matron Grace, AWM41/1059.
Wray, Sister, AWM41/1062.

Personal Record

Watson, Sister Linda, AANS, PR01246.

*Barbara Bates Center for the Study of the History of Nursing, University of Pennsylvania, Philadelphia, USA*

Goodrich, Annie Warburton, Papers, MC 4, Box 1.
McCarron, Sarah, Collection: Diaries, papers, and photographs, MC10.

*Claude Moore Health Sciences Library (Historical Collections), University of Virginia, Charlottesville, USA*

Papers of Base Hospital 41, 1905–2009, Accession Number MS-17

*Between Convoys*, 1 (Dec. 1918).
Cowling, Margaret Brand, File 5, Box 3.
Cowling, Margaret, 'A Red Cross Nurse', incorporated into Deming J. Shear, 'Historical Sketch of Base Hospital #41', File 2, Box 1.
Letter written by Julian M. Cabell to Dr Stephen Watts, 10 Jan. 1919, File 2, Box 3.

*Eleanor Crowder Bjoring Center for Nursing Historical Inquiry, University of Virginia, Charlottesville, USA*

Wills, Camilla Louise, Letters, Camilla Louise Wills Collection.

*Essex Record Office, Colchester, UK*

Luard Family Papers, Files 55/13/1–4, D/Dlu 58.

*Imperial War Museum, London, UK*

Anon., *Australian Nursing Services During the First World War*, Misc 47, Item 790.

Barclay, Miss M., Private Papers: Letter, documents.4320, 82/1/1.

Bickmore, Miss, Private Papers: 'Life on an Ambulance Train in France, 1914–1917', documents.3814, 85/51/1.

Brown, M. A., Private Papers: Three MS diaries covering her service in Egypt, Palestine, and on hospital ships *Devanha* and *Delta*, documents.1001, 88/7/1, Diary 1.

Clarke, Mary, Diary, 84/46/1.

Essington-Nelson, A., Private Papers: Documents.2784, 86/48/1.

Farmborough, Florence, Private Papers: Diaries, documents.1381.

Fussell, Mrs, Early account of the Australian Army Nursing Service, Un-numbered file.

Greg, Miss Elizabeth Agnes, Private Papers: Letters, documents.8337, 01/17/1.

Hodges, Miss K., Private Papers: Documents.1974, 92/22/1.

Jeffery, Miss Mabel, Private Papers: Draft of the book, 'Auntie Mabel's War', containing original documents relating to Miss Jeffery's service as a qualified nurse, documents.6461, 81/38/2&2A.

Lea, Sister E. W. B., Private Papers: Letters, documents.510 Con Shelf.

Manning, R., Private Papers: Account, documents.4763, 80/21/1.

Moor, Mrs E. B., Private Papers: Diary and Letters, documents.7779, 98/9/1.

Paterson, Sister Jentie, Private Papers: Diaries, documents.378, 90/10/1.

Proctor, Evelyn, Private Papers: Manuscript letters, documents.1039, 88/16/1.

Reeves, S., Private Papers: Account, documents.133, 89/10/1.

Scott, Miss F., Private Papers: Documents.6977, 77/15/1.

Seymour, Dorothy, Private Papers: Diary and Letters, documents.3210, 95/28/1.

Seymour, Winifred, Private Papers: Documents.7165, 97/34/1.

Starr, Marjorie, Private Papers: Documents.4572, 81/12/1.

Vernon Allen, Miss M. D., Private Papers: Diary and extracts from letters, documents.4575, 81/13/1.

Woodroffe, Vera, Private Papers: Letters, documents.3262, 95/31/1.

Oral History Interviews

Farmborough, Florence, IWM312.

Johnson, Mrs Louie, IWM330.

Lemere-Goff, Winifred, IWM9523.

Rumney, Mary Millicent, IWM739.

*John Rylands Library, University of Manchester, UK*

Bennett, Catherine Eva, *Record of the Patients of Stamford Hospital, April 24th 1917–Jan 24th 1919, written for the Earl of Stamford*, Archives of the Stamford Family, Dunham Massey Hall, Cheshire.

*Library and Archives Canada, Ottawa*

Cotton, Dorothy, Diary, available online at <www.collectionscanada. gc.ca/nursing-sisters/025013-2200-e.html> [last accessed 17 May 2013].

*Liddle Collection, Brotherton Library, University of Leeds, UK*

Farmborough, Florence, Papers, including oral history interview, conducted by Peter Liddle, July 1975 (tape 302), RUS 11.

Speedy, Fanny, Five diary transcripts (1915–1919), ANZAC (NZ).

*Maryland Historical Society, Baltimore, USA*

Alice Fitzgerald, Unpublished Memoirs incorporating War Diary, Alice Fitzgerald Papers, MdHR M2633 and MdHR M2634 (unpaginated).

*The National Archives, Kew, UK*

Brown, Mary Ann, Service Record, WO 399/1023.

Luard, Kate, Service Record, WO 399/5023.

McCarthy, Maud, Official War Diary of Maud McCarthy, WO95/3988, WO95/3989, WO95/3990, WO95/3991.

Paterson, Jentie, Service Record, WO 399/6503.

*Red Cross Archives, London, UK*

Album of mementoes of the London/28 detachment (Kensington) of the VAD, 1914–1925, 2423/1.

Cannan, May W., *Recollections of a British Red Cross Voluntary Aid Detachment No 12, Oxford University, March 26th 1911–April 24th 1919*.

Egerton, Florence, Papers, 812/1–11.

Miller, Janet Irene, *Recollections of a Military Hospital, Manchester*, AACC 0459, 92/19, T2 (MIL).

Sapwell, Joyce, 'The Reminiscences of a VAD in Two World Wars', T2 SAP.

Van Straubenzee, Margaret, Account, X/142, LIB 88/595, T2(STR).

*Robinson, Dick: Private Collection*

Appleton, Edith, *Diaries.*

*Royal Museum of the Armed Forces and of Military History, Brussels*

Bieswal, Estelle and Thérèse, *Journal: Années 1914 à 1918.*

## Primary Published Sources

Abrahams, Adolphe, 'The Later Effects of Gas Poisoning', *The Lancet*, 200/5174 (28 Oct. 1922), 933–4.

Anon., 'The Work of the St John Ambulance Association', *British Journal of Nursing* (5 Sept. 1914), 189.

Anon. [Kate Luard], *Diary of a Nursing Sister on the Western Front* (Edinburgh: William Blackwood and Sons, 1915).

Anon., 'Sinking of the Marquette', *Marlborough Express*, 49/278 (24 Nov. 1915), 5.

Anon., 'The Anglo-Russian Hospital', *Nursing Times*, 12 (1916), 181.

Anon., 'Another Story of the Flight', *Nursing Times*, 12 (1916), 61.

Anon., 'Arrival of Nurses from Serbia', *Nursing Times*, 12 (1916), 11–15.

Anon., 'Back from Serbia: An Interview with Miss Caldwell', *Nursing Times*, 12 (1916), 291.

Anon., 'British Nurses in Serbia', *Nursing Times*, 12 (1916), 63.

Anon., 'For VAD Probationers', *Nursing Times*, 12 (1916), 48.

Anon., 'A French Military Hospital', *Nursing Times*, 12 (1916), 60.

Anon., 'French Flag Nursing Corps', *British Journal of Nursing* (1 Apr. 1916), 290.

Anon., Column, *British Journal of Nursing* (15 Apr. 1916), 336.

Anon., 'French Flag Nursing Corps: Meeting at the Indian Empire Club', *British Journal of Nursing* (20 May 1916), 437–8.

Anon., 'An Edith Cavell Memorial Nurse', *British Journal of Nursing* (4 Mar. 1916), 214.

Anon., 'News from the Front: Thrilling Experiences in Serbia', *Nursing Times*, 12 (1916), 269.

Anon., 'Nursing and the War', *British Journal of Nursing* (15 Apr. 1916), 335–6.

Anon., Column, *British Journal of Nursing* (22 July 1916), 68.

Anon., 'Return of Two Scottish Units from Serbia: Adventure and Imprisonment', *Nursing Times*, 12 (1916), 210–13.

Anon., 'Care of the Wounded', *British Journal of Nursing* (14 Apr. 1917), 253.

Anon., *The Edith Cavell Nurse from Massachusetts: A Record of One Year's Personal Service with the British Expeditionary Force in France; Boulogne–The Somme,*

*1916–1917; With an Account of the Imprisonment, Trial and Death of Edith Cavell* (Boston: W. A. Butterfield, 1917).

Anon., 'Nursing at La Panne', *British Journal of Nursing* (10 Mar. 1917), 169.

Anon., *History of the Pennsylvania Hospital Unit (Base Hospital No. 10, USA) in the Great War* (New York: Paul B. Hoeber, 1921).

Anon., *Medical Department of the United States Army in the World War* (Washington, DC: US Surgeon General's Office, 1921–9).

Anon. (ed.), *Reminiscent Sketches, 1914 to 1919 by Members of Her Majesty Queen Alexandra's Imperial Military Nursing Service* (London: John Bale, Sons and Danielsson, Ltd, 1922).

Anon., 'Miss J. C. Child's Career', *South African Nursing Journal* (Sept. 1939), 594.

Anon., 'Echoes of the Great War: The Chivalrous Poilu', *British Journal of Nursing*, 88 (Mar. 1940), 39.

Anon., *Twenty Months a VAD* (Sheffield: J. Northen, n.d.).

Anon., Column, *British Journal of Nursing* (9 Oct. 1915), 294.

Anon., Column, *Auckland Weekly News* (11 Nov. 1915), cited at <http://freepages. genealogy.rootsweb.ancestry.com/~sooty/awnppnov1915.html>.

Anon. Column, *British Journal of Nursing* (22 Apr. 1916), 358.

Anon., Column, *British Journal of Nursing* (16 June 1917).

Anon., Letter, *British Journal of Nursing* (18 Mar. 1916), 244.

Bagnold, Enid, *A Diary Without Dates* (1918; London: Virago, 1978).

Barber, Margaret H., *A British Nurse in Bolshevik Russia: The Narrative of Margaret H. Barber, April 1916–December 1919* (London: A. C. Fifield, 1920).

Baroness de T'Serclaes, *Flanders and Other Fields* (London: George G. Harrap and Co. Ltd, 1964).

Barton, E. C., *Hints to VAD Members in Hospitals* (London: *Nursing Times* Publishing, 1915).

Bell, Douglas, *A Soldier's Diary of the Great War* (London: Faber and Gwyer, 1929).

Black, J. Elliot, Glenny, Elliot T., and McNee, J. W., 'Observations on 685 Cases of Poisoning by Noxious Gases Used by the Enemy', *British Medical Journal* (31 July 1915), 165–7.

Blunden, Edmund, *Undertones of War* (1928; London: Penguin, 2000).

Borden, Mary, *The Forbidden Zone* (London: William Heinemann Ltd, 1929).

British Medical Association, *British Medicine in the War, 1914–1917: Being Essays on the Problems of Medicine, Surgery and Pathology Arising Among the British*

*Armed Forces Engaged in This War and the Manner of Their Solution* (London: British Medical Association, 1917).

Britnieva, Mary, *One Woman's Story* (London: Arthur Baker, 1934).

Brittain, Vera, *Chronicle of Youth* (1981; London: Phoenix Press, 2000).

Brittain, Vera, *Testament of Youth: An Autobiographical Study of the Years 1900–1925* (1933; London: Virago, 2004).

Butler, Arthur G., *Official History of the Australian Army Medical Services, 1914–1918*, i. *Gallipoli, Palestine and New Guinea* (2nd edn., Melbourne: Australian War Memorial, 1938).

Butler, Arthur G., *Official History of the Australian Army Medical Services, 1914–1918*, ii. *The Western Front* (Canberra: Australian War Memorial, 1940).

Butler, Arthur G., *Official History of the Australian Army Medical Services, 1914–1918*, iii. *Special Problems and Services* (Melbourne: Australian War Memorial, 1943).

Cator, Dorothy, *In a French Military Hospital* (London: Longman, Green and Co., 1915).

Chalmer, May, Letter, *Kai Tiaki* (Jan. 1917).

Chalmer, May, Letter, *Kai Tiaki* (Apr. 1917).

Chalmer, May, 'NZ Hospital at Walton: A New Extension', *Kai Tiaki* (Apr. 1917).

Crile, George W., *George Crile: An Autobiography* (Philadelphia: J. B. Lippincott, 1947).

Cushing, Harvey, *From a Surgeon's Journal, 1915–1918* (Boston: Little, Brown and Company, 1936).

De Launoy, Jane, *Infirmières de guerre en service commande (Front de 14 à 18)* (Brussels: L'Édition universelle, 1937).

Dock, Lavinia, 'The Progress of Registration', *American Journal of Nursing*, 6/5 (Feb. 1906), 297–305.

Dock, Lavinia L., Pickett, Sarah E., Noyes, Clara D., Clement, Fannie F., Fox, Elizabeth G., and Van Meter, Anna R., *History of American Red Cross Nursing* (New York: Macmillan Company, 1922).

Dock, Lavinia, and Stewart, Isabel, *A Short History of Nursing* (4th edn., New York: G. P. Putnam's Sons, 1938).

Ellison, Grace, 'Nursing at the French Front', in Gilbert Stone (ed.) *Women War Workers: Accounts Contributed by Representative Workers of the Work Done by Women in the More Important Branches of War Employment* (London: George G. Harrap and Co., 1917), 155–80.

Farmborough, Florence, *Nurse at the Russian Front: A Diary 1914–1918* (London: Book Club Associates, 1974).

Farmborough, Florence, *With the Armies of the Tsar: A Nurse at the Russian Front in War and Revolution, 1914–1918* (New York: Cooper Square Press, 2000).

Goodnow, Minnie, *War Nursing: A Text-Book for the Auxiliary Nurse* (Philadelphia and London: W. B. Saunders Company, 1917).

Graves, Robert, *Goodbye to All That* (1929; London: Penguin, 2000).

Haldane, Elizabeth S., *The British Nurse in Peace and War* (London: John Murray, 1923).

Hemingway, Ernest, *A Farewell to Arms* (New York: Charles Scribner's Sons, 1929).

Herringham, Sir Wilmot P., 'Gas Poisoning', *The Lancet*, 195/5034 (21 Feb. 1920), 423–4.

Horton, Charles, H., *Stretcher Bearer! Fighting for Life in the Trenches* (Oxford: Lion Hudson, 2013).

Hungerford, Edward, *With the Doughboy in France* (New York: Macmillan Company, 1920).

La Motte, Ellen N., *The Backwash of War: The Human Wreckage of the Battlefield as Witnessed by an American Hospital Nurse* (New York: G. P. Putnam's Sons, The Knickerbocker Press, 1916).

Latham, F. E., 'With the First British Field Hospital in Serbia', *Nursing Times*, 12/557 (1916), 93–4.

Lewis, Thomas, *The Soldier's Heart and the Effort Syndrome* (London: Shaw and Sons, 1918).

Luard, Kate E., *Unknown Warriors* (London: Chatto and Windus, 1930).

Maclean, Hester, *Nursing in New Zealand—History and Reminiscences* (Wellington, NZ: Tolan Printing Co., 1932).

Macnaughtan, Sarah, *A Woman's Diary of the War* (London: Thomas Nelson, 1915).

Macpherson, Sir William Grant, *History of the Great War Based on Official Documents by Direction of the Historical Section of the Committee of Imperial Defence; Medical Services: General History*, i, ii, and iii (London: Macmillan, 1921, 1923, 1924).

Macpherson, W. G., and Mitchell, W. J. (eds.), *History of the Great War based on Official Documents; Medical Services, General History*, iv. *Medical Services on the Gallipoli Peninsula; in Macedonia; in Mesopotamia and North-West Persia; in East*

*Africa; in the Aden Protectorate, and in North Russia; Ambulance Transport during the War* (London: Macmillan, 1924).

Marie, Queen of Roumania, *Ordeal: The Story of My Life* (New York: Charles Scribner's Sons, 1935).

Masefield, John, *Gallipoli* (London: W. Heinemann, 1916).

Medical Research Committee, *Report on the Anaerobic Bacteria and Infections: Report on the Anaerobic Infections of Wounds and the Bacteriological and Serological Problems Arising Therefrom* (London: HMSO, 1919).

Messer, Mary, 'Is Nursing a Profession?', *American Journal of Nursing*, 15/2 (Nov. 1914), 122–5.

Millard, Shirley, *I Saw Them Die: Diary and Recollections of Shirley Millard*, ed. Adele Comandini (London: George G. Harrap and Co., 1936).

Millicent, Duchess of Sutherland, *Six Weeks at the War* (London: *The Times*, 1914).

Mitchell, T. J., and Smith, G. M., *History of the Great War Based on Official Documents: Medical Services* (Uckfield, West Sussex: The Naval and Military Press, Ltd with the Imperial War Museum; facsimile of book first published in 1931).

Mitton, G. E. (ed.), *The Cellar-House of Pervyse: A Tale of Uncommon Things from the Journals and Letters of the Baroness De T'Serclaes and Mairi Chisholm* (London: A and E Black, 1916).

Oxford, M. N., *Nursing in Wartime: Lessons for the Inexperienced* (London: Methuen and Co., 1914).

Pasternak, Boris, *Doctor Zhivago*, trans. Max Hayward and Manya Harari (1958; London: Vintage Books, 2002).

Rathbone, Irene, *We That Were Young: A Novel* (1932; New York: The Feminist Press, 1989).

Remarque, Erich Maria, *All Quiet on the Western Front* (1929; London: Vintage, 1996).

Stimson, Julia, *Finding Themselves: The Letters of an American Army Chief Nurse at a British Hospital in France* (New York: Macmillan Company, 1927), 79–80.

Stobart, Mabel St Clair, *The Flaming Sword in Serbia and Elsewhere* (London: Hodder and Stoughton, 1916).

Tayler, Henrietta, *A Scottish Nurse at Work: Being a Record of Four and a Half Years of War* (London: John Lane, 1920).

Thurstan, Violetta, *Field Hospital and Flying Column: Being the Journal of an English Nursing Sister in Belgium and Russia* (London: G. P. Putnam's Sons, 1915).

Thurstan, Violetta, *The People Who Run, Being the Tragedy of the Refugees in Russia* (London: G. P. Putnam's Sons, 1916).

Thurstan, Violetta, *A Text Book of War Nursing* (London: G. P. Putnam's Sons, 1917).

Thurstan, Violetta, *The Hounds of War Unleashed* (St Ives: United Writers, 1978).

Vallow, Harold, 'The Later Effects of Gas Poisoning', *The Lancet*, 200/5175 (4 Nov. 1922), 985.

Van Schaick, John Jr., *The Little Corner Never Conquered: The Story of the American Red Cross War Work for Belgium* (New York: Macmillan Company, 1922).

Willis, L. Ida G., *A Nurse Remembers* (Lower Hutt, NZ: AK Wilson, 1968).

## Secondary Sources

Abel-Smith, Brian, *A History of the Nursing Profession* (London: Heinemann, 1960).

Anon., *New Zealanders in Brockenhurst: The No 1 New Zealand General Hospital 1916–1919*, 2nd edn., with foreword by David Brewster (Brockenhurst: Frost Printers, 2006).

Atkinson, Diane, *Elsie and Mairi Go To War: Two Extraordinary Women on the Western Front* (London: Preface Publishing, 2009).

Baly, Monica, *Florence Nightingale and the Nursing Legacy* (1986; London: Whurr Publishers, 1997).

Bassett, Jan, *Guns and Brooches: Australian Army Nursing from the Boer War to the Gulf War* (Melbourne: Oxford University Press, 1992).

Blodgett, Harriet, 'Stobart, Mabel Annie St Clair', in *Oxford Dictionary of National Biography* (Oxford: Oxford University Press, 2004–13).

Boonefaes, Pierre, and Vilain, Willy, *Eenwig in eben vloed* (De Panne: Municipality of De Panne, 2011).

Bostridge, Mark, *Florence Nightingale: The Woman and Her Legend* (London: Viking, 2008).

Bourke, Joanna, *Dismembering the Male: Men's Bodies, Britain and the Great War* (London: Reaktion Books, 1996).

Bowser, Thelka, *The Story of British VAD Work in the Great War* (1917; London: Imperial War Museum, 2003).

Bradshaw, Ann, *The Nurse Apprentice, 1860–1977* (Aldershot: Ashgate, 2001).

Braybon, Gail, *Women Workers in the First World War: The British Experience* (London: Croom Helm, 1981).

Braybon, Gail (ed.), *Evidence, History and the Great War: Historians and the Impact of 1914–1918* (New York: Berghahn Books, 2003).

Brown, Malcolm, *1918 Year of Victory* (London: Pan Books with Imperial War Museum, 1998).

Brush, Barbara, Lynaugh, Joan, Boschma, Geertje, Rafferty, Anne Marie, Stuart, Meryn, Tomes, Nancy J., *Nurses of All Nations: A History of the International Council of Nurses, 1899–1999* (Philadelphia: Lippincott, Williams and Wilkins, 1999).

Bucur, Maria, 'Women's Stories as Sites of Memory: Gender and Remembering Romania's World Wars', in N. M. Wingfield and Bucur, *Gender and War in Twentieth-Century Eastern Europe* (Bloomington: Indiana University Press, 2006), 171–92.

Butler, Janet, ' "Very busy in Bosches Alley": One Day of the Somme in Sister Kit McNaughton's Diary', *Health and History: Journal of the Australian Society of the History of Medicine*, 6/2 (2000) 18–32.

Butler, Janet, *Kitty's War: The Remarkable Wartime Experiences of Kit McNaughton* (St Lucia, Queensland: University of Queensland Press, 2013).

Byerly, Carol R., *Fever of War: The Influenza Epidemic in the U.S. Army During World War I* (New York: Viking, 1991).

Campbell, Joseph, *The Hero with a Thousand Faces* (1949; London: Fontana, 1993).

Clark, Alan, *The Donkeys* (1961; London: Pimlico, 1991).

Clayton, Ann, *Chavasse Double VC* (1992; Barnsley: Pen and Sword Books, 2008).

Clendon, Jill, 'New Zealand Military Nurses' Fight for Recognition: World War I–World War II', *Nursing Praxis in New Zealand*, 12/1 (Mar. 1997), 24–8.

Cockram, John (ed.), *Brockenhurst and the Two World Wars* (Brockenhurst: Cockram, n.d.).

Conway, Jane, *Mary Borden: A Woman of Two Wars* (Chippenham: Munday Books, 2010).

Cooter, Roger, 'Malingering in Modernity: Psycholocial Scripts and Adversarial Encounters during the First World War', in Cooter, Mark Harrison, and Steve Sturdy (eds.) *War, Medicine and Modernity* (Stroud: Sutton Publishing, 1998), 125–48.

Cowen, Ruth (ed.), *War Diaries—A Nurse at the Front: The Great War Diaries of Sister Edith Appleton* (London: Simon and Schuster, 2012).

Crofton, Eileen, *The Women of Royaumont: A Scottish Women's Hospital on the Western Front* (East Linton: Tuckwell Press, 1997).

Darrow, Margaret, 'French Volunteer Nursing and the Myth of War Experience in World War I', *American Historical Review*, 101/1 (1996), 80–106.

Darrow, Margaret H., 'The Making of Sister Julie: The Origin of First World War French Nursing Heroines in Franco-Prussian War Stories', in Alison S. Fell and Christine E. Hallett (eds.), *First World War Nursing: New Perspectives* (New York: Routledge, 2013).

Das, Santanu, *Touch and Intimacy in First World War Literature* (Cambridge: Cambridge University Press, 2005).

Das, Santanu (ed.), *Race, Empire and First World War Writing* (Cambridge: Cambridge University Press, 2011).

de Munck, Luc, and Vandeweyer, Luc, *Het Hospital van de Koningin: Rode Kruis, L'Océan en De Panne* (De Panne: Gemeetebestuur De Panne en de auteurs, 2012).

Donner, Henriette, 'Under the Cross: Why VADs Performed the Filthiest Tasks in the Dirtiest War: Red Cross Women Volunteers, 1914–1918', *Journal of Social History*, 30/3 (1997), 687–704.

Dubois, Ellen Carol, *Woman Suffrage and Women's Rights* (New York: New York University Press, 1998).

Dyer, Geoff, *The Missing of the Somme* (London: Penguin, 1994).

Engel, Barbara, *Women in Russia, 1700–2000* (Cambridge: Cambridge University Press, 2004).

Erickson, Edward J., *Gallipoli and the Middle East, 1914–1918: From the Dardanelles to Mesopotamia* (London: Amber, 2008).

Erickson, Edward J., *Gallipoli: The Ottoman Campaign* (Barnsley: Pen and Sword Military, 2010).

Evans, Jonathan, *Edith Cavell* (London: The London Hospital Museum, 2008).

Fell, Alison S., ' "Fallen Angels?" The Red Cross Nurse in First World War Discourse', in Maggie Allison and Yvette Rocheron (eds.), *The Resilient Female Body: Health and Malaise in Twentieth-Century France* (Bern: Peter Lang, 2007).

Fell, Alison S., 'Nursing the Other: The Representations of Colonial Troops in French and British First World War Nursing Memoirs', in Santanu Das (ed.), *Race, Empire and First World War Writing* (Cambridge: Cambridge University Press, 2011), 158–74.

Fell, Alison S., 'Afterword: Remembering the First World War Nurse in Britain and France', in Fell and Christine E. Hallett (eds.), *First World War Nursing: New Perspectives* (New York: Routledge, 2013), 173–92.

Fell, A., and Sharp, I. (eds.), *The Women's Movement in Wartime: International Perspectives 1914–1918* (Basingstoke: Palgrave, 2007).

Ferrell, Robert H., *America's Deadliest Battle: Meuse-Argonne, 1918* (Lawrence, Kan.: University Press of Kansas, 2007).

Ferro, Marc, *The Great War 1914–1918*, trans. Nicole Stone (1973; London: Routledge, 2002).

Fitzgerald, Gerard, 'Chemical Warfare and the Medical Response during World War I', *American Journal of Public Health*, 98/4 (Apr. 2008), 611–25.

Fitzpatrick, Sheila, *The Russian Revolution* (3rd edn., Oxford: Oxford University Press, 2008).

Freedman, Ariela, 'Mary Borden's *Forbidden Zone*: Women's Writing from No-Man's Land', *Modernism/modernity*, 9/1 (2002), 109–24.

Friedman, Alice Howell, 'Fitzgerald, Alice Louise, Florence', in Martin Kaufman (ed.), *Dictionary of American Nursing Biography* (New York: Greenwood Press, 1988), 121–3.

Fussell, Paul, *The Great War and Modern Memory* (1975; Oxford: Oxford University Press, 2000).

Gatrell, Peter, 'The Epic and the Domestic: Women and War in Russia, 1914–1917', in Gail Braybon (ed.), *Evidence, History and the Great War: Historians and the Impact of 1914–1918* (New York: Berghahn, 2003), 198–215.

Gatrell, Peter, *Russia's First World War: A Social and Economic History* (New York: Pearson Longman, 2005).

Geddes, Jennian, 'Deeds *and* Words in the Suffrage Military Hospital in Endell Street', *Medical History*, 51/1 (2007), 79–98.

Gillespie, H. S., 'McCarthy, Dame (Emma) Maud (1858–1949)', in *Oxford Dictionary of National Biography* (Oxford: Oxford University Press, 2004–13).

Goodman, Martin, *Suffer and Survive* (London: Simon and Schuster, 2007).

Grant, Susan, 'Nursing in Russia and the Soviet Union: 1914–1941: An Overview of the Development of a Soviet Nursing System', *Bulletin of the UK Association for the History of Nursing*, 2 (2012), 21–33.

Graves, Robert, *The Greek Myths* (1955; London, Penguin, 1992).

Grayzel, Susan, *Women's Identities at War: Gender, Motherhood, and Politics in Britain and France during the First World War* (Chapel Hill, NC: University of North Carolina Press, 1999).

Grayzel, Susan R., '"The Souls of Soldiers": Civilians Under Fire in First World War France', *Journal of Modern History*, 78/3 (2006), 588–622.

Gregory, Adrian, *The Last Great War: British Society and the First World War* (Cambridge: Cambridge University Press, 2008).

Hallam, Andrew, and Hallam, Nicola, *Lady Under Fire on the Western Front: The Great War Letters of Lady Dorothie Fielding* (Barnsley: Pen and Sword Books, 2010).

Hallett, Christine E., 'The Personal Writings of First World War Nurses: A Study of the Interplay of Authorial Intention and Scholarly Interpretation', *Nursing Inquiry*, 14/4 (2007), 320–9.

Hallett, Christine E., *Containing Trauma: Nursing Work in the First World War* (Manchester: Manchester University Press, 2009).

Hallett, Christine E., 'Russian Romances: Emotionalism and Spirituality in the Writings of "Eastern Front" Nurses, 1914–1918', *Nursing History Review*, 17 (2009), 101–28.

Hallett, Christine E., 'Portrayals of Suffering: Perceptions of Trauma in the Writings of First World War Nurses and Volunteers', *Canadian Bulletin of the History of Medicine*, 27/1 (2011), 65–84.

Hallett, Christine E., 'Nursing, 1840–1920: Forging a Profession', in Anne Borsay and Billie Hunter (eds.), *Nursing and Midwifery in Britain Since 1700* (London: Palgrave Macmillan, 2012), 46–73.

Hallett, Christine E., ' "Emotional Nursing": Involvement, Engagement, and Detachment in the Writings of First World War Nurses and VADs', in Alison S. Fell and Hallett (eds.), *First World War Nursing: New Perspectives* (New York: Routledge, 2013), 87–102.

Hallett, Christine E., ' "Intelligent interest in their own affairs": The First World War, the *British Journal of Nursing* and the Pursuit of Nursing Knowledge', in P. D'Antonio, J. Fairman, and J. Whelan (eds.), *Routledge Handbook on the Global History of Nursing* (London and New York: Routledge, 2013), 95–113.

Hallett, Christine E., and Cooke, Hannah, *Historical Investigations into the Professional Self-Regulation of Nursing and Midwifery*, i. *Nursing* (London: Nursing and Midwifery Council, 2011); available at the Archives of the Nursing and Midwifery Council, 23 Portland Place, London.

Hallett, Christine E., and Fell, Alison S., 'Introduction: New Persepectives on First World War Nursing', in Fell and Hallett (eds.), *First World War Nursing: New Perspectives* (New York: Routledge, 2013), 1–14.

Harland, Kathleen, *A History of Queen Alexandra's Royal Naval Nursing Service* (Portsmouth: *Journal of the Royal Naval Medical Service*, n.d.).

Harmer, Michael, *The Forgotten Hospital: An Essay* (London: Springwood Books, 1982).

Harris, Kirsty, *More than Bombs and Bandages: Australian Army Nurses at Work in World War I* (Newport, NSW: Big Sky Publishing, 2011).

Harris, Kirsty, ' "All for the Boys": The Nurse–Patient Relationship of Australian Army Nurses in the First World War', in Alison S. Fell and Christine E. Hallett (eds.), *First World War Nursing: New Perspectives* (New York: Routledge, 2013), 71–86.

Harrison, Mark, *The Medical War: British Military Medicine in the First World War* (Oxford: Oxford University Press, 2010).

Hart, Peter, *Gallipoli* (London: Profile, 2011).

Hector, Winifred, *The Work of Mrs. Bedford Fenwick and the Rise of Professional Nursing* (London: Royal College of Nursing, 1973).

Heys, Steven D., 'Abdominal Wounds: Evolution of Management and Establishment of Surgical Treatments', in Thomas Scotland and Heys (eds.), *War Surgery 1914–1918* (Solihull: Helion and Co. Ltd, 2012), 178–211.

Higonnet, Margaret, 'Authenticity and Art in Trauma Narratives of World War I', *Modernism/modernity*, 9/1 (2002), 91–107.

Hingley, Ronald, *Russian Revolution* (London: Bodley Head, 1970).

Hoehling, A. A., *Edith Cavell* (London: Cassel and Company, 1958).

Holmes, Katie, 'Between the Lines: The Letters and Diaries of First World War Australian Nurses' (unpublished honours thesis, Department of History, University of Melbourne).

Holmes, Richard, *Tommy: The British Soldier on the Western Front, 1914–1918* (London: HarperCollins, 2004).

Howard, Michael, *The First World War* (Oxford: Oxford University Press, 2002), 81–4.

Howell, Joel D., ' "Soldier's Heart": The Redefinition of Heart Disease and Speciality Formation in Early Twentieth-Century Great Britain', in Roger Cooter, Mark Harrison, and Steve Sturdy (eds.), *War, Medicine and Modernity* (Stroud: Sutton Publishing, 1998), 85–105.

Hughes, Michael, ' "Revolution was in the Air": British Officials in Russia during the First World War', *Journal of Contemporary History*, 31/1 (1996), 75–97.

Jensen, Kimberly, 'A Base Hospital Is Not a Coney Island Dance Hall: American Women Nurses, Hostile Work Environment, and Military Rank in the First World War', *Frontiers*, 26/2 (2005), 206–35.

Jensen, Kimberly, *Mobilizing Minerva: American Women in the First World War* (Urbana and Chicago: University of Illinois Press, 2008).

Johnson, Niall, *Britain and the 1918–1919 Influenza Pandemic* (London: Routledge, 2006).

Keegan, John, *The First World War* (1998; London: Hutchinson, 1999).

Keeling, Arlene, *Nursing and the Privilege of Prescription, 1893–2000* (Columbus: Ohio State University Press, 2007).

Keeling, Arlene, ' "Alert to the Necessities of the Emergency": U.S. Nursing during the 1918 Influenza Pandemic', *Public Health Reports: Special Supplement on Pandemic Influenza*, 125 (2010), 105–12.

Kendall, Sherayl, and Corbett, David, *New Zealand Military Nursing: A History of the Royal New Zealand Nursing Corps Boer War to Present Day* (Auckland: Sherayl Kendall and David Corbett, 1990).

Kramer, Alan, *Dynamic of Destruction: Culture and Mass Killing in the First World War.* (Oxford: Oxford University Press, 2007).

Leed, Eric J., *No Man's Land: Combat and Identity in World War I* (Cambridge: Cambridge University Press, 1979).

Leese, P. J., *Shell Shock: Traumatic Neurosis and the British Soldiers of the First World War* (London: Palgrave Macmillan, 2002).

Leneman, Leah, 'Medical Women at War, 1914–1918', *Medical History*, 38 (1994), 160–77.

Leneman, Leah, *In the Service of Life: The Story of Elsie Inglis and the Scottish Women's Hospitals* (Edinburgh: Mercat Press, 1998).

Liddle, Peter, *Captured Memories, 1900–1918: Across the Threshold of War* (Barnsley: Pen and Sword Military, 2010).

Light, Sue, 'British Military Nurses and the Great War: A Guide to the Services', *Western Front Association Forum* (7 Feb. 2010), 4; sourced at <http://www.westernfrontassociation.com> [accessed 30 Oct. 2012].

Louagie-Nolf, Jan and Katrien, *Talbot House Poperinge: De Eerste Halte na de Hel* (Lannoo: Tielt, 1998).

Mallinson, Allan, *Fight The Good Fight: Britain, The Army and The Coming of the First World War* (London: Bantam Press, 2013).

McCarthy, Perdita, 'McCarthy, Dame Emma Maud (1859–1949)', in *Australian Dictionary of National Biography*, available online at <http://adb.anu.edu.au/biography/mccarthy-dame-emma-maud-7306> [accessed 24 Aug. 2013].

Macdonald, Alexander, 'X-Rays during the Great War', in Thomas Scotland and Steven Heys (eds.), *War Surgery 1914–1918* (Solihull: Helion and Co. Ltd, 2012), 134–47.

Macdonald, Lyn, *They Called it Passchendaele* (London: Penguin, 1978).

Macdonald, Lyn, *The Roses of No Man's Land* (1980; London: Penguin, 1993).

Macdonald, Lyn, *Somme* (1983; London: Penguin, 1993).

McDonald, Lynn (ed.), *Florence Nightingale: Extending Nursing* (Waterloo: Wilfrid Laurier University Press, 2009).

McEwen, Yvonne, 'Behind and Between the Lines: The War Diary of Evelyn Kate Luard, Nursing Sister on the Western Front and Unofficial Correspondent', in McEwen and Fiona Fisken (eds.), *War, Journalism and History: War Correspondents in the Two World Wars* (Bern: Peter Lang, 2012).

McGann, Susan, *The Battle of the Nurses: A Study of Eight Women who Influenced the Development of Professional Nursing, 1880–1930* (London: Scutari Press, 1992).

Mackie, Mary, *Sky Wards: A History of the Princess Mary's Royal Air Force Nursing Service* (London: Robert Hale, 2001).

Mann, Susan, *Margaret Macdonald: Imperial Daughter* (Montreal: McGill Queen's University Press, 2010).

Meyer, Alfred, 'The Impact of World War I on Russian Women's Lives', in Barbara Clements, Barbara Engel, and Christine Worobec (eds.), *Russia's Women: Accommodation, Resistance, Transformation* (Berkeley and Los Angeles: University of California Press, 1991).

Ouditt, Sharon, *Fighting Forces, Writing Women: Identity and Ideology in the First World War* (London: Routledge, 1994).

Pakula, Hannah, *Queen of Roumania: The Life of Princess Marie, Grand-daughter of Queen Victoria* (London: Eland Publishing, 1989).

Pakula, Hannah, *The Last Romantic: A Biography of Queen Marie of Roumania* (London: Weidenfeld and Nicolson, 1996).

Pelis, Kim, 'Taking Credit: The Canadian Army Medical Corps and the British Conversion to Blood Transfusion in World War I', *Journal of the History of Medicine and Allied Health Sciences*, 56 (2001), 238–77.

Phillips, Howard, and Killingray, David, *The Spanish Influenza Pandemic of 1918–1919: New Perspectives* (London: Routledge, 2003).

Pickles, Katie, *Female Imperialism and National Identity: Imperial Order Daughters of the Empire* (Manchester: Manchester University Press, 2002).

Pipes, Richard, *The Russian Revolution, 1899–1919* (London: Collins Harvill, 1990).

Potter, Jane, ' "I feel as a Normal Being Should, in Spite of the Blood and Anguish in Which I Move": American Women's First World War Nursing Memoirs', in Alison S. Fell and Christine E. Hallett (eds.), *First World War Nursing: New Perspectives* (New York: Routledge, 2013), 51–68.

Poynter, Denise J., ' "The Report on her Transfer was Shell-Shock": A Study of the Psychological Disorders of Nurses and Female Voluntary Aid Detachments Who Served Alongside the British and Allied Expeditionary Forces during the First World War, 1914–1918' (unpublished PhD thesis, University of Northampton, 2008).

Proctor, Tammy M., ' "Patriotism is not enough": Women, Citizenship and the First World War', *Journal of Women's History*, 17/2 (2005), 169–76.

Quiney, Linda, 'Assistant Angels: Canadian Voluntary Aid Detachment Nurses in the Great War', *Canadian Bulletin of Medical History*, 15/1 (1998), 189–206.

Quinn, Shawna M., *Agnes Warner and the Nursing Sisters of the Great War* (Fredericton, New Brunswick: Goose Lane Editions, 2010).

Rae, Ruth, 'Reading between Unwritten Lines: Australian Army Nurses in India, 1916–1919', *Journal of the Australian War Memorial Canberra*, 36 (4 May 2002).

Rae, Ruth, *Scarlet Poppies: The Army Experience of Australian Nurses during World War One* (Burwood, NSW: College of Nursing, 2004).

Rae, Ruth, *Veiled Lives: Threading Australian Nursing History into the Fabric of the First World War* (Burwood, NSW: College of Nursing, 2009).

Rafferty, Anne Marie, *The Politics of Nursing Knowledge* (London: Routledge, 1996).

Rafferty, Anne Marie, and Solano, Diana, 'The Rise and Demise of the Colonial Nursing Service: British Nurses in the Colonies, 1896–1966', *Nursing History Review*, 15 (2007), 147–54.

Robertson, E. Ann, 'Anaesthesia, Shock and Resuscitation', in Thomas Scotland and Steven Heys (eds.), *War Surgery 1914–1918* (Solihull: Helion and Co. Ltd, 2012), 85–115.

Rodgers, Jan, 'Potential for Professional Profit: The Making of the New Zealand Army Nursing Service, 1914–1915', *Nursing Praxis in New Zealand*, 11/2 (July 1996), 4–12.

Rogers, Anna, *While You're Away: New Zealand Nurses At War, 1899–1948* (Auckland: Auckland University Press, 2003).

Roper, Michael, *The Secret Battle: Emotional Survival in the Great War* (Manchester: Manchester University Press, 2009).

Ruthchild, Rochelle, *Equality and Revolution: Women's Rights in the Russian Empire, 1905–1917* (Pittsburgh: University of Pittsburgh Press, 2010).

Sarnecky, Mary T., *A History of the U.S. Army Nurse Corps* (Philadelphia: University of Pennsylvania Press, 1999).

Schneider, E. F., 'The British Red Cross Wounded and Missing Enquiry Bureau: A Case of Truth-Telling in the Great War', *War in History*, 4/3 (July 1997), 296–315.

Schultheiss, Katrin, *Bodies and Souls: Politics and the Professionalization of Nursing in France, 1880–1922* (Cambridge, Mass.: Harvard University Press, 2001).

Scotland, Thomas R., 'Developments in Orthopaedic Surgery', in Scotland and Steven Heys (eds.), *War Surgery 1914–1918* (Solihull: Helion and Co. Ltd, 2012), 148–77.

Scotland, Thomas R., 'Evacuation Pathway for the Wounded', in Scotland and Steven Heys (eds.), *War Surgery 1914–1918* (Solihull: Helion and Co. Ltd, 2012), 51–84.

Sheffield, Gary, *Forgotten Victory: The First World War: Myths and Realities* (2001; London: Headline Book Publishing, 2002).

Sheffield, Gary, *The Somme* (2003; London: Cassell, 2004).

Shephard, Ben, *A War of Nerves: Soldiers and Psychiatrists, 1914–1994* (2000; London: Pimlico, 2002).

Showalter, Elaine, *The Female Malady: Woman, Madness and English Culture, 1830–1980* (London: Virago, 1993).

Smith, Angela, *The Second Battlefield: Women, Modernism and the First World War* (Manchester: Manchester University Press, 2000).

Smith, Angela, *Women's Writing of the First World War* (Manchester: Manchester University Press, 2000).

Smith, Angela K., ' "Beacons of Britishness": British Nurses and Female Doctors as Prisoners of War', in Alison S. Fell and Christine E. Hallett (eds.), *First World War Nursing: New Perspectives* (New York: Routledge, 2013), 35–50.

Smith, Douglas, *Former People: The Last Days of the Russian Aristocracy* (London: Macmillan, 2012).

Sondhaus, Lawrence, *World War I: The Global Revolution* (Cambridge: Cambridge University Press, 2011).

Souhami, Diana, *Edith Cavell* (London: Quercus, 2010).

Stephenson, David, *1914–1918: The History of the First World War* (London: Allen Lane, 2004).

Stoff, Laurie, *They Fought for the Motherland: Russia's Women Soldiers in World War I and Revolution* (Lawrence, Kan.: University of Kansas Press, 2006).

Stoff, Laurie, 'The "Myth of the War Experience" and Russian Wartime Nursing in World War I', *Aspasia: The International Yearbook of Central, Eastern, and Southeastern European Women's and Gender History*, 6 (2012), 96–116.

Stone, Martin, 'Shellshock and the Psychologists', in W. F. Bynum, R. Porter, and M. Shepherd (eds.), *The Anatomy of Madness: Essays on the History of Psychiatry*, ii (New York and London: Tavistock, 1985), 242–71.

Stone, Norman, *World War One: A Short History* (2007; London, Penguin, 2008).

Strachan, Hew, *The First World War* (2003; London, Pocket Books, 2006), 60–3.

Strachey, Ray, *The Cause: A Short History of the Women's Movement in Great Britain* (Bath: Cedric Chivers, 1928).

Stuart, Denis, *Dear Duchess: Millicent Duchess of Sutherland (1867–1955)* (Newton Abbot: David and Charles, 1982).

Sturdy, Steve, 'War as Experiment: Physiology, Innovation and Administration in Britain, 1914–1918: The Case of Chemical Warfare', in Roger Cooter, Mark Harrison, and Sturdy (eds.), *War, Medicine and Modernity* (Stroud: Sutton Publishing, 1998), 65–84.

Summers, Anne, *Angels and Citizens: British Women as Military Nurses, 1854–1914* (London: Routledge and Kegan Paul, 1988).

Tate, Trudi, *Modernism, History and the First World War* (Manchester: Manchester University Press, 1998).

Taylor, A. J. P., *The First World War* (1963; London, Penguin, 1966).

Telford, Jennifer Casavant, 'American Red Cross Nursing during World War I: Opportunities and Obstacles' (unpublished PhD thesis, University of Virginia, 2007).

Todman, Dan, *The Great War: Myth and Memory* (London: Hambledon Continuum, 2005).

Toman, Cynthia, ' "Help us, serve England": First World War Military Nursing and National Identities', *Canadian Bulletin of Medical History*, 30/1 (2013), 156–7.

Torrey, Glen E., 'L'Affaire de Soissons, January 1915', *War in History*, 4/4 (1997), 398–410.

Travers, T., *The Killing Ground: The British Army, the Western Front and the Emergence of Modern Warfare, 1900–1918* (London: Allen & Unwin, 1987).

Tunstall, Graydon A., *Blood on the Snow: The Carpathian Winter War of 1915* (Lawrence, Kan.: University of Kansas Press, 2010).

Tylee, Claire, *The Great War and Women's Consciousness: Images of Militarism ad Womanhood in Women's Writings, 1914–1964* (Houndmills: Macmillan, 1990).

van Bergen, Leo, *Before My Helpless Sight: Suffering, Dying and Military Medicine on the Western Front, 1914–1918*, trans. Liz Waters (Farnham: Ashgate, 2009).

Van Emden, Richard, *The Trench: Experiencing Life on the Front Line, 1916* (London: Corgi Books, 2002).

Villard, Henry Serrano, and Nagel, James, *Hemingway in Love and War: The Lost Diary of Agnes von Kurowsky, Her Letters and Correspondence of Ernest Hemingway* (Boston: Northeastern University Press, 1989).

Wade, Rex A., *The Russian Revolution, 1917* (Cambridge: Cambridge University Press, 2000).

Watson, Janet S. K., 'Wars in the Wards: The Social Construction of Medical Work in First World War Britain', *Journal of British Studies*, 41 (2002), 484–510.

Watson, Janet S. K., *Fighting Different Wars: Experience, Memory and the First World War in Britain* (Cambridge: Cambridge University Press, 2004).

Wenzel, Marian, and Cornish, John, *Auntie Mabel's War: An Account of Her Part in the Hostilities of 1914–1918* (London: Allen Lane, 1980).

Winter, Jay, *Sites of Memory, Sites of Mourning: The Great War in European Cultural History* (Cambridge: Cambridge University Press, 1995).

Wolfe, Bertram D., 'Titans Locked in Combat, Part II', *Russian Review*, 24/1 (Jan. 1965).

Zeiger, Susan, *In Uncle Sam's Service: Women Workers with the American Expeditionary Force, 1917–1919* (Philadelphia: University of Pennsylvania Press, 1999).

## Online Resources

<http://www.scarletfinders.co.uk/25.html> [last accessed 24 Aug. 2013].

<www.collectionscanada.gc.ca/nursing-sisters> [last accessed 17/ May 2013].

*Reveille: Lancaster Military Heritage Group*; available at <http://lancaster warmemorials.org.uk/essays/e27.htm> [last accessed 01 Oct. 2013].

# Index